Palliative Care - Current Practice and Future Perspectives

Edited by Georg Bollig and Erika Zelko

Published in London, United Kingdom

Palliative Care - Current Practice and Future Perspectives
http://dx.doi.org/10.5772/intechopen.1000392
Edited by Georg Bollig and Erika Zelko

Contributors
Adel Moideen, Aia Naksho, Alexander Woodman, Ali Abdolrahmani, Amon Banturaki, Ana Mateus, Asad Merchant, Denise Andrea Harris, Elahe Akbari, Erika Zelko, Eva Niedermann, Firoozeh Samim, Georg Bollig, Ian Duncan, Jose Luis Braga De Aquino, Kalkidan Solomon, Karthik Chandrasekaran, Klaus Wegleitner, Liqing Yao, Luz Marina Cano Molano, Maja Ebert Moltara, Mariuska Forteza Sáez, Marìa del Carmen Llantà, María Sabina Ah. Chu Sánchez de Spengler, Michael Silbermann, Mirgissa Kaba, Navim Mobin, Nicholas Gregory Brown, Patrick Schuchter, Pedro Ponce, Qian Liu, Rok Mihelič, Sah Tatsing Félix Désiré, Sandra Radinger, Gulcin Senel, Siobhan Neylon, Stefanie V. Rieger, Tamim Ahmed, Teresa Velosa, Vania Aparecida Leandro-Merhi, Xueting Chen, Xue Yang, Yoseph Mamo Azmera

First published in London, United Kingdom, 2024 by IntechOpen
IntechOpen is the global imprint of INTECHOPEN LIMITED, registered in England and Wales, registration number: 11086078, 167-169 Great Portland Street, London, W1W 5PF, United Kingdom

British Library Cataloguing-in-Publication Data
A catalogue record for this book is available from the British Library

Additional hard and PDF copies can be obtained from orders@intechopen.com

Palliative Care - Current Practice and Future Perspectives
Edited by Georg Bollig and Erika Zelko
p. cm.
Print ISBN 978-0-85466-050-6
Online ISBN 978-0-85466-049-0
eBook (PDF) ISBN 978-0-85466-051-3

For EU product safety concerns:
IN TECH d.o.o., Prolaz Marije Krucifikse Kozulić 3, 51000 Rijeka, Croatia,
info@intechopen.com or visit our website at intechopen.com.

Meet the editors

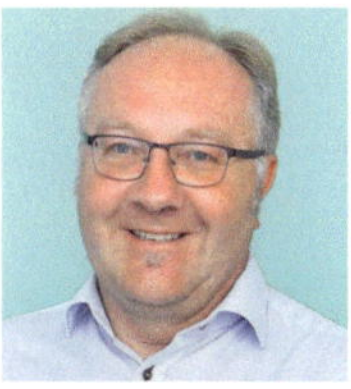

Dr. med. Georg Bollig, MAS (Palliative Care), Ph.D., DEAA is a physician, researcher and social entrepreneur. After completing medical studies at the University of Cologne, Germany; University of Vienna, Austria; and University of Seattle, USA, Dr. Bollig became a specialist in anaesthesiology, pain therapy, and palliative care. Currently, he is a senior consultant in palliative medicine and the head of palliative medicine at the academic teaching hospital Helios Klinikum Schleswig, Germany. In addition to his clinical work, he is a research fellow at the Department of Palliative Medicine, Faculty of Medicine and University Hospital, University of Cologne. Dr. Bollig developed the idea of a Last Aid Course and is the leader of the International Last Aid working group and the Last Aid Research Group International (LARGI).
His main research interests are public palliative care education (PPCE), Last Aid Courses and telepalliative care.

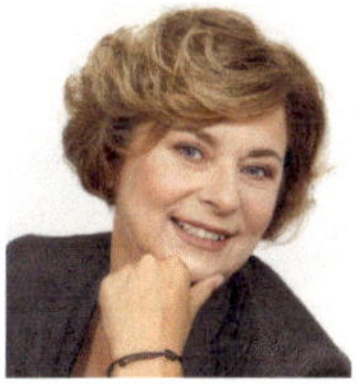

Prof. Dr. Erika Zelko obtained a master's degree in 2007 and a Ph.D. in 2015. Currently, she is a lecturer at the Faculty of Medicine in Maribor and Ljubljana, as well as at the University of Health Sciences in Maribor and Celje, Slovenia. Presently, she is employed at Johannes Kepler University Linz, leading the Institute of General/Family Medicine. With a bibliography boasting more than 250 papers, Dr. Zelko completed the EUPCA course for leadership in palliative care in 2019. Since then, she has been coordinating and managing the international Last Aid program in Slovenia and co-founded the Last Aid Research Group International (LARGI). Active in various professional associations and committees, Dr. Zelko finds leisure in foreign languages, mountaineering, travel, literature, and music.

Contents

Preface

Demographic shifts and advancements in medicine have extended the lifespan of individuals, even in cases of incurable diseases. However, as people approach the end of their lives, there is an increasing emphasis on maintaining quality of life and preserving dignity. Our book, *Palliative Care – Current Practice and Future Perspectives*, offers an insightful introduction to this subject, presenting a multidisciplinary perspective and diverse insights from a team of authors from various disciplines and regions across Europe, Asia, and Africa. Structured into five sections, the book delves into fundamental concepts, philosophical underpinnings, current practices, and future strategies aimed at enhancing palliative care for all who require it. Through this comprehensive approach, readers gain a nuanced understanding of palliative care, its evolving landscape, and the diverse perspectives that shape its implementation and improvement worldwide.

Section 1 describes and discusses concepts and philosophies in palliative care. Death, grief, and death literacy are addressed from different viewpoints. In addition, the section presents personal reflections highlighting the patient's perspective.

Section 2 describes current practices from around the world with examples of the implementation and practice of palliative care from Slovenia, Saudi Arabia, Ethiopia, and central Africa.

Section 3 discusses multidisciplinary approaches and palliative care practice for different patient populations, for example, in pulmonology, gastroenterology, and nephrology. Furthermore, the section examines the role of dental care and physiotherapy for palliative patients.

Section 4 is about well-being and spirituality. It presents the importance of spirituality and different religions in palliative care. It also addresses spiritual distress and depression and the role of pets in the well-being of palliative patients.

Section 5 on future perspectives invites a discussion of the role of machine learning and artificial intelligence use in palliative care. It also highlights the importance of public palliative care education (PPCE) in palliative care practice.

This book contributes to the practice of providing palliative care for those who need it most and is useful for educating the public about how to participate in public health care and palliative care provision in the community.

We hope that readers will gain insights into the current practice of palliative care and find inspiration for the future development of the field. We also hope that the book sparks discussions and contributes to ongoing dialogues about the advancement of palliative care on a global scale.

Georg Bollig
Department of Anesthesiology, Intensive Care,
Palliative Medicine and Pain Therapy,
Helios Klinikum,
Schleswig, Germany

Faculty of Medicine and University Hospital,
Department of Palliative Medicine,
University of Cologne,
Cologne, Germany

Last Aid Research Group International (LARGI),
Schleswig, Germany

Erika Zelko
Last Aid Research Group International (LARGI),
Schleswig, Germany

Medical Faculty,
Institute for General Medicine,
Johannes Kepler University Linz,
Linz, Austria

Medical Faculty,
Institute for Palliative and Hospiz Medicine,
University Maribor,
Maribor, Slovenia

Section 1

Concepts, Patient Perspective and Philosophy

Chapter 1

A Brief Literature Review of Conceptual Models in Palliative Care

Xue Yang, Xueting Chen, Qian Liu and Liqing Yao

Abstract

Receiving palliative care has been shown to be effective in older adults with serious illnesses and reducing the healthcare burden and cost. To improve further research on old adults suffering from serious illness, we summarize the currently available theoretical models of palliative care, which could improve care strategies. Notably, few studies have focused on the conceptual models or theoretical frameworks of palliative care. In this review, we summarize the conceptual models or theoretical frameworks based on empirical data or quantitative research in the end-of-life field. We reviewed the theoretical models in the current literature regarding the field of palliative care. A structured data extraction form was used to record whether a study proposed a theoretical/conceptual model. Several conceptual models or theoretical frameworks were presented and summarized. Future endeavors should explore the conceptual models or theoretical frameworks from a holistic perspective in the field of end-of-life care.

Keywords: older adults, palliative care, palliative care knowledge, theoretical models, serious illness

1. Introduction

The increase in the aging population worldwide has resulted in the rise of people living with multiple chronic illnesses. It is estimated that the number of Americans aged over 65 years old will be more than 98 million by 2060, approximating 24% of the population in the latter part of the century [1]. Individuals with life-threatening illness pose a substantial burden on healthcare systems and can have a detrimental impact on family caregivers. Advancements in medical technology, particularly in the areas of the detection, pathological diagnosis, and treatment of life-threatening illnesses, have resulted in a growing population of older adults with advanced incurable, and progressively fatal conditions. This trend underscores the urgent need to address the complex challenges associated with the care and support of these individuals, as well as to explore innovative approaches to alleviate their suffering and enhance their quality of life. As a result, patients with advanced illness show poor response to treatment and poor quality of life, and suffer from physical and psychological ailments.

This has attracted the attention of authorities and necessitated the development of strategies to improve the care of these patients.

The concept of palliative care has been proposed as an effective intervention that provides active treatment, holistic care, and services for dying patients who have no hope of treatment and whose life expectancy does not exceed 3–6 months. Such an intervention allows the patients to face death calmly, alleviate their pain, and improve their quality of life [2]. Palliative care consists of a multidisciplinary team, comprising primary care physicians, specialty physicians, palliative care specialists, and a supportive ancillary team. Palliative care was first developed by the United Kingdom, which provided a solid theoretical foundation and has a high degree of public participation. Palliative care can alleviate disease and negative psychological emotions, and obtain peace in patients with advanced illness, and provide comfort and dignity in the last days of their life. To promote the development of these domains, the National Institutes of Health (NIH) introduced the concept of developing end-of-life conceptual models in 2004. Subsequently, in the United States, palliative care was predominantly regarded as applicable only during the final 1–2 weeks of life, while medical insurance coverage was limited to hospice care for the last 6 months of life [3]. As of 2017, 48.2% of patients received hospice care [4]. Over the past 30 years, palliative care has shifted from basic hospital care to home care where about a quarter of patients die at home [5]. However, the palliative care remains under-used in the developed nations.

There is a need to develop conceptual models or theoretical frameworks for evaluating research outcomes. The existing body of literature on conceptual models or theoretical frameworks in palliative care is notably limited. Consequently, the objective of this study is to address this research gap by providing a comprehensive summary of conceptual models or theoretical frameworks derived from empirical data or quantitative research in the field of end-of-life care. In this literature review, we aim to enhance the understanding and application of theoretical perspectives in palliative care, facilitating further advancements in the field.

2. Methods

2.1 Search strategies

The search was performed to identify studies published in English in several electronic databases including PubMed, Cochrane Library, EMBASE, Web of science. Two reviewers independently evaluated eligible papers from inception to July 1, 2023 and any discrepancies were resolved by a third investigator. To avoid omission, search terms comprising the following terms were used (e.g., Medical Subject Headings (Mesh)): (palliative care (Mesh) or Care, Palliative or Palliative Treatment or Palliative Treatments or Treatment, Palliative or Treatments, Palliative or Therapy, Palliative or Palliative Therapy or Palliative Supportive Care or Supportive Care, Palliative or Palliative Surgery or Surgery, Palliative) and (Models, Theoretical (Mesh) or Model, Theoretical or Theoretical Model or Theoretical Models or Models, Theoretic) and (Aged (Mesh) or elderly).

The complete search strategy was shown below:

((((((((((((("Palliative Care"[Mesh]) OR (palliative care [Title/Abstract])) OR (Care, Palliative [Title/Abstract])) OR (Palliative Treatment [Title/Abstract])) OR (Palliative Treatments [Title/Abstract])) OR (Treatment, Palliative [Title/Abstract])) OR (Treatments, Palliative [Title/Abstract])) OR (Therapy, Palliative [Title/Abstract]))

OR (Palliative Therapy [Title/Abstract])) OR (Palliative Supportive Care [Title/Abstract])) OR (Supportive Care, Palliative [Title/Abstract])) OR (Palliative Surgery [Title/Abstract])) OR (Surgery, Palliative [Title/Abstract])) AND ((((("Models, Theoretical"[Mesh]) OR (Models, Theoretical [Title/Abstract])) OR (Model, Theoretical [Title/Abstract])) OR (Theoretical Model [Title/Abstract])) OR (Theoretical Models [Title/Abstract])) OR (Models, Theoretic [Title/Abstract]))) AND ((("Aged"[Mesh]) OR (Aged [Title/Abstract])) OR (Elderly [Title/Abstract]))

2.2 Article screening and selection

Endnote X9 was employed to effectively manage all the collected data in this study. Two reviewers conducted independent searches for eligible articles and meticulously screened the titles, abstracts, and full texts for inclusion. In the event of any discrepancies, a third investigator (XY) was involved to resolve conflicts. A detailed overview of the literature screening process is illustrated in **Figure 1**.

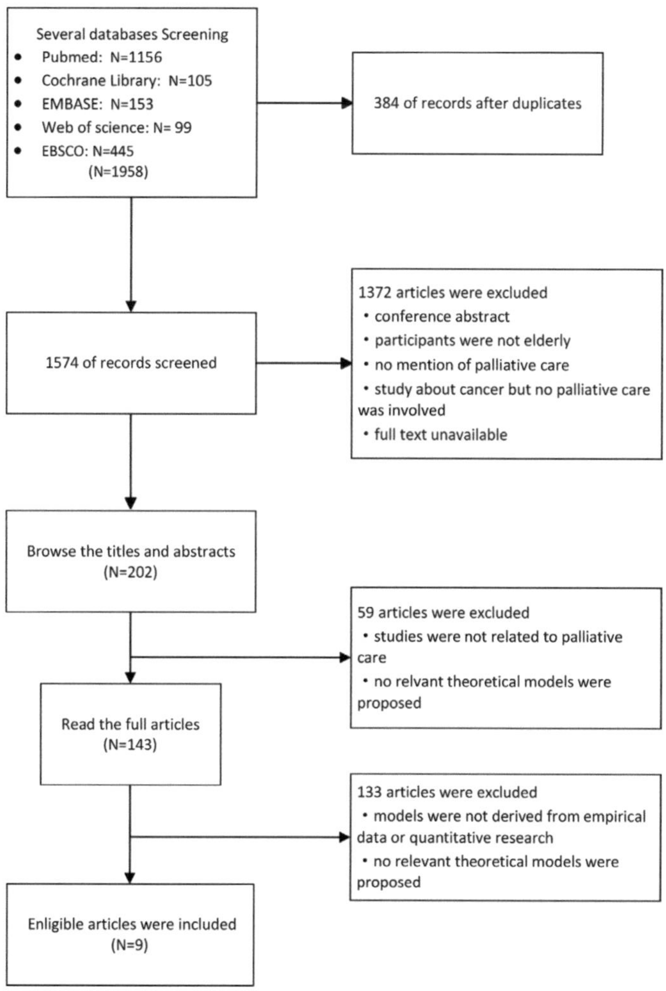

Figure 1.
The flow chart of literature screening.

3. Results

The conceptual models or theoretical frameworks are presented in **Table 1**. In addition, the components or indicators applied in the models were displayed as follows:

3.1 Framework of a good death

This framework improved our understanding of the dying experience and the quality of care in the end-of-life field [6]. It comprised four components: the fixed characteristics of the patients; the modifiable dimensions of the patient's experience; care-system interventions; and outcomes. This framework helped clinicians to conduct comprehensive assessments for end-of-life patients. Additionally, the framework could help promote the relevant research at the end of life.

3.2 Geriatric cancer experience at the end of life

An adapted model named "the geriatric cancer experience at the end of life" was established on the basis of the Framework of a Good Death. Buck et al. reported that the framework of a good death had two limitations: the absence of measurable outcome indicators and their linear relationships among various components. He suggested that linear relationships between clinical status, physiological, psychological, and spiritual components, and quality of life [7]. Finally, he emphasized the significance of physical and spiritual domains in evaluating the quality of life in geriatric end-of-life care.

3.3 The model for the family caregivers' experience in providing care

This model primarily examines the experience of family caregivers, encompassing various aspects of their caregiving journey, including challenges, consequences, and motivations. It proposed that caregiving was the key factor influencing the family caregivers' experience [8]. A comprehensive understanding of family caregivers' experience was presented in a structured way. Elsewhere, Meeker et al. investigated patients' and caregivers' experiences during with the management of advanced illness [9]. He depicted a transitional process involving suffering, struggling, and settling phases. Additionally, scholars have developed an explanatory model to understand the potential mechanisms behind communication deficits among family caregivers, patients, and clinicians [10].

3.4 The Markov multistate model of performance status

Multistate models were primarily used to summarize the complex changes associated with disease progression [11, 12]. Sutradhar et al. used the Markov multistate model to explore relevant and important information for the utility of the palliative care services [11].

3.5 Management models for palliative care

Short-term integrated palliative and supportive care (SIPS) was developed for frail older people in the community to improve symptom management [13].

No.	Authors	Years	Type	Design	Sample	Models or theory	Method	Endpoint	Instruments
1	Buck et al.	2009	Article	Quantitative study	Participants (n = 403)	Symptom experience-- > QoL; Spiritual experience-- > QoL; Emanuel and Emanuel's (1998) framework of a good death	Structural equation model	Quality of life (QoL)	Scales
2	Harding et al.	2019	Article	Interview	Family caregivers (n = 100); Patients (n = 24)	Communication--family--patients	Grounded theory	Outcomes of actions as responses to an event	Coding
3	Meeker et al.	2013	Article	Face-to-face, semi-structured interviews	Family surrogates (n = 100); Patients (n = 12)	Suffering-struggling--setting	Grounded theory	Outcomes of actions as responses to an event	Coding
4	Moorhouse et al.	2012	Article	Quantitative study	Participants (n = 150)	Palliative and therapeutic harmonization (PATH)	Grounded theory	Outcomes of actions as responses to an event	Scales+coding
5	Bone et al	2016	Article	Quantitative study	Participants (n = 80)	Short-term integrated palliative and supportive care (SIPS)	Observational study design	Outcomes of actions as responses to an event	Coding
6	Jerant et al	2004	Article	Quantitative study	Participants (n = 78)	Timely and team oriented, longitudinal, collaborative, and comprehensive (TLC) Model	A nonblinded, prospective comparison trial	Quality of life (QoL)	Questionnaire
7	Murray et al	2007	Review	None	None	Transitions model of palliative care (TMPC)	None	None	None

No.	Authors	Years	Type	Design	Sample	Models or theory	Method	Endpoint	Instruments
8	Emanuel et al	1999	Review	None	None	Good health model	None	Overall experience of the dying process	None
9	Bull et al	2017	Article	None	None	Community-based palliative care (CBPC)	None	None	None

Table 1.
Summary of conceptual models or theoretical frameworks in the palliative care.

Jerant et al. proposed the TLC model, which comprises timely, team-oriented, longitudinal, collaborative, and comprehensive [14]. The TLC model was defined as the palliative care which is in line with the SIPS model. In 2003, the Four Seasons community-based palliative care (CBPC) program was established. It aimed to develop a longitudinal delivery model that integrates an interdisciplinary team to provide comprehensive care for patients with life limiting [15].

3.6 Palliative and therapeutic harmonization (PATH) model

Additionally, PATH model was constructed to assess frailty when making medical decisions [16]. This model showed good performance in various scenarios.

4. Discussion

This brief review summarizes empirical studies on theoretical or conceptual models in geriatric end-of-life care. In future, researchers should pay careful attention to various theoretical and conceptual issues.

4.1 Theoretical issues

Theoretical frameworks are important for guiding the development of knowledge or the explanation of a phenomenon. These theoretical models can guide clinical research, but the lack of such models is an issue in end-of-life research. This review obtained theoretical frameworks primarily focusing on the transition of disease state, experience of family caregivers or patients, and holistic approaches to palliative care management.

4.1.1 The model of disease state

Multistate models have been used to describe the complex changes during the course of a disease [17]. In previous clinical research, a common approach was to conduct survival analysis using two outcome indicators: "alive" and "dead." This represents the simplest form of a multistate model. Another well-known multistate model is the illness-death model, also known as the disability model, which comprises three states: disease-free, diseased, and dead [18]. Multistate models are versatile tools for assessing the probability of patient transitions between different states. These models offer valuable biological insights to physicians, aiding them in making informed clinical decisions [19].

4.1.2 The model focused on patients or family caregivers

The essence of end-of-life care is to relieve patients' suffering, which needs to be a transition from cure-focused interventions to comfort-focused care. Therefore, palliative care is essential to be people-oriented services involving several domains, such as physical, psychosocial, and spiritual domains. Scholars have proposed conceptual models to enhance our understanding of patients' or caregivers' experience. However, limited research exists on conceptual models in palliative care, hindering the development of theoretical frameworks in this area. More quantitative and qualitative research should be needed to investigate the potential influence factors on participants in the whole process of end-of-life care, aiming to develop feasible comfort-focused interventions.

4.1.3 The model focused on incorporating with multidisciplinary

End-of-life care, characterized by holistic, interdisciplinary, and comfort-focused services, is crucial for individuals facing advanced illnesses. Therefore, the implementation of palliative care services is faced with several challenges for older people with life-threatening illness. Scientists acknowledge the importance of investigating the provision of feasible and appropriate palliative care for individuals with advanced illness [13]. An ideal theoretical framework for multidisciplinary management can offer valuable guidance to enhance the quality of life for older individuals.

4.2 Methodological issues

Grounded theory approach is the most common method for qualitative research, which can be widely used to explore theory building or conceptual thinking [20]. This method is an inductive process since a theory is derived from data, rather than a deductive reasoning process. The grounded theory is drawn from sociology, which focuses on studying human behavior on a specific topic by conducting a series of interviews. The interviews contain several forms, such as structured interviews, semi-structured interviews, group interviews among others. Another leading analytical strategy is the structural equation model (SEM), which is useful in empirical research [21]. SEM models can be applied in sociology, psychology, economy, and marketing research. SEM outperforms other statistical approaches owing to its ability to analyze complex, multidimensional, and empirical data inclusive of abstract concepts or theoretical constructs. Prior to constructing SEM models, researchers must ensure that all necessary theoretical assumptions have been established in the analysis. Therefore, the utilization of theoretical frameworks or conceptual models derived from empirical data is essential for implementing the SEM approach.

5. Conclusion

While significant progress has been made in implementing palliative care for advanced illness, further research is required to explore holistic conceptual models and theoretical frameworks in the end-of-life field. Specially, there is a need for empirical studies aimed at alleviating suffering.

Acknowledgements

In addition, I wish to acknowledge the following funds: 1. Yunnan Rehabilitation Clinical Medical Center, zx2019-04-02; 2. Research on a new Model of comprehensive Intervention in Rehabilitation and Psychology of Brain and Heart, 202203AC100007-6; 3. Jia Jie Expert Workstation, 202305AF150032.

Author details

Xue Yang, Xueting Chen, Qian Liu and Liqing Yao*
Department of Rehabilitation Medicine, the Second Affiliated Hospital of Kunming Medical University, Kunming, Yunnan, China

*Address all correspondence to: yaoliqing98731@163.com

References

[1] Roth AR, Canedo AR. Introduction to hospice and palliative care. Primary Care. 2019;**46**:287-302

[2] Walter AC, Gunderson CC, Vesely SK, et al. Central nervous system metastasis in gynecologic cancer: Symptom management, prognosis and palliative management strategies. Gynecologic Oncology. 2015;**136**:472-477

[3] Lim RB. End-of-life care in patients with advanced lung cancer. Therapeutic Advances in Respiratory Disease. 2016;**10**:455-467

[4] Tatum PE, Mills SS. Hospice and palliative care: An overview. The Medical Clinics of North America. 2020;**104**:359-373

[5] Teno JM, Gozalo P, Trivedi AN, et al. Site of death, place of care, and health care transitions among US medicare beneficiaries, 2000-2015. JAMA. 2018;**320**:264-271

[6] Emanuel EJ, Emanuel LL. The promise of a good death. Lancet (London, England). 1998;**351**(Suppl. 2): SII21-SII29

[7] Buck HG, Overcash J, McMillan SC. The geriatric cancer experience at the end of life: Testing an adapted model. Oncology Nursing Forum. 2009;**36**:664-673

[8] Kristanti MS, Effendy C, Utarini A, et al. The experience of family caregivers of patients with cancer in an Asian country: A grounded theory approach. Palliative Medicine. 2019;**33**:676-684

[9] Meeker MA, Waldrop DP, Schneider J, et al. Contending with advanced illness: Patient and caregiver perspectives. Journal of Pain and Symptom Management. 2014;**47**:887-895

[10] Harding R, Nair S, Ekstrand M. Multilevel model of stigma and barriers to cancer palliative care in India: A qualitative study. BMJ Open. 2019;**9**:e024248

[11] Sutradhar R, Seow H, Earle C, et al. Modeling the longitudinal transitions of performance status in cancer outpatients: Time to discuss palliative care. Journal of Pain and Symptom Management. 2013;**45**:726-734

[12] Hanly JG, Urowitz MB, Gordon C, et al. Neuropsychiatric events in systemic lupus erythematosus: A longitudinal analysis of outcomes in an international inception cohort using a multistate model approach. Annals of the Rheumatic Diseases. 2020;**79**:356-362

[13] Bone AE, Morgan M, Maddocks M, et al. Developing a model of short-term integrated palliative and supportive care for frail older people in community settings: Perspectives of older people, carers and other key stakeholders. Age and Ageing. 2016;**45**:863-873

[14] Jerant AF, Azari RS, Nesbitt TS, et al. The TLC model of palliative care in the elderly: Preliminary application in the assisted living setting. Annals of Family Medicine. 2004;**2**:54-60

[15] Bull J, Kamal AH, Harker M, et al. Standardization and scaling of a community-based palliative care model. Journal of Palliative Medicine. 2017;**20**:1237-1243

[16] Moorhouse P, Mallery LH. Palliative and therapeutic harmonization: A model for appropriate decision-making in frail

older adults. Journal of the American Geriatrics Society. 2012;**60**:2326-2332

[17] Hougaard P. Multi-state models: A review. Lifetime Data Analysis. 1999;**5**:239-264

[18] Meira-Machado L, Sestelo M. Estimation in the progressive illness-death model: A nonexhaustive review. Biometrical Journal. 2019;**61**:245-263

[19] Sutradhar R, Barbera L, Seow H, et al. Multistate analysis of interval-censored longitudinal data: Application to a cohort study on performance status among patients diagnosed with cancer. American Journal of Epidemiology. 2011;**173**:468-475

[20] Khan SN. Qualitative research method: Grounded theory. International Journal of Business and Management. 2014:**9**(11)

[21] Tarka P. An overview of structural equation modeling: Its beginnings, historical development, usefulness and controversies in the social sciences. Quality and Quantity. 2018;**52**:313-354

Chapter 2

Death and Grief: A Complex Thought Point of View

Luz Marina Cano Molano

Abstract

The ultimate goal of palliative care is to alleviate the suffering of both the patient and his family, through the proper understanding, detection, and control of physical, psychosocial, and spiritual symptoms experienced by patients at the end of life, regardless of diagnosis. But, while it is true that death is a natural phenomenon, the process of dying is treated as a disease, and today, we are experiencing the medicalization of death. As a consequence, many people die in hospitals in the most extreme loneliness and pain. In other cases, service provision models have been dichotomized to the point of providing aggressive curative treatment and establishing palliative measures in the face of therapeutic failure. The consequence of this reality is that patients and families are left in the middle of an economic and social conflict, since they do not find a team that allows them to understand the nature of the disease, the diagnosis, and the prognosis, this being a crucial aspect for the decision-making at the end of life.

Keywords: death, grief, complex thought, palliative care, interdisciplinary team

1. Introduction

The validation of complexity in biopsychosocial processes forces educational institutions to train new professionals with a high degree of comprehensiveness, Palliative Care—Current Practice and Future Perspectives with programs that allow reality to be constructed from multidimensionality, with clear and innovative ideas, objective judgments, assertive decisions, metacognitive skills, which can articulate the previous knowledge with the new one, and understand the multiplicity in the unit. This implies a wide-ranging reconstruction of the curricular structure. On the other hand, the art of caring is an action whose destiny is the good of a human being and his family in a society. Although physicians dedicate much of their training and assistance to the reproduction and maintenance of life, the end of life is relegated to a few pain specialists and spiritual practices that allow patients and their families to accept and resign from the death process. Precisely, the center of palliative care is the human being, and his family to whom palliative care is directed, care at the end of life. The foregoing means that for an effective implementation, a deep knowledge of human reality is required, not only in its somatic or biological aspects but in all the environmental, psychological, social, and spiritual dimensions of the individual. Additionally, death constitutes one of the fundamental themes of philosophy, psychology, and medicine.

Questions about the meaning of death, its reason for being, and the other questions that arise around it are a constant topic in human history. But beyond death, one of the most studied and least multidisciplinary intervened aspects is the meaning of suffering.

Caring for a human being means accompanying him/her/them, being with him, ensuring him/her/them autonomy, and assisting him in his vulnerability. Palliative care is a specific way of applying this care. Likewise, from the transdisciplinary point of view that the work of caring for a patient can acquire, we can refer to the fact that it is about accompanying the human being in their process of illness and death. Here, death not only becomes a problem but life itself and, therefore, entails a series of bioethical and multidimensional issues. When the human being lives in the vicinity of death, he feels and perceives it with greater impetus. He becomes aware of his radical and challenging character. Therefore, in the care of a person at the end of life, the perception of death must be considered very seriously, since this perception, the sense or nonsense of it, is directly related to the person's state of mind dying. For this reason, before being with this class of patients, it is pertinent and responsible to theoretically confront one's own death, and that of close beings, in order to intervene around it. This scenario is the engine of this research work. Within the course of life, we do not choose to die, but we have the fundamental right to decide how we will die. Therefore, a qualified team is required to provide comprehensive, loving, and compassionate care at the end of life. This chapter describes the phenomenon of dying from a complex thought point of view. Literature gives a wide definition of death. We know what death is, we have experience the loss of a love one. So, this chapter will introduce the key elements of the phenomenon of dying, starting with understanding what complexity is and why this stage of life must be assessed by a transdisciplinary palliative care team [1, 2].

1.1 What is death?

Death is an inevitable part of life, and yet dying remains one of the most complex and emotional journeys one can undertake. At the heart of dying complexity lies the many different factors that shape our experience of life's final chapter. Medical, cultural, spiritual, ethical, and emotional considerations all play a role in shaping the way we approach mortality both as individuals and as a society. This chapter explores the complexity of dying and the many factors that contribute to this experience. We will examine the physical and emotional aspects of dying, the role of culture and spirituality, the ethical issues that arise, and the impact of technology and legal considerations. Additionally, we will delve into the different types of dying experiences, from those facing terminal illness to those experiencing sudden death or trauma. By exploring these many facets of death and dying, we hope to provide a more comprehensive understanding of this universal human experience. We also hope to promote greater empathy and compassion for those facing the end of life [1].

1.2 The process of dying

Dying is a complex process that involves many changes to the body. When an individual is dying, their body shuts down slowly, eventually leading to organ failure and ultimately death. According to Matzo [3], there are many physical changes during the dying process, including decreased appetite, difficulty swallowing, and difficulty sleeping. Symptoms such as fatigue, confusion, and a change in breathing pattern are also common.

The way a person dies can be affected by the specific illness or injury they are facing. For example, in cases of terminal cancer, the dying process may be prolonged and painful, as the cancer cells continue to rapidly divide and cause widespread damage. In contrast, individuals facing sudden acute injuries, such as severe head trauma or a heart attack, may die more quickly due to the sudden shock to their system. These differences in dying experiences are explored in Chochinov's work [4].

In addition to the physical manifestations experienced during the process of dying, various medical interventions and treatments can be utilized to alleviate these symptoms and enhance the individual's overall well-being. As highlighted by Kamal and Bull [5], palliative care plays a crucial role in end-of-life care by concentrating on effectively managing symptoms, providing emotional and psychological support, and addressing spiritual needs. Moreover, medical interventions such as pain management, oxygen therapy, and adequate hydration can be employed to enhance the patient's comfort and offer support throughout this challenging journey.

Supporting individuals through the difficult and distressing process of dying, both for the person experiencing it and their loved ones, involves several important approaches. For instance, incorporating comfort care interventions such as music therapy, massage, and aromatherapy can help alleviate physical and emotional symptoms commonly associated with the dying process [4]. Additionally, family members and caregivers play a crucial role in providing emotional assistance and ensuring that the individual's preferences for end-of-life care are respected. By gaining an understanding of the physical transformations that take place during the dying process, we can foster greater empathy toward those embarking on this challenging journey and deliver more compassionate and effective end-of-life support.

1.3 The emotional and psychological dimensions of the dying process

The emotional and psychological dimensions of the dying process can present challenges and complexities comparable to the physical transformations. When confronted with the reality of their impending death, individuals often undergo a broad spectrum of emotions, encompassing fear, anger, sadness, and acceptance. MonforteRoyo, Villavicencio-Chávez, Tomás-Sábado, and Balaguer's study [5] revealed that those facing an incurable illness commonly experience a deep sense of vulnerability and a loss of control, which evokes intense emotional responses to the knowledge of their approaching demise. Individuals who are approaching the end of their lives often grapple with the daunting realization of their impending mortality, which can make coping immensely challenging. This awareness may lead to the manifestation of anxiety, depression, and various forms of spiritual and emotional distress. During this time, the support and presence of family members and caregivers become crucial, as they provide much needed emotional solace and aid in navigating these difficulties. Breitbart et al. [6] suggest that implementing supportive care measures such as counseling, spiritual guidance, and art therapy can offer individuals confronting the end of life an opportunity to discover a sense of purpose and find meaning in their remaining days.

An important aspect of providing end-of-life care involves upholding the dying individual's wishes and values. This encompasses considerations such as religious or cultural practices and preferences for the involvement of caregivers. Maintaining consistent communication among the dying person, their loved ones, and healthcare providers is crucial to establishing a shared understanding of the individual's goals for end-of-life care [7]. Open and transparent communication fosters an environment that can alleviate anxiety and instill a sense of control, benefiting both the dying person and their loved ones.

In the end, the emotional and psychological aspects of the dying process are profoundly unique and personal to each individual. Nevertheless, caregivers and loved ones hold a crucial position in offering support and solace throughout this demanding period. By comprehending the intricate emotional responses that individuals may undergo, providing empathetic emotional assistance, and promoting open communication, we can contribute to the attainment of peace and comfort for those approaching the end of their lives [1, 8].

The following are the key aspects that will act as quality-of-life dimensions that interact simultaneously in the dying individual:

1. The physical process of dying: What happens to the body during the dying process? How do various illnesses or injuries affect the way a person dies?

2. The emotional and psychological aspects of dying: How do people typically react emotionally to knowing that death is imminent? How can caregivers and loved ones better support those who are dying?

3. Cultural and historical perspectives on death: How have different cultures and societies approached death, mourning, and bereavement throughout history?

4. Are there differences in how people approach death depending on their cultural background?

5. The complexities of grief and bereavement: What is the grieving process like for those left behind after someone dies? How can people work through their grief in a healthy way?

6. Ethical issues related to death and dying: How do we determine when to stop medical interventions in end-of-life situations? What are some of the ethical considerations that come up when making decisions about death and dying?

7. The role of spirituality in dying: How do different belief systems approach death and the afterlife? How can spirituality supports individuals and loved ones facing end-of-life issues?

8. Legal considerations related to death and dying: What are some of the legal issues that arise in end-of-life situations? How do laws and regulations vary by geographic location?

9. The impact of technology on death and dying: How have medical advancements and technology impacted the way we approach death and dying? What are some of the new ethical dilemmas that arise as technology advances in this area?

10. Caregiver burnout and support: How do caregivers cope with the emotional and physical demands of caring for someone who is dying? What support is available for caregivers during the dying process and beyond?

11. Different types of death: How does the process of dying differ for those who have a terminal illness versus those who experience sudden death or trauma? How do different types of death impact the grieving process and those left behind?

12. Death rituals and funeral practices: How do different cultures approach death rituals and funeral practices? Are there any universal practices that span cultures and religions?

1.4 Edgar Morin's perspective on the complexity of dying and importance of death rituals

Edgar Morin, a philosopher and anthropologist, has extensively explored the subject of death and dying. A central aspect of his perspective is the belief that death is an inherent part of the human journey, and confronting it is essential for a truly meaningful existence [9].

According to Morin, death transcends individual experiences and holds a collective significance, impacting entire communities. He posits that societies develop rituals and traditions surrounding death as a means to navigate the loss of loved ones and find understanding within their own mortality [10].

In his work "Penser la Mort" (Thinking about Death), Edgar Morin presents his perspective that death should not be perceived as an ultimate end but rather as a transformative process that leads to rebirth. According to Morin, death is an integral part of the natural cycle of life, and rather than fearing it, we should embrace its significance [11].

Morin further contends that death is a concept influenced by social and cultural factors. He argues that different societies exhibit distinct approaches to death, each with its own set of rituals and customs. For instance, certain cultures regard death as a natural component of life and commemorate it as a means to pay tribute to the departed, while others view it as a tragic event to be avoided by any means necessary.

Morin emphasizes the interconnection between our perception of death and our comprehension of life. He proposes that cultivating a healthy attitude toward death necessitates a comprehensive understanding of life, encompassing its diverse facets including joys and sorrows, as well as successes and failures [12]. Moreover, Morin posits that our fear of death originates from our limited awareness and knowledge about it. He suggests that we can transcend this fear by expanding our understanding of death through dialog, reflection, and education [13].

Morin underscores the significance of proactive engagement in the presence of death. He proposes that instead of postponing it until the final moments, we should prepare for death by leading lives filled with intention and purpose [14]. Additionally, Morin presents a distinct and thought-provoking viewpoint on death. He advocates for perceiving death as an inherent component of life, urging us to accept and find reconciliation with it. Through his work, he challenges us to critically evaluate our approaches to death and explore how our attitudes toward death shape not only our own lives but also the lives of those around us [15].

Furthermore, Edgar Morin has dedicated extensive work to exploring the significance of death rituals within human societies. In his book "La Rumeur d'Orléans" (The Rumor of Orleans), Morin asserts that death rituals extend beyond cultural expressions and serve a vital psychological role in assisting us in coping with the existential realities of life and death. According to Morin, these rituals play a crucial role in acknowledging our own mortality and reaffirming our connection to the broader community we inhabit. He suggests that through these rituals, we can mourn our losses while simultaneously celebrating the lives that were lived.

According to Morin, death rituals present an occasion for both individuals and communities to unite in contemplating the passage of time and the inevitability of death. He proposes that rituals such as wakes, funerals, and memorials furnish an opportunity to exchange memories, stories, and emotions, establishing a sense of continuity and connection in the face of bereavement. Furthermore, Morin asserts that death rituals play a crucial role in attributing significance to loss. By providing a framework through which we can process and comprehend death, rituals assist us in reconciling with our own mortality and the departure of our loved ones [12, 14, 15].

Morin also underscores the significance of adapting death rituals to align with the evolving needs of contemporary society. He proposes that these rituals must continuously transform to accommodate the demands of a rapidly changing world, while still providing a vital sense of solace and comfort to those in mourning [12, 14, 15].

Moreover, Morin posits that death rituals offer valuable insights into the cultural, historical, and social contexts in which they are observed. He suggests that scrutinizing these rituals can enrich our comprehension of the values, beliefs, and practices embraced by diverse cultures and societies [12, 14, 15]. Additionally, Morin recognizes that death rituals are not universally standardized, and each society has its own distinct approach to death. He proposes that these differences reflect the remarkable diversity of human experiences, which should be celebrated. Morin also emphasizes the close correlation between our perception of death rituals and our understanding of death itself.

He argues that cultivating a healthy connection with death necessitates a holistic comprehension of life, encompassing its joys and sorrows, and successes and failures [13, 15]. Furthermore, Morin proposes that death rituals should embrace inclusivity, welcoming individuals from diverse backgrounds and walks of life. He argues that genuine compassion necessitates extending our mourning rituals to all members of society, irrespective of their social status or identity [13, 15].

Morin's perspective on death rituals accentuates their vital role within human society. He suggests that these rituals serve as a means for us to recognize our mortality, grieve our losses, celebrate life, find meaning in death, and cultivate connections with others. Morin also advocates for the evolution of death rituals to meet the evolving needs of contemporary society, promoting inclusive and compassionate approaches, and analyzing these rituals as reflections of cultural and societal values [14, 15].

Throughout history, cultures and societies have exhibited diverse approaches to death, mourning, and bereavement. Varied religious and cultural beliefs have influenced individuals' perceptions of death and shaped the rituals and customs surrounding the dying process. In certain cultures, death is regarded as a natural and serene transition, while in others, it is considered a tragic event that necessitates intricate mourning practices to honor the departed [16], highlighting that many Eastern cultures, such as China, place significant emphasis on the afterlife within their belief systems regarding death. Ancestor worship and filial piety play central roles in mourning rituals within these cultures.

1.5 Sociocultural aspects of the end of life

An individual's cultural heritage can have a substantial influence on their attitudes toward and coping mechanisms for death. For instance, cultural practices surrounding mourning and grief can exhibit significant variations, encompassing factors such as the duration of the mourning period and the acceptable range of emotions to be expressed. In certain cultures, mourning is considered a private affair, while in others, it is embraced as a more communal experience. As noted by Zhai and Du [17], cultural values, beliefs, and practices pertaining to grief can impact both the bereavement experience and the efficacy of therapeutic interventions.

Over the course of history, cultures and societies have undergone significant transformations in their attitudes toward death. For instance, during the medieval period in Europe, death was omnipresent and frequently perceived as a divine retribution. Mourning customs were elaborate and often carried out in public, with social status exerting a notable influence on the associated rituals.

In contrast, contemporary Western culture tends to perceive death as a medical occurrence that should be regulated and controlled. As observed by Helm [18], these societal changes have had an impact on individuals' perspectives and coping mechanisms when it comes to death. In essence, cultural and historical outlooks on death underscore the wide array of human beliefs, values, and customs, and how they shape the end-of-life journey.

By comprehending the cultural variations in death and mourning traditions, healthcare providers can deliver more empathetic and culturally sensitive end-of-life care. This involves collaborating with patients and their families to ensure that end-of-life care decisions align with their cultural and spiritual convictions. Additionally, it entails providing customized emotional support that takes into account the cultural norms surrounding bereavement [19].

1.6 The grieving process

When faced with the loss of a loved one, one pivotal aspect to confront is grief—a complex and highly personalized journey. The grieving process encompasses an array of emotional, physiological, and psychological reactions that can differ significantly based on an individual's unique connection with the deceased. Emotional responses often encompass feelings of shock, disbelief, anger, guilt, and sadness, while physical manifestations may include fatigue, insomnia, and loss of appetite. Stroebe and Schut [20] emphasize the significance of recognizing that grief is not a linear progression but rather a dynamic and multifaceted experience that can fluctuate and evolve over time.

For individuals, it can be arduous to navigate their grief in a constructive manner, especially when facing more intricate forms of bereavement, such as sudden or traumatic deaths. Adopting healthy coping mechanisms becomes crucial in such cases. These can include seeking solace from loved ones, participating in support groups or therapy sessions, and practicing self-care activities such as exercise or meditation. Nevertheless, certain individuals may necessitate additional interventions or specialized care to address more complex responses to bereavement, such as post-traumatic stress disorder (PTSD) or prolonged grief disorder (PGD).

Apart from individual factors, the social and cultural environment surrounding bereavement can also shape how individuals navigate their grief. Cultural norms pertaining to mourning, such as the duration of the mourning period or the acceptable modes of expressing grief, can influence individuals' perceptions of their own grief and the support they seek. For instance, in certain cultures, grief is regarded as a deeply personal journey to be processed privately, whereas in others, mourning is a communal experience characterized by more open expressions of grief [20].

In general, the intricate nature of grief and bereavement underscores the significance of adopting a compassionate and comprehensive approach to end-of-life care. By recognizing the individual and societal aspects that impact grief, healthcare providers can offer more nuanced and culturally sensitive care, addressing the varied needs and experiences of individuals mourning a loss [20].

1.7 Ethical considerations at the end of life

In recent years, ethical considerations pertaining to end-of-life care have grown increasingly intricate due to advancements in medical technologies and the expanded choices available to individuals regarding medical interventions. One pivotal question that clinicians and families grapple with in end-of-life situations is determining the appropriate time to cease medical interventions. Numerous factors can influence this decision, including the patient's expressed desires, the severity of their illness, the prospects of recovery, and the potential risks and benefits associated with the interventions [21].

Nonetheless, ultimately, the final decision about when to discontinue medical treatment rests with the individual patient and their loved ones [20].

When faced with decisions concerning death and dying, an array of ethical considerations must be carefully evaluated. One of the foremost factors to consider is the principle of autonomy, which grants individuals the right to make decisions regarding their medical care and treatment. However, autonomy must be balanced with other ethical principles such as non-maleficence, which stipulates that healthcare providers must refrain from causing harm to their patients, and beneficence, which mandates that healthcare providers act in the best interests of their patients.

As an illustration, certain end-of-life scenarios may present challenges in reconciling these principles when the patient's wishes conflict with the recommendations of healthcare providers [22]. The principle of justice, a crucial ethical consideration, mandates the equitable distribution of healthcare resources. In certain instances, the utilization of extensive medical interventions in end-of-life scenarios might be perceived as an unjust allocation of resources, particularly when other patients could potentially benefit from the same medical technologies. Furthermore, economic factors can also influence decision-making regarding end-of-life care, as certain treatments may entail substantial costs, placing a financial burden on the patient or their family [22].

In general, navigating ethical issues surrounding end-of-life care can be complex. By considering the diverse ethical principles at play and adopting a patient-centered approach to decision-making, healthcare providers can offer more nuanced and compassionate care, ensuring that patients' preferences are honored, and their dignity is preserved.

1.8 Spirituality, belief systems, and death

Spirituality is a fundamental aspect of the human experience that can provide solace, hope, and a sense of purpose as individuals approach the end of their lives. The role of spirituality in the dying process is intricate and multifaceted, shaped by diverse belief systems and cultural contexts. From traditional religious beliefs to secular philosophies, various approaches to spirituality can significantly influence how individuals and their loved ones confront death and contemplate the concept of an afterlife [23].

Numerous belief systems encompass the concept of an afterlife or spiritual realm, which can evoke feelings of hope or fear contingent upon an individual's beliefs and personal encounters. Certain religious traditions, such as Christianity and Islam, espouse firm convictions regarding heaven and hell, wherein the departed undergo judgment and are assigned their eternal destination based on their earthly actions. Conversely, other traditions such as Buddhism and Hinduism perceive death as an inherent component of the life cycle, wherein the soul either reincarnates into a new existence or ultimately attains liberation from the cycle of rebirth [8, 24].

Spirituality can have a vital impact on providing support to individuals and their loved ones as they confront end-of-life concerns. Establishing connections with a spiritual community or partaking in personal spiritual practices can bestow solace and furnish a sense of direction and significance in the presence of mortality. Religious and spiritual customs, such as prayer, meditation, and ritual, can serve as avenues for connecting with a higher power or attaining inner tranquility.

Furthermore, spiritual beliefs and practices can assist individuals in finding meaning in their experiences and offer solace and hope to grieving loved ones [25]. In general, the influence of spirituality on the dying process is profoundly personal and influenced by a multitude of factors, encompassing cultural and religious beliefs, individual experiences, and social support systems. By recognizing the significance of spirituality in the journey toward death and honoring the diverse beliefs and practices of individuals and their loved ones, healthcare providers can extend more compassionate and comprehensive care to those grappling with end-of-life matters [26].

1.9 Legal considerations at the end of life

As individuals approach the final stages of their lives, they may confront various legal matters and inquiries pertaining to their care, treatment, and final wishes. Legal considerations related to death and dying can exhibit wide-ranging disparities contingent upon an individual's geographical location and the specific laws and regulations governing end-of-life care and decision-making.

One of the legal matters that may arise in end-of-life circumstances involves the assessment of decision-making capacity. As individuals approach death, they may become incapable of making decisions regarding their care and treatment, prompting legal inquiries regarding who holds the authority to act on their behalf. Such inquiries can encompass topics related to power of attorney, healthcare proxy, and guardianship laws.

Another legal consideration in end-of-life situations involves the utilization of advanced directives, which are documents that enable individuals to express their preferences regarding the end-of-life care and treatment. Advanced directives can include living wills, which outline specific medical interventions and procedures, as well as durable power of attorney for healthcare, which designates someone to make medical decisions on behalf of the individual. Laws regarding advanced directives can vary across states and countries, underscoring the importance of familiarizing oneself with local regulations.

In certain instances, legal matters pertaining to end-of-life care may involve disagreements between family members or healthcare providers concerning the most appropriate course of action. These disputes can encompass conflicts over decision-making authority, issues surrounding medical consent, and questions regarding the legality of specific treatments or procedures. In such situations, seeking legal counsel may be necessary to resolve conflicts and ensure the individual's wishes are honored [27, 28].

Laws and regulations concerning end-of-life care and decision-making can exhibit significant variations based on geographical location, reflecting cultural, religious, and social distinctions. For instance, in some countries, euthanasia or physician-assisted suicide may be legally permissible under certain circumstances, while in others, these practices are strictly prohibited. Similarly, laws relating to organ donation, funeral and burial arrangements, and estate planning can differ substantially among states or countries [27, 28].

In general, the legal aspects pertaining to death and dying are intricate and diverse, contingent upon factors such as an individual's specific situation, cultural heritage, and geographical setting. By comprehending the array of legal issues and regulations, healthcare providers and family members can offer enhanced support to patients, ensuring that their preferences are acknowledged and upheld [27, 28]. Conversely, the progress of technology has exerted a substantial influence on our perception and handling of death and the dying process. Medical breakthroughs and emerging technologies have facilitated enhanced diagnoses, treatments, and palliative care, resulting in extended life expectancies and better quality of life for individuals with terminal illnesses. However, this advancement has also introduced novel ethical predicaments as we navigate end-of-life care, relying on progressively sophisticated machines and interventions.

1.10 Technology and the end of life

One of the primary consequences of technology in the realm of death and dying is the capacity to extend life through medical interventions. The progress made in medical technology has led to employ life-sustaining measures such as mechanical ventilation and artificial nutrition and hydration, enabling individuals to survive despite serious illness or injury. While these interventions may grant patients additional time for potential recovery or important decision-making, they can also potentially prolong suffering and may not align with the individual's personal wishes or values.

The emergence of novel technologies has facilitated the introduction of inventive palliative care interventions, such as virtual reality encounters and therapeutic robots. These resources have the potential to alleviate pain and anxiety, enhance the quality of life for patients, and minimize the requirement for high-risk medical interventions.

Nevertheless, ethical quandaries can emerge when patients favor these technologies over human interaction, or when uncertainty arises regarding whether their implementation aligns with the individual's personal wishes or values.

Another consequence of technology in relation to death and dying is the capability to preserve bodily functions and genetic data for potential future applications. Practices such as cryonics, which involve freezing the human body with the aspiration of revival in the future, and genetic technologies, which enable embryo selection and gene editing, evoke ethical concerns regarding the intrinsic value of life and the boundaries of medical intervention. As these technologies progress, it becomes crucial to address these dilemmas and ensure that the utilization of technology in end-of-life care adheres to ethical principles.

The utilization of technology in the context of death and dying gives rise to concerns regarding privacy and consent. Electronic health records, online medical platforms, and telemedicine have facilitated convenient access to healthcare services and remote communication with healthcare providers. However, these technologies may also expose patients to a higher risk of data breaches or compromised privacy.

Furthermore, as technology reshapes the dynamics of the doctor-patient relationship and the delivery of medical care, it becomes essential to address matters pertaining to informed consent and the autonomy of patients and their families.

In general, the influence of technology on death and dying has been substantial and diverse. As we progress in the development of new technologies, it becomes crucial to thoroughly examine their ethical ramifications and guarantee that they are utilized in a manner that aligns with ethical principles and safeguards individuals involved [29].

2. Caregivers

In addition to the above aspects, caregiver burnout is a prevalent occurrence among individuals providing care for those nearing the end of their lives. The emotional and physical demands of caregiving can lead to persistent stress, fatigue, and feelings of isolation. It is vital for caregivers to recognize and effectively address these challenges in order to provide the best possible care for their loved ones.

One effective approach to addressing caregiver burnout is to make use of support services. Palliative care teams, social workers, and hospice volunteers can provide emotional support, offer education about end-of-life care, and assist with practical tasks and medication management. Furthermore, joining support groups, either in-person or online, can create a sense of community and validation for caregivers who may feel overwhelmed or isolated by their responsibilities.

Caregivers can also benefit from implementing personal coping strategies, such as mindfulness, engaging in regular exercise, or seeking therapy. These practices can help in managing stress, reducing feelings of anxiety and depression, and promoting overall well-being. Additionally, practicing self-compassion and establishing realistic expectations are important for caregivers, as they acknowledge that caregiving is a demanding and emotionally charged experience [29].

As the end-of-life journey progresses, caregivers may find it necessary to seek specialized support. For instance, as a patient's condition worsens, caregivers may require guidance and assistance in managing symptoms or making difficult decisions. Hospice care teams are available to offer this specialized care, providing pain management and guidance on advanced directives. Moreover, hospice care providers can support caregivers during the bereavement period, offering grief counseling and additional resources to help them navigate the challenging transition following the death of their loved one [29].

It is important to recognize that caregiver support extends beyond the end-of-life stage. Many communities provide ongoing support groups, counseling services, and other resources for bereaved caregivers. Additionally, caregivers must prioritize self-care and attend to their own physical and emotional well-being after the death of their loved one. This may involve seeking therapy, maintaining connections with support groups or other community resources, and practicing self-compassion and forgiveness as they navigate their grief.

Caring for someone who is approaching the end of life is a challenging and intricate responsibility, often accompanied by a range of emotions, thoughts, and obligations. However, with appropriate support and effective coping strategies, caregivers can provide compassionate and competent care for their loved ones while prioritizing their own health and well-being [29, 30].

Different circumstances surrounding death can have varying impacts on the individual nearing the end of life and their loved ones. The dying process can differ based on factors such as a terminal illness, sudden death, or traumatic circumstances. In cases of terminal illness, the dying process may unfold gradually, allowing the person and their family to emotionally and spiritually prepare for death. Terminal illness can involve symptoms such as pain and fatigue, and palliative care services can provide assistance and support to both the person approaching the end of life and their families [29, 30].

On the other hand, experiencing sudden death or trauma can be abrupt and overwhelming for the individuals left behind. Witnessing the sudden loss of a loved one can trigger feelings of shock, disbelief, anger, and guilt. Seeking counseling and support may be necessary to cope with the profound loss. The grieving process for those left behind can be influenced by the specific circumstances of the death. For instance, losing someone to suicide can introduce complex grief issues. Stigma and feelings of blame may accompany these types of deaths, intensifying the challenges faced during the grieving process [30].

The cultural or spiritual beliefs held by individuals and their families can shape their perspectives on death and dying. While some cultures view the dying process as a natural and inevitable stage of life, others may have a tendency to avoid discussions or contemplations on death altogether [8].

3. Culture and the end of life

Death, being an unavoidable aspect of life, is honored in various ways across different cultures. Although death rituals may differ based on cultural and religious beliefs, their underlying purpose remains the same: to pay tribute to and commemorate the life of the deceased. In many cultures, funerals or memorial services play a vital role in the grieving and healing journey of the bereaved family [8, 30].

Death is perceived and dealt with differently across various cultures, reflecting their unique beliefs and customs. For instance, in Hinduism, death is considered a natural phase of the life cycle. The body is cremated, and the ashes are scattered in a sacred body of water, symbolizing the soul's ultimate liberation. In Judaism, the deceased is ritually cleansed, wrapped in a simple white burial garment, and buried within a day, emphasizing the importance of timely burial. Conversely, traditional Chinese culture involves intricate rituals and practices that span multiple days, including the burning of offerings and adherence to Feng Shui principles [8, 31].

While cultural and religious customs vary, certain universal practices are observed across different cultures. Lighting candles or incense and offering prayers for the departed are common ways to guide the soul's journey to the afterlife. Wearing black as a symbol of grief and mourning is a customary practice during mourning periods in many cultures. Additionally, expressing condolences and sending sympathy cards are shared gestures of support and compassion seen across various cultures and religions [8].

4. Conclusion

In summary, while death is a shared aspect of the human condition, the cultural perspectives and practices surrounding it can greatly differ. However, common threads of paying tribute to the departed and providing solace to the grieving are observed universally. Recognizing and respecting cultural diversity in end-of-life customs is crucial for facilitating a serene and respectful passage from life to death [1, 8].

The ultimate goal of palliative care is to alleviate the suffering of both the patient and his/her family, through the proper understanding, detection, and control of physical, psychosocial, and spiritual symptoms experienced by patients at the end of life, regardless of diagnosis. But, while it is true that death is a natural phenomenon, the process of dying is treated as a disease, and today, we are experiencing the medicalization of death. As a consequence, many people die in hospitals in the most extreme loneliness and pain. In other cases, service provision models have been dichotomized to the point of providing aggressive curative treatment and establishing palliative measures in the face of therapeutic failure. The consequence of this reality is that patients and families are left in the middle of an economic and social conflict, since they do not find a team that allows them to understand the nature of the disease, the diagnosis, and the prognosis, this being a crucial aspect for the decision-making at the end of life. Total pain, conceived as the sum of physical pain, psychological pain, and spiritual pain, constitutes one of the origins of suffering. The most relevant triggers in addition to physical pain are the process of dying itself, loss of autonomy, and resignification of life.

The foregoing requires a transdisciplinary team with relevant training to intervene in these realities of patients and family members in palliation. Palliative patients need to develop a closure and forgiveness mechanism to die in peace.

As the end of life approaches, the management of symptoms necessitates comprehensive palliative strategies. Similarly, as interventions become more intense, service delivery processes must be enhanced. It should be emphasized that end-of-life care does not conclude with the patient's death; instead, the focus of the caregiving team shifts toward supporting the family and facilitating the grieving process.

In the context of a complex world, Western culture, rooted in tradition and orthodox values, is encountering an emerging society characterized by diverse and evolving lifestyles, shifting values, and less universally shared perspectives. This transition brings forth new challenges and barriers, such as coexistence in divergent and multicultural settings, changes in identity, marginalization, and the exclusion of social, ethnic, religious, sexual, professional, and academic groups [32].

Recognizing the intricate nature of biopsychosocial processes necessitates educational institutions to equip new professionals with a comprehensive understanding. This entails developing programs that embrace multidimensionality, foster the construction of reality through clear and innovative ideas, enable objective assessments, facilitate assertive decision-making, and cultivate metacognitive skills that allow for the integration of existing knowledge with new information while appreciating the unity within multiplicity [15].

The act of providing care is a purposeful endeavor that serves the well-being of individuals and their families within a societal context. While physicians devote a significant portion of their training and practice to preserving and prolonging life, end-of-life care is often entrusted to a select few pain specialists and spiritual practitioners who facilitate acceptance and surrender to the dying process. Palliative care, however, is specifically aimed at the individual, the human being, and their family during the final stages of life [1, 33].

This implies that for successful implementation, a comprehensive understanding of human existence is necessary, encompassing not only the somatic or biological aspects but also the environmental, psychological, social, and spiritual dimensions of individuals. Furthermore, death is a fundamental subject in the realms of philosophy, psychology, and medicine. Inquiries into the significance of death, its purpose, and the various associated questions have persisted throughout human history. However, beyond death, one of the most extensively examined yet least multidisciplinary aspects is the meaning of suffering [8, 34].

Providing care for a person involves being by their side, supporting their autonomy, and assisting them in their vulnerability. Palliative care embodies a particular approach to delivering this care. Furthermore, from a transdisciplinary perspective, the act of caring for a patient entails accompanying them throughout their journey of illness and death. In this context, death becomes more than just a problem; it encompasses the complexities of life itself. Consequently, it gives rise to a range of bioethical and multidimensional considerations.

When an individual faces the proximity of death, they experience a heightened sense of its presence and significance. They become acutely aware of its profound and challenging nature. Consequently, in the care of someone nearing the end of life, it is crucial to take their perception of death seriously, as it directly influences their psychological state [35, 36]. Thus, it is pertinent and responsible for caregivers to first confront their own understanding of death, as well as that of their loved ones, in order to effectively provide support in this context. This research work is motivated by this very scenario [36].

In the course of life, we do not have the choice to avoid death, but we do possess the fundamental right to determine how we will face it. Therefore, it is essential to have a qualified team that can deliver comprehensive, compassionate, and empathetic are at the end of life [36].

Author details

Luz Marina Cano Molano
Juan N Corpas University, Bogota, Colombia

*Address all correspondence to: luz.cano@juanncorpas.edu.co

References

[1] Cano L. Modelo pedagógico y diseño de currículo en Cuidados Paliativos fundamentado en la Transdisciplina. Ediciones FEDICOR ed. Tunja: Fundación Universitaria Juan N. Corpas. Centro Editorial; 2020

[2] Morin E. Para un Pensamiento del Sur. 2011. Available form: https://www.revistasonline.org/public/pdf/MorinPenseeduSudFR.pdf

[3] Matzo M, Sherman DW. Palliative Care Nursing: Quality Care to the End of Life. New York, NY: Springer Publishing Company; 2006. p. 317. 9780826157935. Available from: https://books.google.com.co/books?id=VTM7BniF-tEC

[4] Chochinov HM. Dignity and the essence of medicine: The A, B, C, and D of dignity conserving care. British Medical Journal. 2007;**335**(7612):184-187. DOI: 10.1136/bmj.39244.650926.47

[5] Tomás-Sábado J, Villavicencio Chávez C, Monforte-Royo C, Guerrero M, Fegg M, Balaguer A. What gives meaning in life in palliative care patients? A comparison between Spanish, German and Swiss populations. Journal of Pain and Symptom Management. 2016;**50**(6):861-866. DOI: 10.1016/j.jpainsymman.2015.06.015

[6] Breitbart W, Rosenfeld B, Gibson C, Pessin H, Poppito S, Nelson C, et al. Meaning-centered group psychotherapy for patients with advanced cancer: A pilot randomized controlled trial. Psycho-Oncology. 2015;**24**(12):1583-1587

[7] Bruera E, Suarez-Almazor M, Velasco A, Bertolino M, MacDonald SM, Hanson J. The assessment of constipation in terminal cancer patients admitted to a palliative care unit: A retrospective review. Journal of Pain and Symptom Management. 1994;**9**(8):515-519

[8] Cano LM. La noología de la muerte. Bogota, Colombia: FEDICOR; 2023. p. 88. ISBN: 978-958-9297-74-2

[9] Morin E. La rumeur d´órleans. L'Histoire immédiate. Éditions du Seuil; 1991

[10] Morin E. Seven Complex Lessons in Education for the Future. Traduction Medellin-Colombia: UNESCO; 2001

[11] Morin E. Culture and Crisis. Urbana, IL: University of Illinois Press; 2002

[12] Morin E. On Complexity. Paris, France: Hampton Press; 2011

[13] Morin E. Homeland Earth: A Manifesto for the New Millenium. Cresskill, NJ: Hampton Press; 2014

[14] Morin E. Ethics: On the Condition of Being Human. Paris, France: Routledge; 2015

[15] Morin E. Penser Global: l'humain et son Univers. Paris, France: L'Herne; 2017

[16] Morin E. "Sociologie de la Mort" (Sociology of Death). Paris: Éditions du Seuil; 1990

[17] Ma J, Chi S, Buettner B, Pollard K, Muir M, Kolekar C, et al. Early palliative care consultation in the medical ICU: A cluster randomized crossover trial. Critical Care Medicine. 2019;**47**(12):1707-1715. DOI: 10.1097/CCM.0000000000004016

[18] Zhai Y, Du X. Loss and grief amidst COVID-19: A path to adaptation and resilience. Brain, Behavior, and

Immunity. 2020;**87**:80-81. DOI: 10.1016/j.bbi.2020.04.053. Epub 2020 Apr 23

[19] Helm. The Death of a Person Has Been Analysed as the 'Reason' Na'aman Forthcoming for Grief, and the Element of Love Has Been Called its 'Background Condition' (Na'aman Forthcoming) or its 'Focus'. Vol. 8, No. 3. Landslide: American Bar Association; 2016

[20] Chen CH, Chen YC. The meanings of death beliefs, dying meanings, and death attitudes. OMEGA-Journal of Death and Dying. 2015;**70**(3):223-237

[21] Stroebe M, Schut H. The dual process model of grief: Past, present, and future. Death Studies. 2015;**39**(4):210-218

[22] Morin E. "Penser la Mort" (Thinking about Death). Paris: Éditions du Seiul; 1995

[23] Canadian Nurses Association. Ethics in Practice: A Guide for Ethical Decision Making. Ottowa, ON: Canadian Nurses Association; 2017

[24] Truog RD, Robinson WM. Role of brain death and the dead-donor rule in the ethics of organ transplantation. Critical Care Medicine. 2003;**31**(9):2391-2396

[25] Robinson MR, Thiel MM, Backus MM, Meyer EC. Matters of spirituality at the end of life in the pediatric intensive care unit. Pediatrics. 2006;**118**:e719-e729. DOI: 10.1542/peds.2005-2298

[26] Eliopoulos C. Gerontological Nursing. 9th ed. Philadelphia, PA: Wolters Kluwer; 2018

[27] Puchalski CM, Vitillo R, Hull SK, Reller N. Improving the spiritual dimension of whole person care: Reaching national and international consensus. Journal of Palliative Medicine. 2014;**17**(6):642-656. DOI: 10.1089/jpm.2014.9427

[28] American Bar Association Commission on Law and Aging. ABA Consumer's Tool Kit for Health Care Advance Planning. American Bar Association Commission on Law and Aging; 2020. Available from: https://www.americanbar.org/groups/law_aging/

[29] Kamal AH, Wolf SP, Troy J, Leff V, Dahlin C, Rotella JD, et al. Policy changes key to promoting sustainability and growth of the specialty palliative care workforce. Health Affairs (Millwood). 2019;**38**(6):910-918. DOI: 10.1377/hlthaff.2019.00018

[30] American Cancer Society. Caregiver Resources. American Cancer Society; 2022. Available from: https://www.cancer.org/content/cancer/en/cancer/coping-with-cancer/caregiversupport.html_Center_to_Advance

[31] Crooms RC, Gelfman LP. Palliative care and end-of-life considerations for the frail patient. Anesthesia and Analgesia. 2020;**130**(6):1504-1515. DOI: 10.1213/ANE.0000000000004763

[32] Smithsonian Magazine. Eight Enduring Traditions on Death and Dying. Smithsonian Magazine; 2017. Available from: https://www.smithsonianmag.com/

[33] Toh SG, And E, Devi MK. Systematic review on the relationship between the nursing shortage and job satisfaction, stress and burnout levels among nurses in oncology/hematology settings. International Journal of Evidence-Based Healthcare. 2012;10(2):126-141

[34] Torralba F. Hacia una Filosofía de los cuidados Paliativos. Revista Seleccionesde Bioética. 2007;**6**:17-23

[35] BBC News. How Different Cultures around the World Deal with Death. England: BBC News; 2016. Available from: https://www.bbc.com/news/world-35706238

[36] O'Boyle et al. Quality of life issues in palliative medicine. Journal of Neurology. 1997;**244**(suppl. 4):18-25

Chapter 3

Perspective Chapter: Last Questions – How Philosophical Practice Contributes to Developing Death Literacy

Patrick Schuchter, Stefanie V. Rieger, Sandra Radinger and Klaus Wegleitner

Abstract

Dealing with existential questions is a constitutive part of palliative care. Interestingly, if we admit that borderline situations at the end-of life give rise to philosophical questions, in the contexts of practice, these questions are perceived (nearly) without any reference to explicit philosophical traditions or to Philosophical Practice. Philosophical Practice is a modern movement for a non-elitist philosophy. It aims to enable people—in the Socratic tradition—to reflect on their experiences in a philosophical way in everyday life. In the recently launched research project *Philosophical Practice in Palliative Care and Hospice Work*, we are investigating the opportunities and limits of Philosophical Practice for the development of death literacy. Building on previous theoretical work, we analyse, discuss, and illustrate concrete models of Philosophical Practice in this chapter. Our conclusions refer to practical indications for relating Philosophical Practice productively to relevant contexts of death literacy development, such as caring communities, Last Aid courses, and everyday ethics.

Keywords: Philosophical Practice, death literacy, palliative care, end-of-life care, public health palliative care, hospice work, philosophy

1. Introduction

In the context of end-of-life care, there are many questions which lead directly to action and concrete solutions, for example, which care services are missing in our community? And how can we communicate and consider concrete wishes for the end-of life? Some everyday questions can be answered through "empirical" knowledge, i.e., through information or e.g., palliative medical expertise. For instance, those questions can be: How can pain and symptoms be treated? Or what complementary options are there? Finally, there are several questions arising around the end-of life, which neither require immediate solutions and action nor can they be answered by experts. These questions demand responses from us in contexts of end-of-life care, but also in life generally. There can be questions such as: What makes a "fulfilled" life and what does it mean to not live it? What does it mean to need help and to "accept help" (from a friend, from a stranger)? What is trust—how is it built, how is it lost? In what ways am I responsible for others?

The latter kind are examples of ultimate or last questions, on which everyone has to personally develop an opinion or has (implicitly) already developed one. The philosopher Immanuel Kant characterises them by an unsurpassed articulation: "Human reason has the peculiar fate of being harassed by questions which it cannot reject, but which it also cannot answer" [1]. Still, last questions can awaken a desire to delve into them deeply, which is an expression of philosophical interest in everyday life.

Attempting to formulate last questions is itself a first philosophical act. Usually, it is not obvious to us what moves us at a deeper human level. Thus, targeting our conversations and (joint) thinking towards last questions is more than an exchange of words. As we tell each other about what moves us and articulate associated feelings, such "conversations" may bear clarity and deeper insight into the issues of our last questions. We may then together engage in gathering concepts of life and their critical examination. Formulated simply, this kind of engagement is the sphere of philosophy and the pursuit of the philosophical interest.

The philosophical interest and desire to philosophise is particularly likely to arise in "borderline-" or "ultimate situations". Following Karl Jaspers, becoming aware of ultimate situations is the deeper origin of philosophising. They are "[s]ituations we can't get beyond, we can't change [...] I have to die, I have to suffer, I have to fight, I get inevitably entangled in guilt [...]. In mere existence we often avoid them by closing our eyes and living as if they weren't there. We forget that we have to die" ([2], p. 18). But does Jaspers refer to academic studies when he speaks of philosophising? In this context, Jaspers refers to ancient philosophy, especially to the Stoics and Epictetus, for whom, philosophising springs from the experience of finitude: "The origin of philosophy is awareness of one's own weakness and powerlessness" ([2], p. 17). Thus, when we think of limits, we do not necessarily think of death alone: "To philosophise is at once to learn to live and to be able to die. Because of the uncertainty of existence in time, life is constantly trying" ([2], p. 18).

The interrelationship between philosophical traditions of thought and society's approach to death and dying is reflected in the Lancet Commission on the Value of Death [3]. It makes clear how much society's approach to dying, death, and mourning is reflected in philosophical traditions of thought. Moreover, it emphasises that end-of-life care, which wants to (re-)integrate dying and death into life and society, indispensably has to take philosophical and spiritual dimensions into account in its practices and cultures. For a life-integrating approach to dying and death ("bringing death back into life"), the following element of a realistic utopia is formulated: "Conversations and stories about everyday death, dying, and grief become common" ([3], p. 870). Strengthening death literacy and also rooting end-of-life care in philosophy and spirituality is considered significant. The question of which everyday care practices could succeed in building bridges here is answered above all with references to conversations about dying and loss, to Death Cafés and/or the Last Aid courses. However, Philosophical Practices are not considered—which marks the beginning of our research interest.

Our research interest is based on two elementary observations. First, the notion "to philosophise is to learn to die" has been at the core and heart of philosophy ever since its beginnings [4]. Secondly, philosophy or Philosophical Practice is virtually absent in the context of palliative care and hospice work—at least not as a structurally anchored practice or as a self-evident conceptual reference.

In this chapter, we, therefore, illuminate how strongly last philosophical questions shape dying and end-of-life care and outline forms of Philosophical Practice for addressing last questions. Our contribution aims to provide exemplary insights and a general orientation on this topic.

2. What is Philosophical Practice? Attempting an overview

All philosophical questions are preceded by the question of philosophy itself: What is philosophy? What at first translates as "love of wisdom" is nevertheless much more than reserved for "the wise": philosophy deals with the fundamental questions of being human.

2.1 A short introduction to philosophy in general

In the history of philosophy, various theses can be found at the beginning of philosophising or philosophy. The ancient philosophers Plato and Socrates identified wonder as the beginning of philosophy. Today, academic philosophy is organised as a scientific discipline amongst others, i.e., it is oriented towards scientific standards and disciplinary frameworks of relevance. This orientation makes it difficult for lay people to access philosophical insights and reflections. Without mediation, insights of relevance to everyday life rarely reach beyond university walls—let alone individual persons. It is not surprising thus that philosophy is often experienced as something irrelevant and not very useful for everyday practice. Yet, it is the original idea of philosophy that philosophising emerges from and is located in everyday life experience.

To capture the various ways in which philosophy can be practised and to define the characteristics of Philosophical Practice, Ute Gahlings [5], inspired by Georg Boehme, differentiates four categories. These build on Boehme's concepts of four manifestations of philosophy: philosophy as a science, as worldly wisdom, as a way of life, and as a Philosophical Practice. **Table 1** gives an overview.

Philosophy	Denotes
Science	An academic subject at university and in organisational form of scientific research and teaching, with corresponding publications, specialist jargon, the social role of the professor, etc.
World wisdom	An intellectual who contributes intelligently and wittily in public to current issues of the time, society, and life, for example, in the *feuilleton*, on television, as a well-known speaker, or "in the street".
Way of life	The orientation of one's own life in confrontation with philosophical sources of inspiration and philosophical exercises. The philosophical life teachings and communities of the Stoics and Epicureans, for example, stand for philosophy as a way of life.
Philosophical Practice	A relatively new, semi-institutionalised offer of thought and discussion for people who want to place their life questions in a broader context and do so in encounter and discussion with a philosopher in concrete forms that are philosophical counselling in the "practice" of a philosopher, philosophical cafés, and more.

Table 1.
Manifestations of philosophy, based on Gahlings [5].

The fact that philosophy does not only belong to academically trained persons becomes particularly visible in the development of philosophy as a form of life since antiquity [6]. The ancient philosophers, especially in the Hellenistic era way before the Christian pastoral care, understand philosophy as care for the soul and the community at the same time, as the art of living and dying, as practising a personally sustaining attitude to life, and a common culture of life. The great role model Socrates philosophises in the marketplace, does not write any lines and is known for the fact that his thinking corresponds to his actions. So, in an elementary and original sense, philosophy is not necessarily an elitist affair. It is simply the expression of thinking about and discussing essential questions of life, of questioning one's own and collective principles and attitudes to life, and of subjecting them to a thoughtful examination.

2.2 Philosophical Practice in the present day

The kind of philosophy which aims at continuing the Socratic tradition today is frequently summarised by the umbrella term "Philosophical Practice" ("*Philosophische Praxis*"). Sometimes, the term "philosophical counselling" is used. It is based on the view that philosophy is relevant to everyday life and that it is a certain form of care for the "soul" and "community".

Historically [7–10], the movement's beginnings are often ascribed to the initiative of Gerd Achenbach who opened his Philosophical Practice in Bergisch Gladbach, Germany, in 1981. Between the late 1980s and early 2000s, Philosophical Practice flourished. The inaugural International Conference on Philosophical Practice took place in 1994 in Vancouver. Since then, various international and national associations of Philosophical Practice have been founded whilst the body of literature has remained modest still. It has been growing more recently, however, since more and more philosophical practitioners are beginning to discuss and publish their approaches [5, 7, 11, 12]. Regarding actual practices, the *café philosophique* initiated by Marc Sautet in Paris in the 1990s, and various approaches to "philosophy for children" are forms of Philosophical Practice which are known to a wider public today.

Next to the wider known forms of Philosophical Practice, it can be found in a variety of formats and contexts (**Table 2**):

Philosophical Practice is found in the following formats:
Individual offers of Philosophical Practice

- Philosophical Counselling "Philosophical counselling",
- Philosophical Supervision,
- Philosophical Biography Work,
- Philosophical Correspondence,
- etc.

Group offers of Philosophical Practice

- Philosophical Cafés,
- Philosophical Salons,
- Philosophical Workshops,
- Philosophical Walks,
- etc.

Table 2.
Formats of Philosophical Practice.

The formats of Philosophical Practice (**Table 2**) indicate that it is—by its very name—oriented towards being active. In the case of Philosophical Practice, this means in-depth thinking together. Philosophical Practice can become visible wherever there is a concrete, active encounter between philosophers. However, the pursuit of philosophical interest can also glimmer in everyday life and in everyday conversations.

2.3 Philosophical Practice and end-of-life care: observations and reflections

Although Philosophical Practice is far from being structurally anchored or established in the practice of end-of-life-care, palliative care, and hospice work (in contrast to, for example, psychotherapy, supervision, coaching, ethical case discussions, pastoral care, or concepts such as spiritual care), there are approaches in which it can be found within these contexts too.

Some philosophical practitioners report experiences with issues typical in palliative care and hospice work: they reflect the possibilities of Philosophical Practice in the context of "illness as an inevitable life topic" [13], use Socratic dialogue to empower rehabilitating cancer patients [14], discuss personal examples of "how philosophy can help us grieve" [15], or have long-term experience in creating "Socratic communities" working with professionals in the field such as nurses, priests, and social workers [16].

Birnbacher [17] reports potentials and limitations of the Socratic method in teaching medical ethics. "Ethics-from-the-bottom-up" [18], our own project from previous research, experimentally explored various aspects of the transition from ethics consultation to philosophical conversation.

Schuchter [19] observes that in spiritual care discourse, philosophical traditions and approaches to spirituality hardly occur at all and consequently describe four philosophical exercises appropriate to the context. An example of "philosophical care" in the context of spiritual care can be found in Krüger [20]. Schuchter et al. [21] furthermore develop "Speed-Philo", a model that is intended to facilitate elementary philosophising. The model has been established in the children's hospice and family support service of Malteser Berlin.

Wegleitner et al. [22] elaborate on the relevance of philosophical settings in the reflection of Caring Community model projects—both in "existential" (spiritual) terms and in a participatory political dimension. This largely corresponds to the Lancet Report mentioned at the beginning of our article [3]. In this context, Leonard et al. [23] define different knowledge dimensions of death literacy, each of which is connected to a philosophical deepening. Philosophical knowledge can prevent death literacy from becoming too "technical".

There is furthermore a remarkable initiative which does not originate in the "hospice and palliative scene" at all but is significant as a way of organising Philosophical Practice within the development of Caring Cities and thus of death literacy. The *DenkZeitRaum* (literally: "thinking-time-space") is a project based at the Institute of Philosophy at the University of Graz, which started in 2011 [24]. The events link the university with the public space and the professional discourse with informal learning processes of citizens. In 2019 and 2020, the *DenkZeitRaum* was dedicated to the question: "Who or what does Europe belong to?". Due to the Corona pandemic and related crises, two philosophical cafés were organised on the topic of death. The *DenkZeitRaum* organises events on three levels: firstly, in the form of academic discourse at the university; secondly, in the form of opening the university to a broad public; and thirdly, in public space. The Philosophical Practice is thus embedded in a cooperative, communal network. Network partners are primarily the city of Graz (mayor's office, cultural office), various institutions depending on the topic (museum, society for political education and others) and, in the case of the philosophical café, the "*Grätzeltreff*" (neighbourhood meeting place, district office). In this context, the topic of death is not addressed from within palliative care, which has the potential of generating surprising perspectives on end-of-life issues. The *DenkZeitRaum* thus realises a participatory, networked structure in the sense of the Compassionate City idea for democratic, philosophical impulses that promote death literacy from the bottom up [25].

It must be said, however, that not all activities of Philosophical Practice relevant to end-of-life care are published. On the contrary, Philosophical Practitioners usually do not operate in the field of philosophy-science and therefore do not necessarily publish. To give examples from the German-speaking world: the philosophical practitioner Judith Tech (together with Bernd Groth) has been offering philosophical cafés and talks as "philosophising in the hospice" and in nursing homes for years [26]; Dietlinde Schmalfuß-Plicht engages in Philosophical Practice in the context of hospice volunteering and mourning work [27].

3. Paradigmatic styles in Philosophical Practice with examples

If we take a closer look at the field of Philosophical Practice, at least three paradigmatic styles can be distinguished. We speak here of "styles" because, in practice, the distinction is not always clear. Our overview is therefore not comprehensive but attempts an initial systematisation with regard to end-of-life care.

To describe each style, we add experiences from our own Philosophical Practice, i.e., from a series of philosophical cafés from the field of hospice and palliative care. These experiences illustrate a particular focus of the different basic styles of Philosophical Practice and build a bridge to the thematic field of palliative care.

Authors of this paper have offered philosophical cafés (or other similar formats) in very different contexts. We focus here on a series of philosophical cafés at the Kardinal König Haus in Vienna [28]. The Kardinal König Haus is an adult education institution with a significant role in the development of hospice and palliative work in Austria. Since 2020, it has offered the "Philosophicum", a philosophical café, at irregular intervals but on an ongoing basis. The café takes place in the evening and lasts about 2 hours. The basic idea of the "Philosophicum" is to philosophically explore and discuss topics that arise in end-of-life care but may also relate to other social fields. The "Philosophicum" has taken place 14 times since 2020.

3.1 The dialogical style

3.1.1 Description

It is typical of the dialogical style that its representatives refuse to ascribe to one single method: "[...] the idea that what is happening can be approached programmatically-methodologically is misleading" ([5], p. 138). Philosophy stands for the freedom of thought, from which methods develop if necessary, and the methods cannot and must not be determined in advance. Therefore, the Philosophical Practitioner plays a special role. "The strength of Philosophical Practice lies in the fact that it is an art […]", the Philosophical Practitioner is therefore challenged in their creativity. Emphasis is therefore placed on the dialogical relationship, which Gahlings calls "solidary participation" ([5], p. 62). As already described by Plato, the spark of thinking between people arises through continuing community of life and thought. A guest (a person attending Philosophical Practice) talks with the Philosophical Practitioner about their history, experiences, and questions. The Philosophical Practitioner listens and helps the guest with recognising their own concepts of life and with thinking and clarifying their thoughts by reference to philosophy. Gerd Achenbach [8] understood Philosophical Practice in this way. In this style, people do not seek out the Philosophical Practitioner with ready-made questions, but share their experiences, often in the form of stories from life. It is then the responsibility of the Philosophical Practitioner to identify together with the guest the philosophical part in the stories. What is told becomes the subject of the conversation. This conversation does not proceed in a psychological or psychotherapeutic manner, but strives for universality, for increasing the understanding of what is experienced, for approaching a shared truth. Philosophical Practice is hence strongly characterised by the art of listening.

On the basis of wonder, philosophers try to identify the life theme [9, 29] that moves the guest in their narrative. Life themes are unavoidable themes—they are of such generality and so fundamental that the experience of the themes cannot be avoided. Lindseth [9] reports that one theme recurs in his own Philosophical Practice, namely the themes of reconciliation. Reconciliation is also a common end-of-life theme that sufferers and carers encounter multiple times in the context of palliative care.

The Philosophical Practitioner and the guest are on a completely symmetrical level in front of the topic of life. That is why the person, the listening, and the wondering play such a role—the Philosophical Practitioner asks themself the question that is at stake in the guest's story. Gerd Achenbach describes the basic dialogue-philosophical situation like this [8, 30]: "One puts a question before me. What do I do? I take it up and ask it to myself as if I had asked it myself […]. By accepting his question as a question to me, I make it my own […]. And now he [the guest] may watch what his question does to me" [31].

It is often stressed that Philosophical Practice is an offer for people seeking support in crises. Nevertheless, the conversation itself is not oriented towards help. According to Achenbach, this ambivalence is to be understood in this way: help is not sought, but often results from the Practice ([8], p. 21).

3.1.2 An example

In the "Philosophicum" titled "What does dignity mean?", a participant tells a story. When he was a child, his father beat him with a belt because he thought his son broke a clock. But that was not true. Despite the beatings, the little boy does not betray his truth and sticks to it, insisting that he is innocent. The story moves the participants of the Philosophical Café; it is empathically received. Sharing the story makes the group that is listening a community (at least for the moment). Then they explore what dignity means in this example—it is no longer about the narrator, but about the theme of life using his story as an example. The participants try to name characteristics of dignity. All sentences are to be understood as attempts to grasp the phenomenon of dignity. It is important not to react too quickly whether this is true or not. The sentences have to be heard first to have an effect on the group and on the thinking. There were sentences like:

- "The belt does not touch the dignity of the boy"—that is, the violence cannot violate dignity or the sense of dignity (which was further discussed and challenged later with other examples, like human trafficking, torture).
- Dignity is a matter of choice, in the sense that the child who sticks to the truth does not accept injustice. The boy feels that there is something in him that gives him the power to keep to his dignity.
- Dependence on others is not the crucial trait about dignity.
- Those who have a sense of dignity can endure many things.
- The victim was stronger—the lack of dignity is in the perpetrator.

At the same time, the guest, telling the story, is dignified with his story and has found an audience. The group shared the thinking effort about the boy's story.

3.2 The analytical style

3.2.1 Description

Philosophical Practice does not only mean to proceed hermeneutically and phenomenologically, as in the dialogical approach. There are also methods of Philosophical Practice that place clear emphasis on a very rational analysis. Oscar Brenifier's style of conducting a philosophical consultation shows an example of this.

The immediate opinions, questions, ideas that a guest brings to the philosophical consultation are subjected to a thoroughly rigorous, critical analysis. Whilst in the dialogical approach, the Philosophical Practitioner takes on a role as a friendly, philosophically educated good listener, in the analytical approach, the philosopher takes on the role of the troublesome Socrates or that of a "detective" ([32], p. 31). Often humorous and playful, nevertheless rigorously and sometimes at first unpleasantly, they undertake a probing interrogation of the guest's ideas and opinions. At the core of interaction lies the guest's question, not their story, which they bring with them, and which in itself already implies a lot of (unconscious) presuppositions. The guest is asked to bring only one philosophical question per session.

The conversation is characterised by short sentences, for example ([33], p. 301), Oscar Brenifier would ask: "What is your question?", and the guest might respond with another question: "How to find the right distance with my parents?" Then the elements of the question are explored, like: "What does 'right distance' mean?" As the conversation progresses, the guest's attempts at definition and statements are comprehensively questioned and examined. The unclear initial question is transformed into a clear one, key terms are defined and distinguished, and contradictions are identified or sought through counterstatements.

Whilst in the dialogical approach, the atmosphere of a participating, empathic understanding in the interpersonal encounter prevails, the atmosphere in the analytical approach is rather that of a clear questioning, which can also be hurtful and frustrating if necessary. The guest—for the sake of coherence and rigour of thought—can be contradicted, interrupted and overall, the guest has to endure that their immediately taken-for-granted opinions and questions are very quickly shaken. Since these opinions are not some purely intellectual theoretical building blocks, but rather the lived conceptions and ideas that are "stored" in one's mind, imprinting patterns, spontaneous ways of acting, one's own life is also put to the test with the examination of one's thinking. Philosophical Practice has the task of transforming a person's unconscious and "indisputable postulates" ([32], p. 25) into "simple hypotheses" about a matter and subjecting them to examination. Those who endure the questioning may well experience a liberating effect, an expansion of thought in the Enlightenment sense. The painfulness of the examination is often softened by humour and playful lightness.

3.2.2 An example

In one of our philosophical cafés, on the topic of "How do we want to die?", a participant tells in a very personal way how she experienced death of a relative. From this experience, she goes on to describe her wish to die peacefully, in the circle of the closest relatives, without pain, with a clear consciousness, and at peace. The atmosphere in the group is now decidedly quiet and a certain emotion is palpable. But, since the group agreed at the beginning that they want to look at the stories with philosophical interest and also question the statements behind them, the moderator asks: "What is the thesis behind this? I would say it is the thesis of peaceful, reconciled dying. Isn't that the ideal and cliché death of the hospice movement? Let's try to question this thesis of dying well. Who can refute it?" In the following sequence—after a short thinking silence—first thoughts come up, like: It is a very quiet, a well-behaved, perhaps all too disciplined death; dying, which is originally supposed to be brought out of the taboo, is after all silenced again; there is no resistance, no revolt in dying, no outcry against the imposition that is death; Suffering must be kept a secret in society, it must not disturb everyday life. The pointed articulation and questioning (even refutation) of a thesis that implies the unspoken, lived, embodied theory of a reconciled, peaceful death "stored" in feelings, spontaneous reactions, and also external structures allows the excluded, repressed to become conscious, expands thinking, and perhaps even leads to—at that moment, in any case, strongly perceptible—"conversion".

3.3 The contemplative style

3.3.1 Description

A contemplative style can be found in the work of the Israeli-American philosophical practitioner Ran Lahav. His style is called Deep Philosophy and is motivated by "love, yearning, wonder" [34]. In common with all other styles of Philosophical Practice, Lahav also states that Philosophical Practice dives into deeper meaning: "In Deep Philosophy we contemplate on basic life issues from our inner depth, in togetherness with our companions and with historical philosophical texts" ([34], p. 14).

By this inner depth, he and the members of the Deep Philosophy Group form a source of understanding that is accessible to any interested person even without prior philosophical knowledge. In order to enter this state of inner understanding, members of the Deep Philosophy Group invite you to join sessions, which can take place preferably in presence, but also online. The 1–2 hour Deep Philosophy unit follows certain moderated rituals based on the joint reading of short text excerpts from a philosophical work. In this way, the participants elicit thoughts prompted by the text, but not necessarily truths.

The session usually begins with a meditative exercise to get into the right mood for the philosophy lesson. The joint reading of the text follows; it can be the exercise of "interpretive reading". Each participant reads a certain passage and adds their own interpretation in the form of individual words or short sentences to the text. The next person then interprets the same passage again. The exercise is repeated in several rounds and, if necessary, only interrupted by reading without adding one's own thoughts. The Deep Philosophy Group is applying the principle of *Ruminatio*, which might be already known from religious contexts. Another method of the Deep Philosophy Group is "precious speaking", meaning all participants say only those terms that came to them as ideas after reading the text. It is important to say just enough to let the others participate in one's own thoughts and to choose the words carefully.

At the end-of the session, the facilitator usually invites the participants to reflect on the whole text. In his book *What is Deep Philosophy?,* Lahav describes the emergence of a "philosophical polyphony" through this particular way of doing Philosophical Practice. Deep Philosophy does not aim to develop something new, but to come back to one's own thoughts.

3.3.2 An example

In the "Philosophicum" titled "Experiencing Mortality", the participants begin by introducing themselves and their initial associations with the topic. There is still a certain hustle and bustle in the room—the waitress is still taking orders for drinks, the pace of everyday life has not been completely discarded. Gradually, with time and a calm manner, the philosophical practitioner facilitates a break from everyday life urgencies. The atmosphere becomes calmer, concentrated, listening, all participants are very present—it becomes "meditative" to a certain degree. For a while, the associations are strung together, and over time the spoken contributions begin to (implicitly) revolve around a leitmotif. A leitmotif or reference point in this specific conversation is that of "commonality in the face of death", posing a question: What makes us feel connected in the shared fate of mortality? The experience of mortality turns into an exploration of the riddle of life with its bonds and divisions. Another leitmotif has an almost philosophical, epistemological character: What does it actually mean to "experience" death or one's own mortality? A nurse says he was often present with dying people, but did not really experience death because he had to function (go on). One mode is "being there without experiencing" or feeling the death. A woman tells how, when her husband died, she had to organise many things and simply "function", which is why she did not consciously experience mortality, grief, and the feeling of her own finiteness at the first moment. But "functioning" kept her alive. Narratives of the perceived sacredness at the time of a dying person's death, where sadness and beauty would touch, are answered by narratives of subsequent family conflicts around the funeral. The experience of the greatest depth and the banality of everyday life meet. Without it being said quite explicitly—in an intellectual way—the notion of experience (and therefore different ways of being and acting as a human being in the world) was differentiated along a crystallising distinction of superficial-deep or everyday-"sacred". The participants struggle for suitable words, for language, for verbalisation of the experiences, which are often relapses. They "understand" without naming the "perfect terms". Instead, philosophical insights are wrapped up in stories. Access to philosophical understanding is created not through the intellect, but from one's own affected existence, from a space of inner and shared depth. It feels as if fundamental meanings, which are precisely not objectified for the intellect, float, as it were, in the common thinking space or settle amongst people.

4. Some conclusions and practical recommendations

Generally speaking, there is a need for further research, practical experience, and experimentation on Philosophical Practice in the field of palliative care. We are pursuing this in our research project *Philosophical Practice in Palliative Care and Hospice Work*. The aim of this chapter is to provide an initial overview and first attempts at giving points of orientation. Limitations are that we make no claim to completeness, and that conclusions have a hypothetical character at this early stage of our research.

4.1 Philosophical Practice as a cultural technique for end-of-life care

The various elements of the different styles taken together give an idea of the potential of Philosophical Practice and characterise it as a cultural technique. Philosophical Practice is based in dialogue; it is an encounter and mutual participation of people who share their experiences not merely for the point of narration, but for understanding a life problem from different sides. Thereby, philosophising essentially emerges between people. The dialogical style points to the community-building potential and empowering potential of Philosophical Practice, especially in the face of questions and in the face of experiencing borderline situations. Philosophical Practice further critically examines the implicit theories that determine our personal and collective lives (analytical approach), which unfolds political-critical potential for the development of a caring society. Finally, Philosophical Practice connects one's own thinking with the thoughts that had already appeared in history in a resonance from the depths (contemplative approach) and elevates and connects the human being with the many voices of life and reality. The focus here is on the spiritual potential of Philosophical Practice.

4.2 The philosophical care: to philosophise is to learn to die

Philosophising can mean learning to die, which is an old *topos* in the history of philosophy and can also be identified in the basic styles of Philosophical Practice. The typical philosophical path of abstraction here lies in distancing oneself from the immediacy of one's own feelings, one's own experience, and one's own unquestioned opinions. This moment of distancing thus characterises the starting point of philosophising and can be regarded as a way of consolation and learning to die. By moving onto the general level, the individual may enjoy a break from the problems of "earthly" life, whilst being very actively engaged in shared thinking and placing one's own questions and experience in a universal context that connects us with life in general. The soul does not find comfort by solving its problems too quickly (which are often unsolvable anyway), but, paradoxically, by deepening these problems. One's thinking opens up to the plethora of many different voices of reality.

Thus, when asked whether philosophy "helps", two paradoxes must be reckoned with. The first paradox is that Philosophical Practice does not aim at helping, but at investigating a matter—but the help is usually a result. The second paradox is that philosophy helps by moving away from the individuality of the participants and aiming at the general level. Instead of detaching, moving towards the general "raises" the individual beyond themselves and connects them with whole life and reality. Philosophising is called learning how to die not so much because one talks about death, but because the movement of philosophical thinking is itself a kind of exercise through which the finiteness of the *individual person* is transcended.

4.3 Everyday philosophising in care practice

From a philosophical perspective, professionals in everyday care could be empowered and encouraged to develop a sense of wonder [16, 30], to consider existential experiences, to share them with one another, and to deepen understanding. We can ask ourselves: What moves me more deeply? Why? What does this mean for care and selfcare? In some ethical approaches, wonder is considered the appropriate moral feeling towards the other person [35]. It would be useful to create spaces for discussing existential experiences by Philosophical Practice.

4.4 Last Aid and last questions

Philosophical Practice could be combined with Last Aid courses. Last Aid courses [25] teach basic knowledge and practical skills in a short time, touching on existential questions and providing space for conversation. Participants who are interested in deepening existential questions could attend a philosophical format afterwards (e.g., "Speed-Philo", "Philosophicum"). The combination of Last Aid and Last Questions would be a holistic and still manageable and effective concept to further develop death literacy of communities.

4.5 Caring communities and death literacy

The public health approach in end-of-life care contains a philosophical core and mission. It is ultimately immoral when experts influence "behaviour and conditions" (according to their ideas and ultimately key figures of health and good dying, etc.) without enabling people themselves to come to and articulate insights on what good life and good dying actually mean to them [36]. These questions go beyond the competence of individual sciences and specialists and require people involved to think for themselves and to think together. The first or at least an essential task of end-of-life-care developments in the population would therefore have to be:

a. To initiate and organise an open process of reflection, conversation, and networking that allows and empowers citizens to think about what matters in life, what are concerns and hopes, what constitutes good living and dying, and

b. To organise that citizens—across different roles, life, and work worlds—can share experiences and insights with each other in a deeper sense so that compassion, care, and empathy are to be real structural elements of social life.

Caring Communities would accordingly begin in a thoroughly philosophical sense as a social and existential, *maieutic* learning process in the social system of the "community". This is where philosophy comes into play in its original (ancient) meaning as: "midwifery in everyday life" ([37], p. 26). Philosophical Practice has potentials for exploring further: from the programmatic reflection of the Lancet Commission on the Value of Death [3] to concrete practices in the midst of society.

Acknowledgements

This research was funded by the Austrian Science Fund (FWF) P 35627-G. For the purpose of Open Access, the authors have applied a CC BY public copyright licence to any Author Accepted Manuscript (AAM) version arising from this submission.

Conflict of interest

The authors declare no conflict of interest.

Thanks

We thank our colleague Urša Marinšek for her support with proofreading and feedback.

Author details

Patrick Schuchter*, Stefanie V. Rieger, Sandra Radinger and Klaus Wegleitner
University of Graz, Austria

*Address all correspondence to: patrick.schuchter@uni-graz.at

References

[1] Kant I. Kritik der reinen Vernunft. Herausgegeben von Ingeborg Heidemann. Stuttgart: Reclam; 1966, A VII

[2] Jaspers K. Way to Wisdom: An Introduction to Philosophy. Translated by Ralph Manheim. New Haven, London: Yale University Press; 1964

[3] Sallnow L, Smith R, Ahmedzai SH, Bhadelia A, Chamberlain C, Cong Y, et al. Report of the lancet commission on the value of death: Bringing death back into life. The Lancet. 2022;**399**(10327):837-884

[4] Montaigne M. Essais. Erste moderne Gesamtübersetzung von Hans Stilett. Erstes Buch. Frankfurt: Goldmann; 1998. pp. 126-147

[5] Gahlings U. Philosophische Praxis. Baden-Baden: Verlag Karl Alber; 2023

[6] Hadot P. Qu'est-ce que la philosophie antique? Paris: Gallimard. Hansen; 1995

[7] Staude D, editor. Methoden Philosophischer Praxis: Ein Handbuch. Bielefeld: transcript Verlag; 2010

[8] Achenbach G. Zur Einführung der philosophischen Praxis. Vorträge, Aufsätze, Gespräche und Essays, mit denen sich die philosophische Praxis in den Jahren 1981 bis 2009 vorstellte: eine Dokumentation. Köln: Dinter; 2010

[9] Lindseth A. Zur Sache der Philosophischen Praxis. Philosophieren in Gesprächen mit ratsuchenden Menschen. Freiburg/München: Karl Alber; 2005

[10] Romizi D. Philosophische Praxis: Eine Standortbestimmung. Information Philosophie. 2019;**4**:84-94

[11] Weiss MN, editor. The Socratic Handbook. Dialogue Methods for Philosophical Practice. Wien: LIT; 2015

[12] Krauß J. Perspektiven Philosophischer Praxis. Eine Profession zwischen Tradition und Aufbruch. Baden-Baden: Alber; 2022

[13] Lindseth A. Being ill as an inevitable life topic. Possibilities of Philosophical Practice in health care and psychotherapy. In: Weiss MN, editor. The Socratic Handbook. Dialogue Methods for Philosophical Practice. Wien: LIT; 2015. pp. 45-66

[14] Knox JBL. "Tell me, what is it you plan to do with your one wild and precious life?" Socratic dialogue in a dramatic setting. In: Weiss MN, editor. The Socratic Handbook. Dialogue Methods for Philosophical Practice. Wien: LIT; 2015. pp. 269-282

[15] Diaz-Waian M. How philosophy can help us grieve: Navigating the wake(s) of loss. International Journal of Applied Philosophy. 2014;**28**(1):19-48

[16] Finn TH. The call and practices of wonder. How to evoke a Socratic community of wonder in professional settings. In: Weiss MN, editor. The Socratic Handbook. Dialogue Methods for Philosophical Practice. Wien: LIT; 2015. pp. 217-244

[17] Birnbacher D. The Socratic method in teaching medical ethics: Potentials and limitations. Medicine, Health Care and Philosophy. 1999;**2**:219-224

[18] Schuchter P, Heller A. The care dialog: The "ethics of care" approach and its importance for clinical ethics consultation. Medicine, Health Care and Philosophy. 2018;**21**:51-62

[19] Schuchter P. Was ist mit der Philosophie in Spiritual Care?: What about philosophy in spiritual

care? Spiritual Care. 2020;**9**:25-36. DOI: 10.1515/spircare-2019-0112

[20] Krüger C. Philosophical care: Philosophical care. Spiritual Care. 2022;**11**:62-65. DOI: 10.1515/spircare-2021-0034

[21] Schuchter P, Rueger-Hochheit A, Thissen S. Speed-Philo. In: Wegleitner K, Schuchter P, Groebe B, Blümke D, editors. Zu jung fürs Thema Sterben?! Junge Menschen für Hospizkultur in Gesellschaft #interessieren #stärken #beteiligen. Esslingen: hospiz Verlag; 2022. pp. 233-239

[22] Wegleitner K, Schuchter P. Caring communities as collective learning process: Findings and lessons learned from a participatory research project in Austria. Annals of Palliative Medicine. 2018;**7**(Suppl. 2):84-S98. DOI: 10.21037/apm.2018.03.05

[23] Leonard R, Noonan K, Horsfall D, Kelly M, Rosenberg JP, Grindrod A, et al. Developing a death literacy index. Death Studies. 2022;**46**(9):2110-2122. DOI: 10.1080/07481187.2021.1894268

[24] Meyer L, Reiter B, Konrad H, editors. Wem und was gehört Europa? Graz: Unipress Verlag; 2022

[25] Bollig G, Brandt F, Ciurlionis M, Knopf B. Last aid course. An education for all citizens and an ingredient of compassionate communities. Healthcare (Basel). 2019;**7**(1):19. DOI: 10.3390/healthcare7010019

[26] Philosophical Practice – Philosophizing in Conversation [Internet]. Available from: https://philosophieren-im-gespraech.de/ [Accessed: July 11, 2023]

[27] Philosophical practice MILAN [Internet]. Available from: https://www.philosophie-milan.de/ [Accessed: July 11, 2023]

[28] Kardinal König Haus [Internet]. Available from: https://www.kardinal-koenig-haus.at/[Accessed: July 11, 2023]

[29] Denken und Staunen. Available from: https://www.denken-und-staunen.de/ [Accessed: July 11, 2023]

[30] Schuchter P. Sich einen Begriff vom Leiden Anderer machen: eine praktische Philosophie der Sorge. Bielefeld: transcript Verlag; 2016

[31] Achenbach G. Kann Denken trösten. In: Vom Richtigen im Falschen. Wege philosophischer Lebenskönnerschaft. Freiburg im Breisgau/Wien: Herder; 2003

[32] Brenifier O. Philosophical consultation: Principles and difficulties. Journal of Human Cognition. 2021;**5**(2):17-35

[33] Brenifier O. Philosophical Consultation. Independently published: Editions Alcofribas; 2020. Available from: http://www.pratiques-philosophiques.fr/wp-content/uploads/2020/01/Philosophical-consultation-last-version.pdf [Accessed: July 12, 2023]

[34] Lahav R. What Is Deep Philosophy? Philosophy from Our Inner Depth. Vermont: Loyev Books; 2021

[35] La Caze M. The encounter between wonder and generosity. Hypatia. 2009;**17**(3):1-19. DOI: 10.1111/j.1527-2001.2002.tb00938.x

[36] Buchanan DR. An Ethic for Health Promotion. Rethinking the Sources of Human Well Being. Oxford: Oxford University Press; 2000

[37] Berger W, Heintel P. Die Organisation der Philosophen. Frankfurt a. M: Suhrkamp; 1998

Chapter 4

Quality in Palliative Care from the Patient Perspective

Gulcin Senel and Michael Silbermann

Abstract

Patients with life-threatening illnesses who face death may suffer physically, psychosocially, and spiritually. The constant presence of illness and episodes of worsening illness is a persistent reminder of forthcoming death and can lead to feelings of fear. Existential issues may arise in addition to the physical suffering. Patients' approaches to life, illness, and ideal quality of life were found to create a sphere of influence that shaped their palliative care experience. Especially at the end of life, patients' preferences for help in living a meaningful life are connected to the aim of palliative care "to improve quality of life," which includes the patients' perspectives of what is considered meaningful and important. Patients' perceptions of their care may be seen as an indicator of quality of care and is considered important for the development and improvement of palliative care.

Keywords: palliative care, quality of health care, patient perspective, dignity, meaning of life

1. Introduction

Contemporary palliative care aims to relieve patients' "total pain" and improve their quality of life, based on the holistic view that suffering is physical, psychosocial, and spiritual [1, 2]. Palliative care includes holistic care principles according to which the individual patient is at the center of care. These principles are respectful and sensitive to the conditions of the patient and take into account the opinion of the family and the team. Life history, preferences, needs, and values, as well as the patient's knowledge, are combined with the abilities of the health personnel in order to provide the patient with the best possible care [3].

Patients may have a wide variety of care needs at the same time, which is related to their personality, education, cultural background, religious and spiritual beliefs, expectations from life, family relationships, financial opportunities, variety and stage of their disease, symptom burden, care environment, and care burden. If palliative care is not well integrated into health systems, it is inevitable to encounter difficulties in meeting these needs. However, if all maintenance environments are ready and maintenance transitions can be made smoothly, continuity can be ensured.

While the number of patients who continue to live with life-threatening diseases increases, efforts to provide palliative care services to everyone equally and to improve existing systems continue. These efforts should continue until ideal quality palliative care organizations are provided in theory and clinical practice.

2. Quality of health care in general

Quality of care in general health services is defined by six dimensions: it must be safe, effective, patient-centered, timely, efficient, and equitable [4]. The two main elements that comprise quality of care are the preferences of the patients and the resource structure of the care organization. It is order and predictability in the rational domain that determines patient preferences, and consideration of their unique situation in the human domain. The resource structure of the care organization is formed by the caregiver team and the infrastructure of the care environment. In this theoretical framework, patients' perceptions of quality of care can be considered in four dimensions: the medical-technical competence of the caregivers, the physical-technical conditions of the care institution, the identity-oriented approach of the caregivers, and the sociocultural atmosphere of the care organization [5].

2.1 Perception of health care quality

Patients' preferences and perceptions of care have been acknowledged as being important components of health care quality [6]. Patients' perceptions of quality of care can be explained by patients' assessments of what they perceive as important about their care, their preferences, and how they perceive their care experience, all of which differ from patient satisfaction, which is defined as an emotion. Patient satisfaction indicates adequate and acceptable care, not perfect care, and is a relative concept so that care that satisfies one patient may not satisfy another [7]. In order to validate patients' perceptions of the quality of care, it is important to ask questions about aspects of care that are important to patients.

Personalities and institutional conditions may affect patients' perceptions of the quality of care. Person-related conditions include patient characteristics related to sociodemographic information such as age, education, and living conditions, as well as health-related information, such as diagnosis and quality of life. Relatively few studies have investigated the association between patients' perceptions of subjective importance and person-related conditions, especially in the palliative care context, and therefore the relationships between them are uncertain. Several studies have investigated the relationship between person-related conditions and patients' perceptions of the care they received. Although the relationship between age and subjective importance is contradictory or unclear [8–10], subjective importance is reported to be higher in women than in men [8, 11].

Person-centered care is an important part of the quality of care. However, we do not yet have data showing the effect of person-centered care on patients' perceptions of quality of care. It may not be possible to change individual circumstances, but it is important to explore them in order to target and individualize care for patients who are at risk of adverse experiences with quality of care. Health care providers should aim to improve conditions that negatively affect patients' perceptions of the organization.

Different results have been reported regarding the importance of patients' subjective perceptions of health status, including both physical and mental health, and the relationship with patients' sense of coherence [8, 10]. In one study, a positive correlation between psychological well-being and subjective importance was found [11]. Studies in the context of palliative care have reported that perceived actual care is better in the presence of a cancer diagnosis compared with nonmalignant diseases [12, 13]. Similarly, patients with chronic obstructive pulmonary disease preferred a lower level of advanced care compared to cancer patients [14].

Although it is known that patients living alone and with a life-threatening illness may experience care differently from those living with someone else [15, 16], there is insufficient data on the perceptions of care of those who live alone and lack the affection of family and friends [17]. While some studies evaluating the perception of care in hospital- and nursing-home environments that did not include palliative care patients found a positive relationship between the number of personnel and the quality of care [18, 19], in another study, the number of nurses in the services and the service occupancy rates were higher, but it was evaluated as a negative situation in terms of the sociocultural atmosphere [20].

2.2 Perception of palliative care quality

Despite global efforts to improve health and palliative care integration, barriers to optimal delivery of palliative care services remain. Referrals to palliative care are unfortunately made too late, when patients are in the final stages of their illness, causing some opportunities to be missed [21–23]. Common barriers to timely referral to palliative care include the inability to accept a diagnosis of an incurable disease, clinicians' unwillingness or inability to communicate bad news and discuss palliative care, negative biases by patients, families, and clinicians toward palliative care, and a lack of information about the purpose or scope of palliative care and palliative care services [24, 25]. Regarding negative perceptions, research shows that patients, families/caregivers, and clinicians still largely associate palliative care with end-of-life care, sometimes viewing it as a "last resort" or "hope lost" [26, 27]. These negative perceptions about palliative care affect the quality of care and prevent patients and caregivers from benefiting from supportive treatments. The development of quality palliative care services requires a broad, multifaceted approach targeting all levels of society, not just patients and clinicians, involving awareness, education, communication, and the implementation of policies that support access to palliative care services [28, 29].

In palliative care, patients are faced with numerous severe symptoms that impair their quality of life. In particular, pain can be perceived as worse than death for patients. Effective pain control is one of the most important indicators of quality palliative care. The pain that prevents patients from living their lives with dignity should be treated immediately. It is inevitable that the perception of care will be negatively affected in cases of uncontrollable symptoms that impair the quality of life of the patient and the caregiver family. Palliative sedation should be discussed with the patient and/or family in cases of uncontrollable symptoms such as treatment-resistant pain, dyspnea, and delirium. A lower symptom burden in patients with advanced incurable disease has been found to be associated with higher quality of care [30]. The use of systematic symptom assessment and documentation provides better symptom control. At the same time, documenting patient information improves the overall quality of care [31, 32]. In palliative care, the use of assessment tools such as the individual care plan, patient care records, and the Edmonton Symptom Assessment Scale (ESAS) for systematic assessment and documentation of specific symptoms are essential for guiding and improving care. Care environment transitions compatible with the nature of the support can be achieved more easily by informing and planning the care in advance. At the same time, emergency service applications that cause stress to the patient and their relatives can be prevented. In the context of palliative care, planning and continuity of care are extremely important for patients [33]. More information is needed on how the organization of medical and nursing care affect patients' perceptions of palliative care.

In a study conducted to determine patients' own definitions of quality of care, the properties used to describe quality of care were patient-centered care, access, communication and information, courtesy and emotional support, care efficiency/ effective organization, technical quality, and structure/facilities [6]. Similarly, in another study, effective communication and joint decision-making, specialized care, respectful and compassionate care, trust and confidence, a suitable environment for care, and minimizing the patient burden were determined as the most important elements of care [34].

Cognitive, emotional, physical, preparatory, social, and spiritual domains, as well as personal autonomy and health care delivery, are important quality of life parameters for people with a life-limiting illness receiving palliative care [35]. In palliative care, patients may experience progressive loss, increasing disability, difficulties in coping with symptoms, and uncertainties about prognosis. The balance between controlling their own lives and putting themselves in the hands of others is important in maintaining the values that make up their identity. When it comes to shared decision-making, it has been found that most patients do not experience inclusion in care according to their preferences [36]. In palliative care, patients should be approached with honesty, respect, and empathy, the planning of services should be conducted cooperatively, and patients' preferences should be considered in providing a safe and enjoyable environment for medical care.

There are several reviews that explore areas of care that are important to patients in the context of palliative care. In a study evaluating the palliative care perceptions of patients, it was found that care needs were met in home-care settings, but spiritual, psychosocial, practical, information, and rest needs were not met, and there was a loss of isolation and autonomy [37]. It has been reported that the environment in hospital palliative care is not suitable due to poor management of symptoms, too many interruptions, and noise [38], but patients who attended palliative day care centers reported that the environment and psychosocial experiences were positive [39, 40]. In two studies focusing on hospital and hospice environments intended for elderly patients receiving palliative support and their families, it was emphasized that patients prefer a home-like environment next to their families, where their privacy is protected [41, 42].

The competence of doctors and nurses in palliative care positively affects the perception of care received [30, 43]. It has been reported that patient families' perceptions of quality of care increase positively when specialized palliative care is provided [44]. Patients and caregivers who received specific palliative care interventions in terms of continuity, coordination, and care-location transitions reported better quality of care [45]. In palliative care, the presence of a specialized team such as psychologists, social workers, occupational therapists, spiritual support specialists, clergy, doctors, and nurses increases the quality of care. However, the relationship between diversity and functionality of team members and perceptions of quality of care is unknown.

3. Death and the perception of a good death

The perception of death, which overlaps with the social and cultural identity of the individual, plays a decisive role in the integration with the society lived in all societies and cultures. Today, with the developments in medicine and technology, death is delayed and is preceded by increasingly longer end-of-life periods. The definition of a good death can comprise awareness of death, preparation for death, abandonment of roles and responsibilities, and farewell. Similar expressions such as "die well," "die peacefully," "proper death," "desired death," or "death with dignity" are used synonymously in the scientific literature. Studies have shown that the concept of a good death is different for patients, caregivers, doctors, and relatives [46, 47]. At this point, the importance of advanced care directives declared by the patient is obvious. However, since there is little research on what is important and what patients think at the end of their lives, discussions on the topic tend to be driven by academic and clinical perspectives [48].

What constitutes a good death for each person is highly individual, may change over time, and is based on personal perspectives, cultural contexts, and experiences gained through life stories. For many, a good death often comprises personal qualities that are considered important such as pain and symptom control, preparation for death, spirituality, a subjective sense of closure at the end of one's life, and maintaining clear judgment [47, 49, 50]. However, what patients consider a "good death" is heavily influenced by culture, religion, age, living conditions, illness, and financial issues.

There are significant differences, and sometimes contradictions, in the preferences and issues that concern people, even if they have similar qualities. As a result of these choices, suffering may be experienced when facing death. For example, control of pain and physical symptoms is universally accepted as contributing to a good death. Consequently, in societies where access to health care or medication is socioeconomically limited, concerns focus on pain relief [51–53]. In societies where access to health is assured, aspects such as participation in treatment decisions seem to be given more importance than pain control [54, 55].

Although the quality death environment that individuals define for themselves may vary, it can be supplemented by a palliative care philosophy. Giving patients a chance to express their experience of aspects of a good death at different points in the illness/death trajectory can help improve the quality of care they receive, thus contributing to the overall quality of death [56]. It is also important to determine the performance and prognosis of the patient related to the disease in order to determine the appropriate time to talk about death and the preferred death environment with the patient. Death is not usually instantaneous; rather, it is a process and choices regarding death need to be carefully monitored throughout the course of the disease. Therefore, end-of-life support and care must address individuals' ideas and wishes in flexible and dynamic ways on an ongoing and individual basis. Health care professionals should be aware of their own value systems and recognize the risks of imposing their own accepted concept of a good or bad death on the patient [57, 58]. In providing care and support to the dying, efforts should always be made to explore the specific societal conditions, problems, conflicts, and social inadequacies that prevent people from dying as they please.

4. Conclusion

Patients' perspectives on their care are extremely important in assessing and further developing quality in health care in general and in palliative care in particular. However, studies involving patients' perspectives on care are still scarce in palliative care research, often due to patient vulnerability and difficulties in obtaining informed consent. For this reason, family members are often used as proxies to investigate patients' views on their care. One advantage of using relatives as proxies is the opportunity to include the views of terminally ill patients who are unable to communicate their perceptions of quality of care. However, subjective aspects of patients' experiences, such as pain, anxiety, depression, and perception of the importance of care, cannot be evaluated with information received from the family. Studies comparing patients' perceptions of important aspects of care with the care actually received are also scarce.

Areas that need improvement for the development of palliative care include relief of symptoms, psychological and moral support, improved relationships with physicians, participation in decision-making, honest communication, planning, cooperation and continuity of care, reduced family burden, and avoidance of life-prolonging interventions when there is no hope of recovery. There is a need for more studies investigating palliative care perceptions in all care settings, especially in hospice settings, home care services, and in patients diagnosed with cancer and non-cancer diseases.

Author details

Gulcin Senel[1] and Michael Silbermann[2]*

1 Pain Clinic and Palliative Care Unit, Ankara Oncology Training and Research Hospital, University of Health Science, Turkey

2 Middle East Cancer Consortium, Haifa, Israel

*Address all correspondence to: michaelsilbermann0@gmail.com

References

[1] Clark D. 'Total pain', disciplinary power and the body in the work of Cicely Saunders, 1958-1967. Social Science and Medicine. 1999;**49**(6):727-736

[2] World Health Organization (WHO). Quality of Care: A Process for Making Strategic Choices in Health Systems. Geneva: World Health Organization (WHO); 2006

[3] Kvåle K, Bondevik M. What is important for patient centred care? A qualitative study about the perceptions of patients with cancer. Scandinavian Journal of Caring Sciences. 2008;**22**(4):582-589

[4] Institute of Medicine. Crossing the Quality Chasm: A New Health System for the 21st Century. Washington DC: National Academy Press; 2001

[5] Wilde B, Starrin B, Larsson G, Larsson M. Quality of care from a patient perspective: A grounded theory study. Scandinavian Journal of Caring Sciences. 1993;**7**(2):113-120

[6] Sofaer S, Firminger K. Patient perceptions of the quality of health services. Annual Review of Public Health. 2005;**26**(1):513-559

[7] Crow R, Gage H, Hampson S, Hart J, Kimber A, Storey L, et al. The measurement of satisfaction with health care: Implications for practice from a systematic review of the literature. Health Technology Assessment. 2002;**6**(32):1-244

[8] Henoch I, Lövgren M, Wilde-Larsson B, Tishelman C. Perceptionof quality of care: Comparison of the views of patients' with lung cancer and their family members. Journal of Clinical Nursing. 2011;**21**(3-4):585-594

[9] Wilde-Larsson B, Larsson G, Kvist LJ, Sandin-Bojö AK. Womens' opinions on intrapartal care: Development of a theory-based questionnaire. Journal of Clinical Nursing. 2010;**19**(11-12):1748-1760

[10] Wilde LB. Patients' views on quality of care: Age effects and identification of patient profiles. Journal of Clinical Nursing. 1999;**8**(6):693-700

[11] Wilde Larsson B, Larsson G, Chantereau M, von Holstein K. International comparison of patients' views on quality of care. International Journal of Health Care Quality Assurance. 2005;**18**:62-73

[12] Brännström M, Hägglund L, Fürst CJ, Boman K. Unequal care for dying patients in Sweden: A comparative registry study of deaths from heart disease and cancer. European Journal of Cardiovascular Nursing. 2011;**11**(4):454-459

[13] Murray SA, Boyd K, Kendall M, Worth A, Benton TF, Clausen H. Dying of lung cancer or cardiac failure: Prospective qualitative interview study of patients and their carers in the community. BMJ. 2002;**325**(7370):929-932

[14] Rocker GM, Dodek PM, Heyland DK. Toward optimal end-of life care for patients with advanced chronic obstructive pulmonary disease: In sights from a multicentre study. Canadian Respiratory Journal. 2008;**15**(5):249-254

[15] Ek K, Sahlberg-Blom E, Andershed B, Ternestedt BM. Struggling to retain living space: Patients' stories about living with advanced chronic obstructive pulmonary

disease. Journal of Advanced Nursing. 2011;**67**(7):1480-1490

[16] Hanratty B, Addington-Hall J, Arthur A, Cooper L, Grande G, Payne S, et al. What is different about living alone with cancer in older age? A qualitative study of experiences and preferences for care. BMC Family Practice. 2013;**14**(1):22-29

[17] Strohbuecker B, Eisenmann Y, Galushko M, Montag T, Voltz R. Palliative care needs of chronically ill nursing home residents in Germany: Focusing on living, not dying. International Journal of Palliative Nursing. 2011;**17**(1):27-34

[18] Aiken LH, Clarke SP, Sloane DM. Hospital staffing, organization, and quality of care: Cross-national findings. Nursing Outlook. 2002;**50**(5):187-194

[19] Kirkevold Ø, Engedal K. The quality of care in Norwegian nursing homes. Scandinavian Journal of Caring Sciences. 2006;**20**(2):177-183

[20] Grøndahl VA, Karlsson I, Hall-Lord ML, Appelgren J, Wilde-Larsson B. Quality of care from patients' perspective: Impact of the combination of person-related and external objective care conditions. Journal of Clinical Nursing. 2011;**20**(17/18):2540-2551

[21] Wentlandt K, Krzyzanowska MK, Swami N, Rodin GM, le LW, Zimmermann C. Referral practices of oncologists to specialized palliative care. Journal of Clinical Oncology. 2012;**30**:4380-4386

[22] Love A, Liversage LM. Barriers to accessing palliative care: A review of the literature. Progress Palliative Care. 2014;**22**:9-19

[23] Maciasz RM, Arnold RM, Chu E, Park SY, White DB, Vater LB, et al. Does it matter what you call it? A randomized trial of language used to describe palliative care services. Support Care Cancer. 2013;**21**:3411-3419

[24] Aldridge MD, Hasselaar J, Garralda E, van der Eerden M, Stevenson D, McKendrick K, et al. Education, implementation, and policy barriers to greater integration of palliative care: A literature review. Palliative Medicine. 2016;**30**:224-239

[25] Shalev A, Phongtankuel V, Kozlov E, Shen MJ, Adelman RD, Reid MC. Awareness and misperceptions of hospice and palliative care: A population-based survey study. The American Journal of Hospice & Palliative Care. 2018;**35**:431-439

[26] Stjernsward J, Foley KM, Ferris FD. The public health strategy for palliative care. Journal of Pain and Symptom Management. 2007;**33**:486-493

[27] Von Roenn JH, Voltz R, Serrie A. Barriers and approaches to the successful integration of palliative care and oncology practice. Journal of the National Comprehensive Cancer Network. 2013;**11**(Suppl. 1):S11-S16

[28] Brereton L, Gardiner C, Gott M, Ingleton C, Barnes S, Carroll C. The hospital environment for end of life care of older adults and their families: An integrative review. Journal of Advanced Nursing. 2012;**68**(5):981-993

[29] Rigby J, Payne S, Froggatt K. What evidence is there about the specific environmental needs of older people who are near the end of life and are cared for in hospices or similar institutions? A literature review. Palliative Medicine. 2010;**24**(3):268-285

[30] Aiken LH, Sloane DM, Bruyneel L, Van den Heede K, Griffiths P, Busse R,

et al. Nurse staffing and education and hospital mortality in nine European countries: A retrospective observational study. The Lancet. 2014;**383**(9931): 1824-1830

[31] Chaudhry B, Wang J, Wu S, Maglione M, Mojica W, Roth E, et al. Systematic review: Impact of health information technology on quality, efficiency, and costs of medical care. Annals of Internal Medicine. 2006;**144**(10):742-752

[32] Kripalani S, LeFevre F, Phillips CO, Williams MV, Basaviah P, Baker DW. Deficits in communication and information transfer between hospital-based and primary care physicians: Implications for patient safety and continuity of care. JAMA. 2007;**297**(8):831-841

[33] Engelberg RA, Downey L, Wenrich MD, Carline JD, Silvestri GA, Dotolo D, et al. Measuring the quality of end-of-life care. Journal of Pain and Symptom Management. 2010;**39**(6):951-971

[34] Virdun C, Luckett T, Davidson PM, Phillips J. Dying in the hospital setting: A systematic review of quantitative studies identifying the elements of end-of-life care that patients and their families rank as being most important. Palliative Medicine. 2015;**29**(9):774-796

[35] Kamel G, Paniagua M, Uppalapati A. Palliative care in the intensive care unit: Are residents well trained to provide optimal care to critically ill patients? The American Journal of Hospice & Palliative Care. 2015;**32**:758-762

[36] Bélanger E, Rodríguez C, Groleau D. Shared decision-making in palliative care: A systematic mixed studies review using narrative synthesis. Palliative Medicine. 2011;**25**(3):242-261

[37] Ventura AD, Burney S, Brooker J, Fletcher J, Ricciardelli L. Home-based palliative care: A systematic literature review of the self reported unmet needs of patients and carers. Palliative Medicine. 2014;**28**(5):391-402

[38] Robinson J, Gott M, Ingleton C. Patient and family experiences of palliative care in hospital: What do we know? An integrative review. Palliative Medicine. 2013;**28**(1):18-33

[39] Bradley SE, Frizelle D, Johnson M. Patients' psychosocial experiences of attending specialist palliative day care: A systematic review. Palliative Medicine. 2011;**25**(3):210-228

[40] Stevens E, Martin CR, White CA. The outcomes of palliative care day services: A systematic review. Palliative Medicine. 2010;**25**(2):153-169

[41] Mccaffrey N, Bradley S, Ratcliffe J, Currow DC. What aspects of quality of life are important from palliative care patient's perspectives? A systematic review of qualitative research. Journal of Pain and Symptom Manage. 2016;**52**(2):318.e5

[42] Hui D, Kim SH, Kwon JH, Tanco KC, Zhang T, Kang JH, et al. Access to palliative care among patients treated at a comprehensive cancer center. The Oncologist. 2012;**17**:1574-1580

[43] Waibel S, Henao D, Aller MB, Vargas I, Vázquez ML. What do we know about patients' perceptions of continuity of care? A meta synthesis of qualitative studies. International Journal for Quality in Health Care. 2011;**24**(1):39-48

[44] Zimmermann C, Riechelmann R, Krzyzanowska M, Rodin G, Tannock I. Effectiveness of specialized palliative care: A systematic review. JAMA. 2008;**299**(14):1698-1709

[45] Dy SM, Aslakson R, Wilson RF, Fawole OA, Lau BD, Martinez KA, et al. Closing the quality gap: Revisiting the state of the science: Improving health care and palliative care for advanced and serious illness. Evidence Report/Technology Assessment. 2012;**208.8**:1-249

[46] Payne SA, Langley-Evans A, Hillier R. Perceptions of a "good" death: A comparative study of the views of hospice staff and patients. Palliative Medicine. 1996;**10**:307-312

[47] Steinhauser KE, Clipp EC, McNeilly M, Christakis NA, McIntyre LM, Tulsky JA. In search of a good death: Observations of patients, families, and providers. Annals of Internal Medicine. 2000;**132**:825-832

[48] Broom A, Cavenagh J. Masculinity, moralities and being cared for: An exploration of experiences of living and dying in a hospice. Social Science & Medicine. 2010;**71**:869-876

[49] Akechi T, Miyashita M, Morita T, Okuyama T, Sakamoto M, Sagawa R, et al. Good death in elderly adults with cancer in Japan based on perspectives of the general population. Journal of the American Geriatrics Society. 2012;**60**:271-276

[50] Vig EK, Davenport NA, Pearlman RA. Good deaths, bad deaths, and preferences for the end of life: A qualitative study of geriatric outpatients. Journal of the American Geriatrics Society. 2002;**50**:1541-1548

[51] Chacko R, Anand JR, Rajan A, John S, Jeyaseelan V. End-of-life care perspectives of patients and health professionals in an Indian health-care setting. International Journal of Palliative Nursing. 2014;**20**:557-564

[52] Kikule E. A good death in Uganda: Survey of needs for palliative care for terminally ill people in urban areas. BMJ. 2003;**327**:192-194

[53] Grant E, Murray SA, Grant A, Brown J. A good death in rural Kenya? Listening to Meru patients and their families talk about care needs at the end of life. Journal of Palliative Care. 2003;**19**:159-167

[54] Willems DL, Hak A, Visser F, Van der Wal G. Thoughts of patients with advanced heart failure on dying. Palliative Medicine. 2004;**18**:564-572

[55] Rietjens JAC, van der Heide A, Onwuteaka- Philipsen BD, van der Maas PJ, van der Wal G. Preferences of the Dutch general public for a good death and associations with attitudes towards end-of-life decision-making. Palliative Medicine. 2006;**20**:685-692

[56] Leung KK, Tsai JS, Cheng SY, Liu WJ, Chiu TY, Wu CH, et al. Can a good death and quality of life be achieved for patients with terminal cancer in a palliative care unit? Journal of Palliative Medicine. 2010;**13**:1433-1438

[57] Hart B, Sainsbury P, Short S. Whose dying? A sociological critique of the "good death". Mortality. 1998;**3**:65-77

[58] Semino E, Demjen Z, Koller V. 'Good' and 'bad' deaths: Narratives and professional identities in interviews with hospice managers. Discourse Studies. 2014;**16**:667-685

Chapter 5

There is More to a Person than Motor Neurone Disease

Denise Andrea Harris

Abstract

When a person is living with motor neurone disease (MND), their temporality comes to the forefront. In the present, the lived-through past takes on new meaning, and the future is anticipated with angst. In contrast to many MND studies, where the focus is on the person in the present and the impact of MND on the body. This chapter explores a research journey and developed papers to propose a model of person-centred care in MND with a focus on individuality, which includes three major elements: 1. presuppositions, 2. acceptance, and 3. temporality.

Keywords: motor neurone disease, person-centred care, presuppositions, acceptance, temporality

1. Introduction

People can live with motor neurone disease (MND) for months before receiving a diagnosis of MND [1]. On diagnosis, a person learns that MND is a progressive neurological terminal illness which results in the degeneration of the motor neurones in the brain and spinal cord [2–5]. While the progressive nature of MND is unpredictable, the terminal aspect of MND is not [6]. The period after receiving a diagnosis of MND is thus experienced as 'devastating' for the person and their family. The prognosis for Progressive Bulbar Palsy (PBP) MND can be months, compared with Amyotrophic Lateral Sclerosis (ALS) MND which is three to five years, and Progressive Muscular Atrophy (PMA) MND which is 10 years. A person with MND and their family will face many challenges during the progression of the disease including physical problems (dysarthria, loss of mobility, respiratory failure, and dysphagia) and psychosocial problems (loss, bereavement, depression, and family distress) [4, 7]. For some people with MND, cognitive and behavioural changes may occur [3]. However, around 50% of people with MND are unaffected by cognitive changes [5], making their experiences of loss more painful. Family members must observe the overwhelming effects of MND on the ever-changing body of their loved one. This chapter is a reflective account of a research journey that began when the researcher (DH) initially studying palliative care teams and best interests' determinations to eventually developing a model of person-centred care.

2. Research journey

The researcher observed her mother being overwhelmed by the effects of MND on her body, resulting in her becoming the 'patient' in the continuing health care (CHC) context. The palliative care professionals involved in the researcher's study were managing continuing health care (24-hour agency nursing care) in her mother's home. The provider of palliative care was also the researcher's employer. To avoid any conflict of interest, the researcher made a resolute decision to assert her role as an informal carer in the care context. The nature of PBP MND meant that her mother had loss of speech and movement within three months following her diagnosis. The researcher understood that her mother was unaffected by cognitive changes because she could still respond by blinking her eyes for 'yes' and shaking her head for 'no.' Thus, best interests' determinations became the focus of care, to support her mother to die, her way. The motivation behind the project described in this chapter stems from concerns, including seeing existential suffering despite the researcher's mother receiving person-centred care as she perceived it.

3. The project

The research project was undertaken in the Northwest of England, UK, by the author and researcher (DH), in fulfilment of a PhD by Published Works. Supervisors and mentors have brought collective knowledge of hermeneutic phenomenology, bricolage and other multi-method approaches to this research, which together have helped the researcher to develop both interpretive thought and voice. This chapter will present five papers and discuss them as an unfolding research journey that resulted in the proposed person-centred care model in MND. Like any other research journey, the process started with a review of the literature on living with MND.

Information on the meaning of living with MND through time is limited. Locock et al. [8] examined whether the concept of biographical disruption is appropriate for people living with a life-limiting illness and found that being diagnosed with MND is a 'biographical abruption' of life, while Brott et al. [9] explored the occupational disruption of living with MND. Brown [10] explored the disparity between patient needs and care delivered and emphasised the need for the professional focus to be on a person rather than their disease. Foley et al. [11] explored the meaning of quality of life when diagnosed with MND and highlighted the importance of faith, control and dignity, and the desire to maintain identity. Brown and Addington-Hall [12] explored how people with MND talk about living and coping with the condition, especially how they live and cope with the loss of movement and speech. Existential concerns of people with MND have been explored in previous studies [10, 13, 14]. Existential suffering has also been observed by those caring for people living with MND towards their end of life [15]. The evidence suggests that people living with MND who are experiencing loss of movement and speech have existential concerns, and carers have observed existential suffering at the end of life; however, despite this, care is focused on the loss of function [10].

These studies have focused on single points in time; thus, knowledge of the meaning of existence with MND through time is limited. The next stage in the research journey was to consider an appropriate methodological approach to study experiences through time.

3.1 Paper 1:interpreting two philosophical positions on existential phenomenology and philosophical hermeneutics

Paper 1 sets out to provide a reflective account of how the researcher interpreted hermeneutic phenomenology. This methodology was appropriate because it brings together Heidegger's [16] existential phenomenology and Gadamer's [17] philosophical hermeneutics. Heidegger asked the question: 'what it means to be?' a person in the world (lifeworld) through temporal time (past, present and future). He understood that a person is born into history, culture, and practice. A person may choose to adopt their forebears' ways of being or project themselves forward into other possibilities [18, 19]. A hermeneutic position holds that stories are interpretations of life ([20], cited in [21]). Gadamer had ideas to illuminate the process of understanding (interpreting) things from someone else's perspective [22]. He understood that presuppositions (preunderstandings and prejudices) cannot be 'bracketed' as if they do not exist; instead, they are part of the interpretive process. In the process of dialogue, a person needs to 'examine and be aware of their presuppositions to be open to the meaning of others' ([23], p. 267). The research methodology therefore began with bringing presuppositions to consciousness, before recruiting and meeting with the participants.

3.2 Paper 2: hermeneutic reflexivity to explore presuppositions

Given the need identified in Paper 1 to be aware of one's own presuppositions to be open to the meaning of others, Paper 2 is a personal reflection on supporting a loved one living with PBP MND throughout her illness trajectory. This reflection is about one individual (the researcher's mother) first noticing something untoward was happening to her body: she was losing the ability to communicate. Each person with MND has their own unique trajectory. The researcher's mother received her diagnosis of PBP MND as an outpatient and was advised that her MND was rapidly progressing. She was recommended to have percutaneous endoscopic gastrostomy (PEG) feeding and accept palliative care to provide a quality of life and consented to both. Life continued until MND took hold of her body, and she became dependent on others for her survival. What followed was a traumatic illness journey to end-of-life Harris [24].

It was important for DH to identify her presuppositions resulting from this lived experience, because this highlighted the issue of prejudice before completing the research proposal and before recruiting and meeting the participants. The reflective process gave closure to events that would not be considered ethically appropriate to research. It helped to decide on the research question. Presuppositions are an evolving process; keeping a research diary meant changes in presuppositions during data collection and interpretation of the data, these were explored through regular discussion with colleagues [25].

3.3 Paper 3: researching the meaning of existence with MND through time

Paper 3 presents the project study aimed at answering the research question: 'What does it mean to be a person living through the illness trajectory of MND?' and considering the phenomenon of existence when given a diagnosis of MND and in the context of receiving health care ([26], p. 1579). In keeping with Heidegger's existential hermeneutic phenomenology and Gadamer's philosophical hermeneutics, the following ideas were developed into processes:

1. The researcher asked the four people living with MND to tell their life story since first noticing something untoward was happening to them, thus focusing on lived experiences.

2. Gaining an understanding of the participants' illness journey through temporal time (the past brought into the present, anticipating the future).

3. Taking the stories back to the participants to ask if they wished to add or remove any part of their story.

4. Interpretation using Heidegger's existential (lifeworld) perspectives: being-in-the-world, being-with-others, thrownness, temporality, spatiality, embodiment, mood, and mortality.

5. Making sense of the whole story.

6. Identification of passages (excerpts) that were representative of shared understanding between the researcher and the participants.

The findings suggest that people with MND experience 'existential loss' of past, embodiment, spatiality, and future. The diagnosis of MND means that a person's mortality becomes the focus of attention, and the once-projected future of supporting family into adult life is lost. The impact of MND on the body means that people can no longer continue with their past ways of being a professional athlete, international businessperson or retired person, ways of being that created meaningful and purposeful identities. In the present, MND affecting on the body is experienced as degrading, humiliating, and cruel because people can no longer do things for themselves, and they feel humiliated; it is experienced as a loss of control because people are reliant on others for their survival. In the present, a person anticipates their own death, knowing that their body will deteriorate further before they die, and they will be unable to move, communicate or breathe without equipment and the support of others to ensure the equipment is in place. The significance of these results suggests that 'the concept of existential loss requires closer attention by healthcare professionals from the time of diagnosis and on through the illness trajectory' ([26], p. 1579). The findings also revealed that people with MND are living with uncertainty, and this needed further exploring.

3.4 Paper 4: exploring the meaning of supporting a loved one with MND to die

The fourth paper aimed to explore the meaning of supporting a loved one with MND to die. The researcher used self-reflection, and her autobiographical story was used to connect with broader cultural, political, and social meaning and understanding of dying as a phenomenon. The research processes involved:

1. Returning to previously published reflections

2. Reflecting and linking those experiences with Heidegger's existential (lifeworld) perspectives

3. Engaging with the literature

Through this process, four themes were found: Loss of person (lived body experienced in silence); loss of relationships (lived relations are challenged); loss of home and loss of time (lived space and lived time take on new meaning); loss of future (dying facing it alone). Lived space became an outreach nursing home, with different nurses coming and going, supplies and equipment. The researcher reflected on lived time: 'the future was anticipated with anxiety, the present was unrelenting, and the past embedded in our memories.' Relationships within the care triad were challenging: 'the commitment to care for the patient with MND was evident, however in the care context the person (as a patient) lost her past identities' ([27], p. 289). The paper concludes that dying with MND is a complex phenomenon, with the body experienced in silence so a can no longer take part in decision-making: thus, relationships between those involved in end-of-life care are challenging. 'A person with MND needs the support from palliative care professionals, and those acting with power of attorney, to make their end-of-life their own' ([27], p. 290). However, not everyone has access to palliative care or has others to support them to die; and this fact shows a need for a different approach to person-centred care in MND.

3.5 Paper 5: exploring the meaning of uncertainty for people with MND

Paper 5 involved returning to the original philosophical framework analysis to explore the meaning of uncertainty for people diagnosed with MND. Three phases of the MND illness trajectory appeared: body failing prematurely and searching for answers; body deterioration and responses to care; body nearing its end and needing to talk. Throughout these three phases, the participants were living with uncertainty, and similarities can be found in the kinds of uncertainty, for example: what condition they might have, how their care would be managed, and how they would be supported to die. Experiences of the first phase and diagnosis varied significantly, resulting in thoughts of assisted suicide for one participant going private, and experiences of loss of control for one participant going through the NHS. Body deterioration was varied, and the focus of care in this phase was on monitoring symptoms and assessing needs. The phase of the body nearing its end meant that people needed to talk to professionals who were prepared to listen, about loss, uncertainty, and other concerns, resulting in referral to palliative care professionals. The paper concluded that 'this study showed that people with MND are living with uncertainty and other concerns throughout their illness trajectory. People are having to turn to palliative care professionals who are more able to meet their concerns than those caring for other aspects of their disease' ([27, 28], p. 2062). However, referral to palliative care professionals in the end stage of the illness trajectory may be too late for people who are experiencing life in crisis.

The project findings suggest that people with MND are living with loss, uncertainty, and other concerns. Person-centred care in MND focuses on monitoring symptoms and assessing needs. People are referred to the palliative care professionals when they are nearing their end-of-life. Palliative care professionals are perceived to be more able to provide a quality of life for the person and family and support a person to die. Thus raising the question as to why are people needing to be referred to palliative care professionals to talk about loss, uncertainty, and other concerns, when they are receiving person-centred care already?

4. What is person-centred care in MND?

The literature on person-centred care suggests that the origins began with Carl Rogers' [29] humanist model, seeing a person as being the expert on themselves and the therapist being the facilitator [30]. Similarly, Heidegger [16] suggests that a person always understands themselves concerning their existence through time. The values of seeing a person as an individual with rights and need for sensitive interaction are the focus of the Nursing Midwifery Council (NMC) professional standard of practice, which states that professionals must: 'make sure that those receiving care are treated with respect, that their rights are upheld and that any discriminatory attitudes and behaviours towards those receiving care are challenged' ([31], p. 6).

Similarly, the values of person-centred care are the focus of the Royal College of Occupational Therapist (RCOT) [32]. Code of ethics and professional conduct, which suggests that professionals must: 'always recognise the human rights of service users and act in their best interests, and enable individuals to preserve their individuality, self-respect, dignity, privacy, autonomy and integrity' ([32], p. 16). However, implementing the values of person-centred care can be a challenge in twenty first Century NHS care settings. The challenges include healthcare organisation culture, processes, and systems; professionals' belief that they already provide person-centred care, and patients beliefs impacting on engagement with their own healthcare [33]. Healthcare is known for doing 'to' and 'for' a person rather than doing 'with' them [34].

The current challenges to the delivery of coordinated interprofessional care in MND have been explored. Hogden et al. [4] highlight that issues may arise between acute care, rehabilitation, and palliative care teams, because of differing philosophies of care. Hardiman et al. [35] suggest that the shift in treatment paradigms from cure to symptom management to palliation is difficult for professionals, patients, and their families. The call is for increased collaboration between neurology and palliation [36, 37]. Hogden et al. ([4], p. 206) suggest a multidisciplinary approach to person-centred care in MND, that addresses a patient's broad range of needs and includes:

> *'Medical practitioners in neurology, respiratory, gastroenterology, rehabilitation, and palliative care; allied healthcare professionals in physiotherapy, occupational therapy, speech and language pathology, nutrition and social work; and health professionals in specialist nursing, genetic counselling and psychology, including neuropsychology.'*

Lannie and Peelo-Kilroe [38] raise concerns about care and culture that is task-focused, is not illuminating person-centredness. Brooker ([30], p. 220) suggests that an individual's perspectives 'are part of person-centred care.' The findings from Paper 5 suggest that MND care and professional culture are focused on monitoring symptoms and do not consider individual perspectives on whether the person wishes to become a patient with needs. Findings from a consensus review by Oliver et al. [37] show that palliative care and a person-centred approach to communication do result in improved care and patient experience. Connolly et al. ([36], p. 435) suggest that the focus of MND care should be to have early and open discussions of end-of-life concerns with patients and families. Allowing time for reflection and planning can 'obviate the introduction of unwanted interventions or procedures, can provide reassurance, and can alleviate fear.' Ng ([7], p. 114) suggests 'a proposed model for service interaction in caring for persons with MND shows the involvement of neurologists and palliative care teams in the acute and terminal phases of care, with a relatively smaller role for rehabilitation physicians.' Person-centred care is not just about monitoring symptoms, a needs-led care approach or advance care planning. We also need to think about how a person can gain a more profound meaning because of the past and, primarily because of the future. We suggest that an alternative person-centred care model in MND is needed, throughout the whole illness trajectory, one developed on hermeneutic phenomenological perspectives.

5. Proposed person-centred care model in MND

The proposed model of person-centred care in MND involves a focus on individuality that includes three major elements: 1. Presuppositions, 2. acceptance, and 3. temporality.

PCC (person-centred care) = P + A + T.

This person-centred care model offers an approach involving both experience and reflection. The focus is on acknowledging that our understanding is not fixed but changing and always open to new perspectives [17]. These elements are explored in more detail below.

5.1 Presuppositions

Professionals need to be aware of their presuppositions (preunderstanding and prejudices), to be open to new perspectives [17]. According to Gadamer, 'prejudice has to be provoked to be realisable' ([25], p. 117). Fleming et al. [25] suggests that one approach to provoke presuppositions is to have a conversation with a professional colleague. The process helps professionals enter the hermeneutic circle of understanding and remain orientated to 'being open' to the opinion of the other, bearing in mind that understanding is never fully achieved because it is constantly evolving. Gadamer [17] recommends not trying to put oneself in the shoes of another, because to do so is to ignore one's presuppositions and historical awareness. It is better to collaborate with a person to reach a shared understanding, otherwise termed as having a hermeneutic difference. The recommendation is to use this approach when understanding what is important to the person with MND and accepting that understanding will change through time.

5.2 Acceptance

Professionals need to accept what shows itself, rather than applying theories [39] or their own professional ideas on what constitutes a person's needs. Professionals need to accept that a person may wish to talk about loss, uncertainty, and other concerns. Such concerns relating to life and death are 'existential concerns.' which are recognised and accepted in the field of cancer care [40]. Existential concerns are not recognised and accepted in the field of MND care until a person is referred to palliative care. The MNDA ([6], p. 24) guidance states that professionals caring for people with MND are at risk of 'compassion fatigue,' defined as emotional, physical, and spiritual exhaustion, because of witnessing and absorbing the problems of others. Professionals need to accept that a person may not want the illness trajectory of MND, and they have the freedom to make choices to refuse treatments, and on how and where to die.

5.3 Temporality

Professionals need to understand (interpret) a person in a wider temporal frame and beyond their illness context. As Heidegger suggests, to ignore a person's past and future, is subordinating that person to the present [41]. Dewing ([42], p. 11) calls for a reassessment of person-centred nursing frameworks to take account of body and time (corporeality and temporality) if claiming an 'allegiance' with personhood. Corporeality and temporality are particularly important for a person as they first notice that something untoward is happening to their body. In the present, a person does not acknowledge their body, because mostly they are going about their daily lives and taking their body for granted. It is only when something untoward happens that they might be more likely to pay attention to their body, as it is not functioning as it did before. This occurrence may be a one-off, or it may be something more sinister; whatever it is, it causes an episode of anxiety. A person contacts their deeper modes of temporality: because of the present and anticipated future, they reinterpret and redefine their past [16, 41, 43]. Asking a person to tell their story about how MND has affected on all aspects of their existence through temporal time brings forward individual experiences and provides a focus for person-centred care in MND.

A person with MND whose cognition is not affected are fully aware of their past; the memories cannot be removed, but the ability to communicate them can. In the care of older people, biographical work is acknowledged as respecting the intrinsic worth of a person [44], particularly in the context of decision-making [45], and can also provide a sense of continuity [46]. In palliative care, life review can improve the emotional well-being of the patient with terminal cancer, especially when a person feels out of control of their situation, is unable to adapt to change or is distressed by earlier life events [47]. The proposed model recognises a person with MND has a unique history, culture, and practice. The care process involves professionals enabling the person to talk about their lived-through past. The expected outcome: a person with MND will be defining their identities and finding meaning in life as lived. It may help a person to talk about their regrets.

A person with MND may experience the present in crisis because life with MND has no meaning. Frankl [48] suggests people who are suffering are unable to move forward into the future. Dame Cicely Saunders [49, 50] understood, through her experiences of caring for people with advanced cancer, that suffering was not only caused by physical pain but also by psychological, social, and spiritual factors. She introduced the concept of 'total pain' to convey that a person's whole being can be affected by a terminal illness due to a lack of meaning [51, 52]. The proposed model respects a person is a self-interpreting being existing in a social and cultural world with others, who include family, friends, colleagues, carers, and the wider community. The care process involves listening to 'what is important for a person.' The expected outcome: a person with MND will be determining their being, thus creating feelings of recognition, respect, and trust.

A person with MND may wish to talk about their anticipated future and how to exert choice over the timing of death and achieve clarity over the legality of these options [6]. The timing of end-of-life discussions and decision-making is a contested area of MND practice. Gale [53] raises concerns because it is asking a person to think ahead to a time of future loss. Others prioritise end-of-life discussion and decision-making because of the risk to verbal communication [54] and decision-making capacity at end-of-life [55, 56]. The proposed model responds to a person's freedom and right to make choices. The care process should involve listening to their loss of once-projected

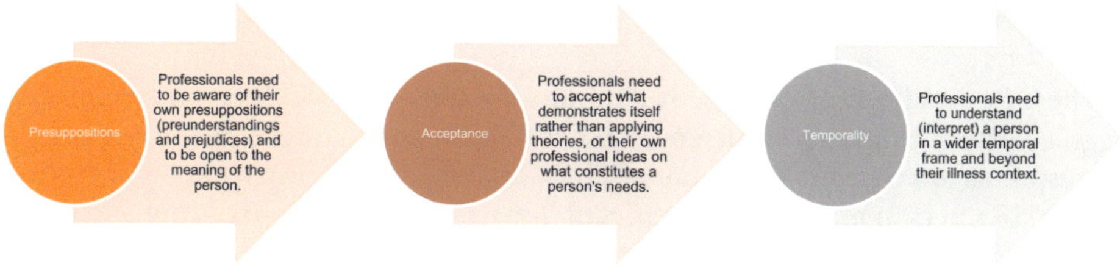

Figure 1.
Person-centred care model in MND.

future, their concerns for a future of being unable to communicate, move and breathe at end-of-life, and their concerns for others. Their needs, priorities and preferences are understood and documented in an advance directive. The expected outcome: a person with MND will be facing death while still being in control (**Figure 1**).

6. Discussion

This chapter presents a reflexive hermeneutic account of a research journey and the development of papers that followed, resulting in a developed model of person-centred care for people with MND. This body of work makes contributions to knowledge as follows: it provides a nuanced account of interpreting two philosophical positions on existential phenomenology [16] and philosophical hermeneutics [17], and applying these as a method. The designed method of data collection and analysis enabled a sensitive approach to researching the meaning of existence with MND through time. The findings uncovered the concept of 'existential loss' of past ways of being-in-the-world, embodiment, spatiality, and the once-projected future. A return to the findings to examine the meaning of uncertainty uncovered how people living with MND are receiving patient-centred care, but in a form where the focus is on the patient in the present. The concern is that this approach to person-centred care is emphasising medical diagnosis and the identification of symptoms that need to be monitored [57]. Becoming a patient within the NHS promote standards of behaviour, such as accepting objectified care. As Gadamer [58] asserted, the individuality of the person gets lost in this context. A person at their end-of-life needs support from palliative care professionals and those holding a power of attorney to reassert their individuality. The proposed model of care will enable professionals to focus on their presuppositions, accept what shows itself, and focus on a person's unique individuality from the time of diagnosis to end-of-life.

7. Conclusion

MND has a significant impact on a person's lifeworld, but the current focus of care is on the patient's MND symptoms. The proposed person-centred care model focuses on understanding (interpreting) a person in a wider temporal frame, and beyond the context of their illness. The expected collaborative outcomes: a person is acknowledged as more than a 'patient with MND'; a professional is providing person-centred care based on 'individuality.' This is a collaborative approach between the person, others, and professionals. Such person-centred care focused on individuality may prevent a person experiencing life in crisis and suffering towards end-of-life.

8. Relevance to practice

These project findings provide insight into the impact of MND on temporality. We suggest a way of thinking about a person with MND, one that recognises, respects, and responds to a person's temporality. Thus, understanding (interpreting) what is essential to a person may have a significant impact on the recipient of care and on the provider of care. This can support a change in person-centred care and culture for people diagnosed with MND, or any other terminal illness.

8.1 What does this chapter contribute to the broader global clinical community?

- The project findings show on-going concern about bringing forward the needs of this group.
- The experiences of MND care can have a detrimental effect on people who are living with loss, uncertainty, and other concerns, and these experiences are often ignored.
- This chapter has recommended a person-centred care model that will support professionals to interpret (understand) a person with MND in a wider temporal frame, and beyond the context of their illness.

Author details

Denise Andrea Harris
Faculty of Health, Psychology and Social Care/Nursing, Manchester Metropolitan University, Manchester, UK

*Address all correspondence to: denise.harris13@outlook.com

References

[1] Donaghy C, Dick A, Hardiman O, Patterson V. Timeliness of diagnosis in Motor Neurone Disease: A population-based study. Ulster Medical Journal. 2008;**77**(1):18-21

[2] Bäumer D, Talbot K, Turner MR. Advances in motor neurone disease. Journal of the Royal Society. 2014;**107**(1):14-21

[3] Goldstein LH, Abrahams S. Changes in cognition and behaviour in amyotrophic lateral sclerosis: Nature of impairment and implications for assessment. The Lancet Neurology. 2013;**12**:368-380

[4] Hogden A, Foley G, Henderson RD, James N, Aoun SM. Amyotrophic lateral sclerosis: Improving care with a multidisciplinary approach. Journal of Multidisciplinary Healthcare. 2017;**10**:205-215

[5] Motor Neurone Disease Association. Motor Neurone Disease: A Guide for GPs and Primary Care Teams. Northampton: Motor Neurone Disease Association; 2015

[6] Motor Neurone Disease Association. A professional's Guide to End of Life Care in Motor Neurone Disease (MND). Northampton: MNDA; 2016

[7] Ng L. The Use of International Classification of Functioning, Disability and Health in Motor Neurone Disease Rehabilitation [Unpublished thesis]. Melbourne: The University fo Melbourne; 2011

[8] Locock L, Ziebland S, Dumelow C. Biographical disruption, abruption and repari in the context of motor neurone disease. Sociology of Health and Illness. 2009;**31**(7):1043-1058

[9] Brott T, Hocking C, Paddy A. Occupational disruption: Living with motor neurone disease. British Journal of Occupational Therapy. 2007;**70**(1):24-31

[10] Brown J. User, carer and professional experiences of care in motor neurone disease. Primary Health Care Research and Development. 2003;**4**:207-217

[11] Foley J, O'Mahony P, Hardiman O. Perceptions of quality of life for persons with motor neurone disease/amyotrophic lateral sclerosis: A qualitative study. In: Rehabilitation and Therapy Research Society 2nd Annual Conference. Dublin: Physical Therapy Reviews; 2006. p. 209

[12] Brown J, Addington-Hall J. How people with motor neurone disease talk about living with their illness: A narrative study. Journal of Advanced Nursing. 2008;**62**(2):200-208

[13] Bolmsjö I. Existential issues in palliative care: Interviews of patients with amyotrophic lateral sclerosis. Journal of Palliative Medicine. 2001;**4**(4):499-505

[14] Ray RA, Street AF. Nonfinite loss and emotional labour: Family caregivers' experiences of living with motor neurone disease. Journal of Clinical Nursing. 2007;**16**:35-43

[15] O'Toole S. A Narrative Analysis of Accounts of Dying with Motor Neurone Disease: Stories of Suffering [Unpublished thesis]. Dublin: University College Dublin; 2011

[16] Heidegger M. Being and Time. Translated by Robinson, E and Macquarrie, J. Oxford: Blackwell Publishing; 1927/1962

[17] Gadamer H-G. Truth and Method. 2nd ed. Translated by Weinsheimer, J. and Marshall, D. New York: Continuum; 1975

[18] Inwood M. Heidegger: A Very Short Introduction. Oxford: Oxford University Press; 1997

[19] Moran D. Introduction to Phenomenology. London: Routledge Taylor and Francis Group; 2000

[20] Widdershoven GAM. The story of life: Hermeneutic perspectives on the relationship between narrative and life hisotry. In: Atkinson R, editor. Qualitative Research Methods. Vol. 44. London: Sage Publications; 1998. pp. 54-74

[21] Atkinson R. The Life Story Interview. Qualitative Research Methods Series 44. Thousand Oaks: SAGE Publications; 1998

[22] Clark A. Philosophy, understanding and the consultation: A fusion of horizons. British Journal of General Practice. 2008;**58**(546):58-60

[23] Harris DA. Doing research drawing on the philosophy of existential hermeneutic phenomenology. Palliative and Supportive Care. 2017b;**15**(2):267-269

[24] Harris DA. Supporting a loved one living with motor neurone disease. Palliative and Supportive Care. 2017a;**15**(1):141-142. DOI: 10.1017/S1478951516000134

[25] Fleming V, Gaidys U, Robb Y. Hermeneutic research in nursing: Developing a Gadamerian-based research method. Nursing Enquiry. 2003;**10**(2):113-120

[26] Harris DA. Lived-through past, experienced present, anticipated future: Understanding "existential loss" in the context of life-limiting illness. Palliative and Supportive Care (UK: Cambridge University Press). 2015;**13**(6):1579-1594. DOI: 10.1017/S1478951515000620

[27] Harris DA, Jack K, Wibberley C. Making her end of life her own: Further reflections on supporting a loved one with MND. International Journal of Palliative Care Nursing. 2018a;**25**(6):284-292

[28] Harris DA, Jack K, Wibberley C. The meaning of living with uncertainties for people with motor neurone disease. Journal of Clinical Nursing. 2018b;**27**(9-10):2062-2071

[29] Rogers CR. On Becoming a Person. Boston: Houghton Mifflin; 1961

[30] Brooker D. What is person-centred care in dementia? Clinical Gerontology. 2004;**13**:215-222

[31] Nursing and Midwifery Council (NMC). The Code. Professional standards of practice and behaviour for nurses, midwives and nursing associates. London: NMC; 2018

[32] Royal College of Occupational Therapists. Code of Ethics and Professional Conduct. London: RCOT; 2015

[33] Moore L, Britten N, Lydahl D, Naldemirci O, Elam M, Wolf A. Barriers and facilitators to the implementation of personcentred care in different healthcare contexts. Scandinavian Journal of Caring Sciences. 2017;**31**:662-673

[34] The Health Foundation. Person-Centred Care Made Simple. London: The Health Foundation; 2016

[35] Hardiman O, Leonard H, van den Berg, Kiernan MC. Clinical diagnosis and management of amyotrophic lateral sclerosis. Amyotrophic Lateral Sclerosis. 2011;(7):639-649

[36] Connolly S, Galvin M, Hardiman O. End-of-life management in patients with amyotrphic lateral sclerosis. The Lancet Neurology. 2015;**14**(4):435-442. DOI: 10.1016/S1474-4422(14)70221-2

[37] Oliver DJ, Borasio GD, Caraceni A, de Visser M, Grisold W, Lorenzl S, et al. A consensus review on the development of palliative care for patients with chronic and progressive neurological disease. European Journal of Neurology. 2016;**23**:30-38

[38] Lannie A, Peelo-Kilroe L. Personcentredness in palliative care. In: Nursing and Health Care: Theory and Practice, by McCormack and McCance. Chichester: Wiley Blackwell; 2017. pp. 248-258

[39] Heidegger M. Zollikon Seminars: Protocols-Conversations-Letters. Edited by Medard Boxx. Translated by Franz Mayr and Richard Askay. Illinois: Northwestern University Press; 2001

[40] Henoch I, Danielson E. Existential concerns among patients with cancer and interventions to meet them: An integrative literature review. Psycho-Oncology. 2009;**18**(3):225-236

[41] Polt R. Heidegger: An Introduction. London: Routledge, Taylor and Francis Group; 1999

[42] Dewing J. Personhood and dementia: Revisiting Tom Kitwood's ideas. International Journal of Older People Nursing. 2008;**3**:3-13

[43] Sartre JP. Being and Nothingness. New York: Philosophical Library; 1956

[44] Ford P, McCormack B. Future directions for gerontology: A nursing perspective. Nurse Education Today. 2002;**20**(5):389-394

[45] McCormack B, McCance T. Person-Centred Nursing Theory and Practice. Oxford: Wiley-Blackwell; 2010

[46] Nolan MR, Davies S, Brown J, Keady J, Nolan J. Beyond 'person-centred' care: A new vision for gerontological nursing. International Journal for Older People Nursing. 2004;**13**(3a):45-53

[47] Lester J. Life review with the terminally ill-narrative therapies. In: Firth P, Luff G, Oliviere D, editors. Loss, Change and Bereavement in Palliative Care. Berkshire: Open University Press; 2005. pp. 66-79

[48] Frankl VE. Man's Search for Meaning: The Classic Tribute to Hope from the Holocaust. London: Rider; 1962

[49] Saunders C. Care of patients suffering from terminal illness at St Joseph's Hospice. Nursing Mirror. 1964:vii-x

[50] Saunders C. Spiritual pain. Journal of Palliative Care. 1988;**4**:29-32

[51] Clarke D. 'Total pain': The work of Cicely Saunders and the maturing of a concept. End of Life Studies. 2014. Available from: http://endoflifestudies.academicblogs.co.uk/total-pain-the-work-of-cicely-saunders-and-the-maturing-of-a-concept/ [Accessed: February 5, 2016]

[52] LeMay K, Wilson KG. Treatment of existential distress in life-threatening illness: A review of manualized interventions. Clinical Psychology Review. 2008;**28**:472-493

[53] Gale C. Assisting patients with motor neurone disease to make decisions about their care. International Journal of Palliative Nursing. 2015;**21**(5):251-255

[54] Preston H, Fineberg IC, Callagher P, Mitchell JD. The preferred priorities for care document in motor neurone disease: View of bereaved relatives and carers. Palliative Medicine. 2012;**26**(2):132-138

[55] Harris D, Fineberg IC. Multidisciplinary palliative care teams'

understanding of Mental Capacity Act 2005 best interests determinations. International Journal of Palliative Care Nursing. 2011;**17**(1):20-25

[56] National Council for Palliative Care (NCPC). End of Life Care in Long-Term Neurological Conditions; a Framework for Implementation. London: The National Council for Palliative Care; 2010

[57] Draper J, Tetley J. The importance of person-centred approaches to nursing care. The Open University; 2019. Available from: https://www.open.edu/openlearn/health-sports-psychology/healthcare-careers/the-importance-person-centred-approaches-nursing-care [Accessed: March 1, 2019]

[58] Gadamer H-G. The Enigma of Health. Translated by ason Gaiger and Nicholas Walker. Stamford, California: Stamford University Press; 1996

Section 2

Current Practice from around the World

Chapter 6

Perspective Chapter: The Development and Integration of Palliative Care at the Institute of Oncology Ljubljana

Maja Ebert Moltara

Abstract

The history of the development of palliative care at the Institute of Oncology Ljubljana dates back to the 1990s when counseling and advisory work in the field of palliative care began. In 2007, the Department for Acute Palliative Care was established with six beds to treat palliative care patients with the most complex symptoms. The beginning of outpatient care and the reestablishment of consular work date back to 2013. The number of patients increased from year to year until 2017, the first critical year when palilalia almost brought the activity to an end. With the support of patients' associations, the activity was nevertheless maintained, sustained through the COVID-19 epidemic, and increased again in recent years. In 2021, the Mobile Palliative Unit and 24-hour telephone support were added to the previous activities.

Keywords: palliative care, cancer center, oncology institute, development, network of services

1. Introduction

The beginning is the hardest thing, but keep your heart, and everything will be fine. (Vincent van Gogh)

The main goal of palliative care is to ensure the quality of life of patients with advanced incurable diseases by alleviating the physical, psychological, sociological, and spiritual needs of patients and with support to their loved ones through all periods of the disease (**Figure 1**). Treatment should be individualized based on the current condition and wishes of the patient. To ensure optimal palliative care, early recognition of needs, timely inclusion of the treatment, and its integration into oncological interventions are important [1].

Patients and their loved ones may have very different needs when dealing with an incurable disease. It is important to recognize those individual needs and appropriately tailor the most suitable management of them with an interdisciplinary approach. Support systems must be dynamic and flexible and adapted to different needs during different periods of palliative care [2].

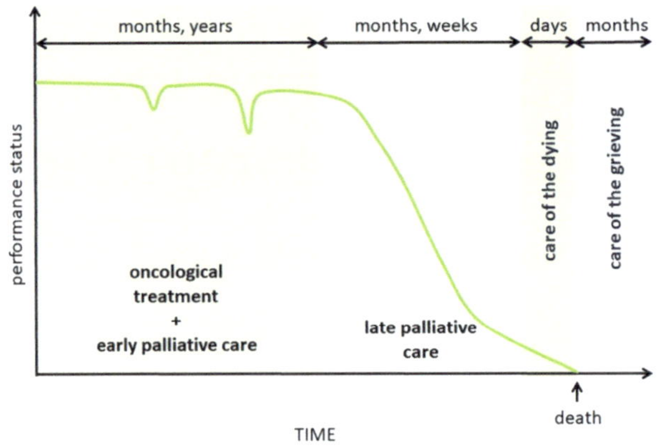

Figure 1.
Palliative care periods.

2. Cancer in Slovenia

Among the 2 million Slovenian citizens, in 2019, there were 16,080 new cancer cases, and 6285 patients died from it. To achieve the most effective cancer control, the National Cancer Control Program was implemented in 2010; it coordinates activities according to international recommendations adapted to the Slovenian healthcare system [3]. Organizationally, there is one major central cancer center and several smaller satellite clinics nationwide. The Institute of Oncology Ljubljana, established in 1937, is a comprehensive national cancer center that carries out services required for cancer prevention, diagnostics, and treatment, as well as rehabilitation and palliative care of cancer patients.

Recently, the Slovenian Cancer Registry has been reporting a trend of increasing cancer incidence and rising numbers of patients who died due to cancer. Nevertheless, over the years, the incidence and mortality trends from cancer are becoming increasingly separated, indicating the more successful treatment of cancer patients [4]. However, according to the Lancet Commission, the proportion of patients who need palliative care in oncology is estimated at 90% of all those who die from cancer [5]. Therefore, Slovenia's estimated needs for good holistic palliative care, just for oncological patients, are massive.

3. History of palliative care in Slovenia

The roots of Slovenian palliative care date back over four decades ago. The pioneering work began in 1980 when anesthesiology teams in all major hospitals organized pain clinics that offered specialized treatment for patients with severe pain [6]. In 1996, the Slovenian Hospice Society, a nongovernmental, nonprofit, humanitarian organization, started offering professional and lay support to dying patients and their relatives [7]. In 2000, at the Institute of Oncology Ljubljana, the first palliative team was established, working as a consultation team that supported hospitalized palliative care patients at the oncological center and offered telephone support to other Slovenian healthcare workers [8]. At the same time, some initiation of palliative care activities also started in some nursing hospitals, health centers, and senior homes. At that time, the majority of the staff had no advanced education on palliative care [9].

After several years of preparation, in 2010, the National Program for Palliative Care was accepted [10]. Nowadays, it offers a foundation for the development of that important field. From the beginning, the development of palliative care differed regionally, influenced mostly by the activism of local individuals [11]. The COVID-19 period also had a major influence on palliative care and the healthcare system in general. Some palliative care services have expanded, while others completely disappeared [12].

The Slovenian Association for Palliative and Hospice Care was founded in 2011, with the primary task of implementing different training programs for various palliative care team members. They became a full member of the European Association for Palliative Care in 2014 [13].

To accelerate research on palliative care, the Institute for Palliative Care was established in 2014 [14].

4. Current model of oncological palliative care in Slovenia

The current model of oncological palliative care for patients with cancer was developed over several years following the National Program for Palliative Care and the National Cancer Control Program.

According to the National Program for Palliative Care, since 2010, palliative care has been provided at two levels: basic palliative care and specialized palliative care [2, 15].

4.1 Basic palliative care

Basic palliative care should cover the needs of 80% of patients with palliative care [16] and should be provided by everyone who cares for the incurably sick. Mostly they are teams at the primary level of the health system (family doctor, community nurse) and any healthcare providers in an institution where such patients are treated (senior homes, general hospitals, general hospital departments, and hospices). All those providers should have knowledge of basic palliative care. Unfortunately, the necessary knowledge is still often missing due to a lack of universal palliative care education; in general, however, there is a trend for a better understanding of palliative care approaches. Also, to overcome this barrier, several educational materials and handbooks in Slovenian language have been published in recent years: Basic concepts and suggested terminology in palliative care, Handbook of palliative care and Palliative care of adult patients in family medicine: a manual for primary care physicians [17–19].

4.2 Specialized palliative care

Specialized palliative care is provided by additionally educated and experienced physicians. They usually work in palliative care most of their working time, some full-time. Specialized palliative care can be provided as dedicated hospital units in the form of acute palliative care departments, consultation work, outpatient clinics for early palliative care, mobile palliative units, and support to the providers at basic palliative care. Specialized palliative care activities are aimed at patients with the most complex needs [2, 15]. According to estimates by international experts, 20% of all patients need specialized palliative care [16]. To support knowledge at this level, an educational handbook in Slovenian language has been published under the title Palliative care of adult cancer patients in Slovenia: basic concepts and recommendations [2].

4.3 Palliative care coordination

Palliative care coordination plays an important role in providing care adapted to the patient's needs. The name of this service can be found in the literature under several expressions, such as "palliative care coordination" or "case manager." The coordinator is the key person who evaluates the individual's holistic needs and plans, facilitates, and advocates through proper communication. The coordinating activity enables the monitoring of patients at home after discharge via telephone. This involves coordinating counseling for patients and relatives at home regarding current problems, measures, and options. The palliative care coordinator is the connecting link between patients and members of the palliative care team and other health and social care institutions. The coordinator connects and integrates different levels of the healthcare system. The purpose of coordination is primarily to ensure optimal palliative care for the individual patient; at the same time, good coordination also ensures optimal use of the available resources in healthcare [15, 20].

Palliative care coordinators must be professionally qualified with appropriate knowledge about symptom management and support of relatives, and also during times of death and mourning [2].

5. Palliative care at the institute of oncology Ljubljana

At the Institute of Oncology Ljubljana, palliative care has been provided for several decades, but it has become an integral part of the comprehensive treatment of cancer patients during the last few years. At first, in 2000, the first palliative team was working as a consultation team that supported hospitalized palliative care patients at the oncological center and offered telephone support to other Slovenian healthcare workers [8]. Since then, several changes and adaptations have been made. In 2006, the first internal recommendations regarding the implementation of palliative care in hospitals were drawn up; the recommendations anticipate palliative care on two levels: basic palliative care provided by health workers in all clinical departments of the hospital and specialized palliative care. The year 2007 was a turning point, with the official establishment of the Department for Acute Palliative Care with six beds. Later, additional specialized services were added: in 2012, an official counseling service; in 2013, an outpatient clinic for early palliative care; and in 2021, mobile palliative care units for patients at home care with 24/7 phone support for patients and healthcare providers elsewhere. Today's scope of work of palliative care team members does not include only patient care, monitoring, and coordination but also educational and research activities (**Figure 2**).

In 2009, the Institute of Oncology Ljubljana was recognized by the European Society for Medical Oncology (ESMO) as a Designated Centre of Integrated Oncology and Palliative Care, an oncology center with the successful integration of palliative care into a comprehensive oncological approach; we have continued to fulfill the criteria since then [21, 22].

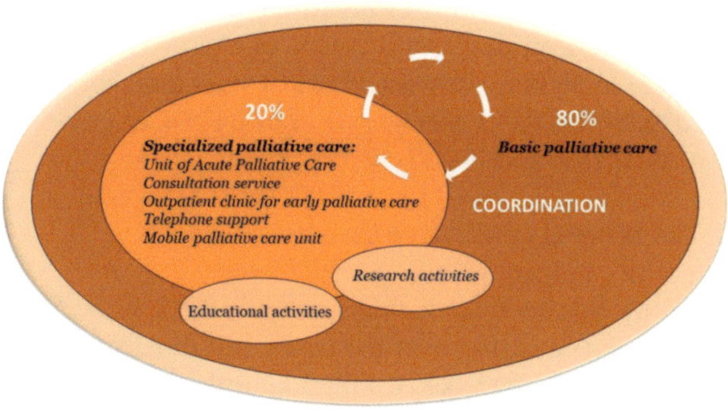

Figure 2.
Palliative care at the Institute of Oncology Ljubljana.

5.1 Unit of acute palliative care

This hospital unit is the oldest ongoing specialized palliative care service at the Institute of Oncology Ljubljana, established in February 2007. Since its foundation, the number of beds was increased from 6 to 12 during the COVID-19 period. Today, it is a seven-bed department in which specialized palliative care is offered with an interdisciplinary approach to the patients with the most complex needs. In addition to physicians and nurses with special knowledge of palliative care, members of the pain management team, psychologists, psychiatrists, physiotherapists, dieticians, pharmacists, spiritual supporters, volunteers, and others are included in the treatment [23].

The annual number of admissions to acute palliative care is increasing, while the average length of hospitalization remains the same over the years. In 2022, 355 patients were admitted to the acute palliative care department, with an average length of stay of 5.4 days. The vast majority of patients were admitted from home as part of the coordination program, and most of them (60.8%) were discharged back home, (5.9%) were transferred to hospice, and (28.4%) died at the department.

5.2 Consultation service

The consultation service has been monitored since 2012. Today, as part of this service, a triage of all referrals to specialized palliative care is done, as well as consultation visits and family meetings of patients from other departments of the Institute of Oncology Ljubljana are carried out. According to a review of available information during triage, a patient is directed to the most suitable services for his case: hospitalization in an acute palliative care unit, consultation visits to other departments, monitoring in the outpatient clinic, 24/7 phone support, or visits with mobile palliative care unit.

From 2014 to 2019, we received, on average, 199 referrals per year; however, in recent years, we have observed a significant increase in referrals to 433 in 2020, 617 in 2021, and 811 in 2022.

In 2022, 56% of referrals came from the Department of Medical Oncology, followed by referrals from the Department of Radiotherapy (24.1%) and the Department of Oncological Surgery (6.3%), as well as a significant increase in external referrals (family physicians, other hospitals in the region) from 2.5% in 2020, 3.4% in 2021, to 13.5% in 2022.

Consultation visits include a review of documentation, a conversation with a patient and his oncologist, a clinical examination of a patient, family meetings' participation, and help in difficult communication and counseling.

From 2012 to 2019, we held, on average, 200 family meetings per year; in 2020, we carried out 214; in 2021, 233; and in 2022, 205 of them.

5.3 Outpatient clinic for early palliative care

The outpatient clinic has been operating since July 2013. Indications for this type of management have been changing over the years, but mostly patients were directed to that service by their oncologist based on their complex needs that required more intensive monitoring and support. Currently, we advise outpatient clinic management for patients with incurable cancer in the period of early palliative care, when they are still receiving specific treatments, and for patients in the late period of palliative care, if they are easily mobile and visiting the clinic does not present unnecessary burdens. The purposes of early palliative management are additional support to the patient during actual specific treatment, help in understanding of the disease, help in dealing with symptoms (physical, psychological, social, and spiritual), providing assistance in decision-making regarding cancer treatment, nutrition, physical activity, and also to ensure the continuity of care, providing support to loved ones, preparation for the last period of life, as well as recognition and addressing of the individual's spiritual needs.

Nowadays, the outpatient clinic is open on working days, several hours per day, also for patients on specific oncological therapy at the Institute of Oncology Ljubljana, regardless of their region of residence. The frequency of visits depends on the patient's problems and is adapted to the wishes and abilities of the patients and their families.

Between 2014 and 2019, in outpatient clinic we treated an average 183 patients/year. In 2022, 513 examinations were carried out (242 first time, 273 control), significantly more than in any previous year. Having own space for an outpatient clinic enabled more visits every day.

5.4 Telephone support

During the early period of the specialized palliative care at the Institute of Oncology Ljubljana, the telephone number of the coordination office was active only during regular working hours every weekday. At that time, on average, around 400 patients were supported in this service annually. Since the COVID-19 period, the telephone number has been available 24/7 and provides support for patients and their relatives in palliative care, as well as counseling for medical professionals. The activity is carried out for all cancer patients regardless of the region of residence and regardless of the period of palliative care. When appropriate, the patient and loved ones are referred to local palliative care teams. For documentation, "phone cases" are recorded; these are individual records of activities to resolve problems; several phone calls per day may be required for one phone case. We also do not record short coordination calls within the hospital.

Since we started to record phone cases, there were 1573 telephone cases in 2020, 2344 in 2021, and 4457 in 2022. Since September 1, 2021, they have been covered by the Mobile Palliative Care Program and are officially recorded in the Register of Specialized Palliative Care at the Institute of Oncology Ljubljana.

5.5 Mobile palliative care unit

The Mobile Palliative Team Program, covered by National Health Insurance, has been taking place at the Institute of Oncology Ljubljana since September 1, 2021 and incorporates palliative care services, such as triage, a consultation service, an outpatient clinic, 24-hour telephone support, and home visits. Most of these services have been carried out at the Institute of Oncology Ljubljana for many years; in contrast, the Mobile Home Visits unit was introduced in 2021. The Mobile Palliative Care Unit complemented the previous activities of specialized palliative care at the Institute of Oncology Ljubljana.

The Mobile Palliative Care Unit visits patients at home during the period of late palliative care and dying. It supports patients with incurable cancer who are less mobile or for whom traveling to the hospital causes a great deal of effort and burden. The Mobile Palliative Unit of the Institute of Oncology Ljubljana covers the Central Slovenia region from Monday to Friday. The team consists of a physician and a registered nurse, with additional staff if necessary.

In 2021, from September to December, the Mobile Palliative Care Team completed 164 visits and 631 visits in 2022, which ranged from 41 to 61 visits per month. One effect of palliative care home support was a drop in the hospital mortality of patients from the Central Slovenian region, from 64% in 2017 to 57% in 2022 [24].

5.6 Educational activities

The specialized palliative team is dedicated to education in the field of palliative care. Members give lectures on palliative care in undergraduate programs. Also, mentorships are offered to residents of oncology, family, and emergency medicine who have obligatory rotations at the Department of Acute Palliative Care.

Once a week, internal lectures are prepared by palliative care team members together with invited external lecturers. Several times a year, intensive training courses in the special skills in palliative care are held, such as the workshops "Communication," "Last Days of Life," and "Pain Treatment".

Team members are also active on the national level of education and are part of the Slovenian Association for Palliative and Hospice Care educational team that performs multidisciplinary educational programs for all palliative care team members, several times a year. Over the last 10 years, more than 650 health professionals completed 60-hour intensive palliative care education. Moreover, more than 1000 participants attended the first four Slovenian Congresses of Palliative Care.

One important aspect of education is publishing educational articles, handbooks, and manuals for health providers; in recent years, several have been released [2, 17–19].

To improve knowledge about palliative care of patients and their relatives in the Slovenian language, the online platform https://paliativnaoskrba.si/ was started in 2014, where leaflets of the Butterfly Project with useful information and advice on palliative care are available. Patients can also find contacts of specialized palliative care team providers from all over the country.

5.7 Research activities

As with all the clinical and educational works, it is sometimes difficult to carry out research activities, but for the time being, the members of specialized palliative care attempt to conduct at least some simple research works and present their results at National and International Congresses or publish them in medical journals. Research topics cover analyses of clinical work, the impact of new interventions and services, and the influences they have on the place of care and death [22, 25].

6. Conclusion

Despite the many advances in oncology, many cancer patients still need palliative care as part of their comprehensive care. The Institute of Oncology Ljubljana, recognized as an ESMO Designated Centre of Integrated Oncology and Palliative Care, has a 16-year tradition of specialized palliative care. Today, the institute can offer several different services according to the need of an individual patient. The structure of palliative care is as complex as the needs of the patients. The mission of the Institute of Oncology Ljubljana is to provide the best possible support network for patients with palliative care needs and to support their relatives. At the same time, we are aware of the responsibility to share and spread our experiences and knowledge to other areas, to nononcological palliative patients, and to patients in all regions of Slovenia.

Author details

Maja Ebert Moltara
Department for Acute Palliative Care, Institute of Oncology Ljubljana, Ljubljana, Slovenia

*Address all correspondence to: mebert@onko-i.si

References

[1] Ebert Moltara M, Bernot M, Benedik J, Žist A, Golob N, Malačič S, et al. Basic Concepts and Suggested Terminology in Palliative Care. Ljubljana: Slovenian Association of Palliative and Hospice Care; 2020

[2] Ebert Moltara M, Bernot M, editors. Palliative Care of Adult cancer Patients in Slovenia: Basic Concepts and Recommendations. 1st ed. Ljubljana: Oncology Institute; 2023. DOI: 10.25670/oi2023-breview1

[3] National Cancer Control Program [Internet]. 2023. Available from: https://www.dpor.si/

[4] Cancer in Slovenia 2019. Epidemiology and Cancer Registry, Slovenian Cancer Registry. Ljubljana: Institute of Oncology Ljubljana; 2022

[5] Sleeman KE, Brito M, Etkind S, Nkhoma K, Guo P, Higginson IJ, et al. The escalating global burden of serious health-related suffering: Projections to 2060 by world regions, age groups, and health conditions. The Lancet Global Health. 2019;7:e883-e892. DOI: 10.1016/s2214-109x(19)30172-x

[6] Krčevski Škvarč N. Academy Awards for 20th Anniversary of Slovenian Association for Pain Management. Slovenian Association for Pain Management. Ljubljana; 2017

[7] Slovenian Hospice Society [Internet]. 2023. Available from: http://www.drustvo-hospic.si

[8] Salobir U. Palliative care. Onkologija. 2002;**2**:87-90

[9] Lunder U, Logar V. Palliative care in Slovenia and future challenges. Zdravstveni Vestnik. 2003;**72**:643-647

[10] National Program for Palliative Care. Ministry of Health. [Internet]. 2010. Available from: https://www.gov.si/assets/Ministrstva/MZ/DOKUMENTI/pomembni-dokumenti/47cbef2cb3/Drzavni-program-paliativne-oskrbe.pdf

[11] Golob N. The state of palliative care in Slovenia. ISIS. 2020;**1**:24-25

[12] Ebert Moltara M, Zakotnik BM. The impact of covid-19 epidemic to the implementation of acute palliative care in oncology. Onkologija: A Medical-Scientific Journal. 2021;**25**(1):18-30. DOI: 10.25670/oi2021-011on

[13] Slovenian Association for Palliative and Hospice Care [Internet]. 2023. Available from: http://www.szpho.si

[14] Institute of Palliative Medicine and Care [Internet]. 2010. Available from: https://paliativa.si/#

[15] Luckett T, Phillips J, Agar M, Virdun C, Green A, Davidson PM. Elements of effective palliative care models: A rapid review. BMC Health Services Research. 2014;**14**(1):136. DOI: 10.1186/1472-6963-14-136

[16] Radbruch L, Payne S. White Paper on standards and norms for hospice and palliative care in Europe: Part 1, part 2. EAPC update. European Journal of Palliative Care. 2009;**16**(6):22-33

[17] Ebert Moltara M, Bernot M, Benedik J, Žist A, Golob N, Malačič S, et al. Basic Concepts and Suggested Terminology in Palliative Care. Ljubljana: Slovenian Association for Palliative and Hospice care; 2020. Available from: https://0501.nccdn.net/4_2/000/000/008/486/temeljni-pojmi-in-predlagano-izrazoslovje-splet.pdf

[18] Ebert Moltara M, Koritnik B, Handbook of Palliative Care. Slovenian Association for Palliative and Hospice care. 2021. Available from: https://0501.nccdn.net/4_2/000/000/008/486/priroc%C3%8C%C2%8Cnik_paliativna_oskrba_-e-verzija-.pdf

[19] Zelko E, Rotar Pavlič D, Rifel J, Petek D. Palliative Care of Adult Patients in Family Medicine: A Manual for Primary Care Physicians. Ljubljana: Institute for the Development of Family Medicine; 2021

[20] Reeves E et al. Care coordination in palliative home care: Who plays the key role? International Journal of Integrated Care. 2020;**20**(3):1-9. DOI: 10.5334/ijic.5466

[21] Institute of Oncology Ljubljana [Internet]. ESMO Designated Centres of Integrated Oncology and Palliative Care. Available from: https://www.esmo.org/for-patients/esmo-designated-centres-of-integrated-oncology-palliative-care/esmo-accredited-designated-centres/institute-of-oncology-ljubljana

[22] Boltezar L, Ebert Moltara M, Jezeršek B. Trends in specialized palliative care referrals at an oncology center from 2007 to 2019. BMC Palliative Care. 2021;**20**:135. DOI: 10.1186/s12904-021-00828-w

[23] Benedik J, Pahole Goličnik J, Ebert Moltara M. Department for acute palliative care at the Ljubljana Oncology Institute. In: Through Knowledge and Experience to Quality Palliative Care. Ljubljana; 2017. pp. 60-61 Available from: https://dirros.openscience.si/IzpisGradiva.php?lang=slv&id=12127

[24] Ebert MM. Palliative care. Onkologija: A Medical-Scientific Journal. 2014;**18**(1):53-55 Available from: http://www.dlib.si

[25] Ebert Moltara M, Bernot M, Ivanetič Pantar M, Golob N, Globočnik Kukovica M, Lahajnar Čavlovič S, et al. Mobile palliative care team of Oncology Institute of Ljubljana. Onkologija: A Medical-Scientific Journal. 2022;**26**(2):30-34. DOI: 10.25670/oi2022-010on

Chapter 7

Challenges Associated with End-of-Life Care in Saudi Arabia

Alexander Woodman

Abstract

There is extensive literature on theoretical arguments and fundamental subjects for the study of bioethics challenges from Saudi healthcare providers' perspective. Some of the core principles of end-of-life care in Saudi Arabia are respect for dignity of both the patient and the caregiver; compassion to the wishes of the patient and family; management of pain; assessment and management of the psychological and social needs of the patient and the family. However, healthcare professionals often neglect good clinical practice by failing to comply with informed consent. This insensibility leads to the reluctance of patients being aware of the procedures, although they have expressed an interest in decision-making process. The collective engagement of family and health care professionals is the ultimate level of success. Future research and education should involve healthcare professionals, patients, and their families in decision-making by providing the knowledge empowering intelligence on how to communicate with sensitivity, dignity, sympathy, and respect.

Keywords: end-of-life care, physician-patient relationship, informed consent, do-not-resuscitate, good clinical practice, Saudi Arabia

1. Introduction

Ethics is the study of the nature of morals and the adoption of specific moral choices. Some of these are common to humanity and transcend cultures, religions, and regions (common morality), while others include responsibilities and professional standards (particular morality) [1–3]. Bioethics comprises principles that focus on medical/clinical ethics (issues in healthcare), research ethics (issues in the conducting and implications of research), environmental ethics (issues that arise due to relationships between human activities and the environment), and public health ethics (issues in public health) [3–5].

Ethics is an inherent and integral part of clinical medicine, where the physician is expected to make decisions that often go beyond selecting an appropriate treatment or intervention. Beneficence, non-maleficence, autonomy, and justice are the four ethical principles. These principles are also part of the Islamic bioethics applicable in Saudi Arabia, where interest in various codes of medical ethics, as a separate area of scientific research, has grown over the past few years [2–4]. In addition, the medical sector in Saudi Arabia is governed by Islamic ethics requiring adherence to Islamic medical ethics, including the observance of fatwas—religious decisions that healthcare providers follow in the Muslim world [3–5]. Despite these well-established principles and fatwas covering a wide range of social, religious, and bioethical topics, healthcare providers in Saudi Arabia often face dilemmas in their daily practice [3–5].

It is well-established that end-of-life care includes physical, emotional, social, and spiritual support for patients and their families. The goal of end-of-life care is to control pain and other symptoms so the patient can be as comfortable as possible [6]. This process also includes various components of the doctor-patient relationship, such as informed consent and the do-not-resuscitate (DNR) order, that are often overlooked or not included as part of the whole treatment. Despite significant advances in end-of-life care in Saudi Arabia, the relevant knowledge of both the general population and practitioners is often limited by the focus on curing [4, 5]. Thus, as shown in the most recent comprehensive systematic review of ethical issues reported in Saudi Arabia, the five most discussed bioethical areas are: 'Medical Ethics Curriculum in Saudi Arabia,' 'Doctor-Patient Relations,' 'Informed Consent,' 'Do-Not-Resuscitate,' 'Organ Donation and Transplantation' [5].

Of these five areas, three constitute one of the most discussed topics in bioethics in Saudi Arabia and around the world, namely end-of-life care. These areas included 'Doctor-Patient Relations,' 'Informed Consent, and 'Do-Not-Resuscitate.' This chapter aims to systematically appraise the research related to the doctor-patient relationship, informed consent, and DNR in the Saudi setting, and discuss their association with disease control and end-of-life care.

1.1 Physician-patient relationship

The doctor-patient relationship is a complex psychosocial interplay of vulnerability, trust and professional authority. It should be understood that the knowledge and skills of physicians are only some of the determining factors in building these relationships [7, 8]. Thus, the duty of the doctor is not only to inform the patient fully about their state of health, provide optimal treatment and refer the patient to the appropriate specialist if required, but also to build effective communication to increase patient satisfaction, reduce patient complaints and positively influence the overall clinical outcomes and mental health of patients.

According to the Saudi Commission for Health Specialties (2015), trust is at the core of any successful doctor-patient interaction, while integrity and honesty are essential for achieving trust [9]. Although patients do not expect perfection from their healthcare providers, they need to know that their doctor is reliable and trustworthy. Earlier in 2006, the Saudi government published the 'Patients' Bill of Rights (PBR)' aimed at improving the experience of patients and healthcare professionals with a focus on quality of care [10]. The PBR defines patients' rights as "accessible health care that meets their needs, to be treated with respect, to receive understandable information, to be involved in treatment options and plans, to file a complaint and to the inviolability of personal privacy." Hence, doctors should effectively facilitate doctor-patient relationships and dynamic exchanges before, during, and after a medical appointment. In addition, healthcare professionals must be upfront with patients regarding their rights and responsibilities, and how those rights are supported through informed consent [9, 10].

At the same time, there are certain established clear boundaries for doctors regarding what is allowed and what is forbidden relating to medical practice and scientific research [2, 9]. The doctor cannot act against the patient's will within these limits. However, the doctor's task in diagnosis and treatment determines the urgency of medical intervention. Therefore, when treatment can save a life in certain cases, doctors have the right to disregard the patients' will and start treatment. The doctor-patient relationship is a complex area made up of several factors, including doctor-patient communication, patient involvement in decision-making, and patient satisfaction. It is expected and recommended that the physician and patient work together to improve psychopathological conditions, giving particular attention to the therapeutic relationship that influences the patient's thoughts, emotions, and behavior [1, 2, 9].

Due to the complex nature of this field and the delicate nature of the doctor-patient communication, this relationship is one of the most studied areas of Saudi bioethics. A general synthesis on the topic over the past decades has shown that, despite well-established provisions and fatwas, people, including medical professionals, knew little about the doctor-patient relationship. In addition, there was little knowledge of the PBR, and those who did know had fragmentary knowledge. Health professionals who were aware of the PBR expressed dissatisfaction with the shortage of staff and the lack of the necessary facilities that would allow full adherence to the PBR in primary healthcare centers. However, there was a strong consensus that every patient should be treated with honesty and dignity. Moreover, healthcare providers knew about patients' rights to respect, privacy, and confidentiality. Patients of a high socioeconomic class should not be treated with extra care, and confidentiality should be maintained in all circumstances [5, 11–13].

The professional status of a doctor was found to be positively associated with patient satisfaction, empathy for the patient, and a better knowledge of bioethics. In addition, the manner of a doctor's communication was influenced by the specialty of that doctor. Thus, family physicians were more closely associated with rapport building, psychosocial exchange, and patient orientation. Physicians working in public hospitals were more likely to enjoy a higher level of patient trust compared to private hospitals [14–16]. This picture suggests that, despite the lack of knowledge, the relationship with patients was generally satisfactory and positive from the perspective of physicians. However, in studies with a target population of patients, rather conflicting data have been obtained.

The overall level of satisfaction in a doctor-patient relationship was found to be less than moderate. Patients reported that lack of training, questionable awareness of cultural norms, patient participation in decision-making, gender differences between patients and physicians and lack of time were major barriers to effective communication skills with patients and their families [17–19]. Furthermore, some patients perceived the nurses to be lacking in responsiveness and compassion. Patients further encouraged doctors and nurses to improve their interpersonal skills and take a more holistic, patient-centered approach when privacy was a major concern for participants, especially women. While most participants supported informed consent in general, some studies reported that informed consent was incorrectly obtained. In addition, there was disagreement among patients/relatives and physicians over treatment decisions, including treating patients with impaired or uncertain decision-making, and conflict with administrative policies and procedures. Finally, participants with higher levels of relationship satisfaction had a stronger sense of self-efficacy in managing their chronic illnesses [5, 17–19].

It is well known that all areas of Saudi bioethics are intertwined with religion to provide a sense of legal-ethical discourse on matters pertaining to biomedical matters [2, 3]. The study of the relationship between the doctor and the patient showed, both patients and doctors noted the positive influence of religion on health and overcoming illnesses. At the same time, religion rarely caused feelings of guilt, anxiety, or other negative emotions that can lead to an increase in the suffering of the patient. Family physicians were more likely to initiate religious discussions, and physicians with intrinsic religiosity were more likely to share their religious views [17–20].

While physicians are trained to maintain health and fight disease, the data presented in this area has shown that Saudi physicians lack detailed knowledge about communicating with patients and their families. This situation can escalate when it comes to end-of-life care. That said, good communication can help minimize pain, avoid fear and suffering, and allow patients' families to suffer less. Conversely, poor communication can lead to suboptimal care, patients and their families may be subjected to undue mental or physical suffering.

As mentioned above, Saudi patients are more likely to seek companionship than treatment. Consequently, most patients are interested in discussing end-of-life care with their physicians, and most feel that physicians should introduce the topic. Physicians must take responsibility for a timely dialog, as many patients will wait for their doctor to raise this issue. Thus, acquiring communication skills during medical education and participating in continuing education courses can lead to a competitive advantage. Medical educators should use the patient's understanding of their care, and focus on areas of study that will help practitioners meet patient expectations when treating common flu or when caring for terminally ill patients at the end-of-life stage.

1.2 Informed consent

Patient rights are one of the most important ethical issues relating to patients, their families, and society, including such important ethical issues as: autonomy, informed consent, privacy, confidentiality, risk information, refusal of treatment, personal safety and protection, and a process for resolving patient complaints [1, 2, 21]. Informed consent is the means by which a healthcare provider informs a patient about risks, benefits, consequences, and alternatives of a given procedure or intervention. According to the Saudi Ministry of Health (1988), before delivering medical treatment or carrying out an operative procedure, the legally competent patient's consent shall be obtained, whether they be male or female. This ethical and legal obligation for medical practitioners in Saudi Arabia stems from the patient's right to direct the treatment process. In addition, the doctor shall adequately explain to the patient or his guardian the nature of the medical treatment or operative procedure he intends to apply [2, 9, 22]. The informed consent procedure involves assessing the patient's understanding of the treatment, providing objective advice, and documenting the process. When providing informed consent, doctors are expected to fully disclose all medical facts related to the disease and intervention so that the patient makes a decision based on a full understanding of all the facts. The disclosure must include the following:

- Explanation of the diagnosis as much as possible to a lay patient
- Explanation of the intended procedure in non-technical terms
- Disclosure of all known side effects and benefits of the procedure

- Enable the patient to make an informed decision
- Disclose alternative procedures and treatments, their benefits and side effects
- Disclose the financial costs of the procedure, but preferably at a later stage, as this may adversely influence the patient's decision [2, 9, 22].

Since the family plays an important role in decision-making in Saudi Arabia, patients cannot be isolated from their families, and often want to consult with family members about the religious and social significance of a given treatment. In addition, the patient often expects a trusted person to make a decision on his/her behalf [2, 9]. It could be argued that this approach to informed consent does not preserve the principle of autonomy as intended, since it often extends to the patient's family rather than an individual's opinion and point of view. However, the family is the central pillar of Saudi society, the basic cell of social organization in traditional and modern Saudi Arabia. Saudis are expected to be loyal and give and receive support for and from their family, especially in protecting their family members [2, 4]. Therefore, in this context, informed consent aims to inform the patient and his family about the expected consequences of the course of a treatment. Consequently, Saudi doctors should recognize the importance of informed consent in their practice, and its relation to the patient's family. While Saudi doctors have a reasonable understanding of this, they need more training, as evidenced by the available data, both from the point of view of doctors and patients [2, 4, 9].

The overall data synthesis shows that Saudi physicians support informed consent, have a positive attitude toward obtaining consent, and know that patients should always be informed about treatment procedures. Moreover, physicians recognize that each new procedure should be consented to and seen as an ongoing process rather than a one-time decision [23, 24]. At the same time, a study among medical trainees from the Eastern Province has found that participants agreed that the surgeon could exceed consent in the case of an emergency and/or the absence of a guardian, and only a few agreed that the patient should be allowed to review their medical records or make copies [25].

Despite this knowledge and the recognition of the importance of informed consent, the quality of informed consent is low regarding experiences with informed consent processes and transparency [23–25]. Thus, some healthcare providers report that, although they have a reasonable knowledge of informed consent for surgery, most do not provide patients with the full information about a procedure before obtaining consent. For instance, a study by Alsaihati et al. among n = 140 surgeons in Saudi Arabia found that, while there is sufficient knowledge about informed consent for surgery and how to obtain it, most surgeons do not fully inform patients about the procedure before obtaining consent [26]. Some see consent as merely a preoperative routine or simply a matter of signing a document. The majority are against the use of consent for all surgical procedures [25, 26].

Physicians believe that consent should be clear and contain the necessary information for patients. One of the main considerations put forward by the doctors is that some consider the process of obtaining consent strange for Saudi psychology and are against the use of consent during the entire surgical procedure. Senior physicians are the primary physicians receiving informed consent from patients, while interns are the least comfortable with obtaining consent [5, 23–26].

Regarding pediatric treatment, physicians consider parental consent mandatory and necessary from the moment the child is admitted to the hospital and throughout treatment. Moreover, the majority prefer both parents to consent, and the parental consent forms are detailed enough to obtain maximum information. In contrast, it is considered that the child's assent form should be kept short to avoid increasing the burden on the child since the decision belongs with the parents [27, 28]. According to Saudi Guidelines for Informed Consent and Saudi Commission for Health Specialties, the age of seven is considered the age when a child can make some decisions. It is prudent to listen to them and consider their views, fully aware that the parents will give consent; children can only assent. However, children below the age of seven have no say in treatment decisions; parents make decisions. Children who have reached puberty are effectively adults, and unless there is evidence of their incompetence, they should be allowed to make decisions about their treatment. Parents may assent to the decision of a fully capable post-pubertal child under the age of majority, currently 18 years old, in Saudi Arabia [9, 27, 28].

Patient safety is a major concern in healthcare, and informed consent is critical. Health professionals are expected to make it clear that the patient is involved in the decision-making process, and not allow the patient to feel compelled to agree with their treatment decision. However, despite having knowledge and understanding of the informed consent procedures, healthcare providers in Saudi Arabia often view the procedure as a routine that can be avoided, as shown by the data provided. Therefore, it is equally important to explore the opinion of Saudi patients about informed consent: how they are informed about the proposed intervention, their role in decision-making on issues, such as a discussion of alternatives to the proposed intervention, and the risks of the proposed intervention.

The general attitude toward informed consent is positive, and this process is important for patients. However, some patients have expressed dissatisfaction with the poor quality of informed consent regarding their experience with information delivery procedures and transparent risk communication. Further synthesis of the data shows a low awareness of the patients' rights. The consent form followed by the registration of a complaint about the service provided is the best-known guarantee of patient rights. However, patients feel that their decision is irrelevant and trust the physician to make decisions on their behalf, and are not interested in obtaining a copy of the informed consent [29, 30].

On the other hand, despite the lack of knowledge about the risks of intervention and alternative treatment, there is a desire for more self-decision-making and better disclosure. Furthermore, the general patterns show that the quality of informed consent is generally low in content and administration, whereas the doctor's explanation predicts a higher quality of informed consent. Finally, issues relating to the lack of or incomplete informed consent attracted attention only when the procedure resulted in adverse events or patient dissatisfaction [27–30].

One of the goals of end-of-life care is to prevent or alleviate suffering as much as possible, while respecting the patient's wishes [1–4]. As important as it is for disease management, informed consent in end-of-life care is especially important. Respect for wishes and decisions at the end of life gives the patient permanent freedom to choose how he/she wants to live. Informed consent demonstrates the commitment of clinicians and researchers to respecting the dignity and autonomy of patients and participants. Therefore, it is important to allow patients and their families to participate in decision-making to protect the rights and dignity of all parties involved in the informed consent process. Thus, the Saudi Council for Health Specialties has developed guidelines on informed consent as part of the ethics of the medical profession to raise awareness by involving patients and their families in health care in all medical facilities in the KSA regions [2, 9]. To ensure that an informed consent is valid, consent must be given by a professional who understands the nature and implications of the procedures. Medical procedures or scientific research require the legal proof of patient consent in Saudi Arabia. While consent can be easily explained to patients and their families, doctors' and patients' awareness and adherence to these guidelines in Saudi Arabia remain unclear and controversial.

1.3 Do-not-resuscitate

Physicians play a vital role by fulfilling patients' rights and providing effective and satisfactory treatment that increases their life expectancy [1, 2, 31]. At the same time, it is equally important to have patient-centered care at the end of life for patients suffering from incurable diseases, and to support patient participation at all stages, including discussing such sensitive topics as do-not-resuscitate (DNR) order, an important decision for critically ill patients [2, 4].

Illness in Islam is considered to be a trial the patient must go through, and the doctor does not have the right to take the patient's life [32]. However, when death becomes imminent, as determined by physicians assigned to terminally ill patients, the Islamic concept regarding the decision of the DNR must be implemented, as was recorded in Fatwa No. 12086, issued on March 28, 1409 (1989), stating: "If three knowledgeable and trustworthy physicians agreed that the patient condition is hopeless; the life-supporting machines can be withheld or withdrawn. The family members' opinion is not included in decision-making as they are unqualified to make such decisions."

According to the fatwa, there are six situations in which DNR is granted: (i) if the patient arrives at the hospital dead; (ii) if a team of doctors determines that the patient's condition is incurable and their death is imminent; (iii) if the patient's condition does not render him or her a suitable candidate for resuscitation; (iv) if the patient suffers from a severe heart or lung condition, or repeated cardiac arrest; (v) if the patient is in a vegetative state; (vi) if resuscitation is considered futile. The fatwa also clarifies that the patient's family should be informed of the decision, but they cannot intervene as they are not considered qualified, which is why the decisions and integrity of these specialists and competent doctors are to be respected. Nevertheless, as with informed consent, medical practice in Saudi Arabia involves families and caregivers when discussing the DNR. If the family still objects the DNR policy after clarifying the fatwa, they should be offered the option of transferring the patient to another hospital that is ready to accept the patient. Despite the existing rules and legislation, a synthesis of the literature shows that the debate about the practice of the DNR continues to vary greatly [32].

Evidence of knowledge of the DNR order and fatwa in studies among healthcare professionals indicates that while most physicians participate in DNR discussions with patients and family members or decision-makers, they cannot confirm whether there is a clear local or national DNR policy [33–35]. However, most Muslim doctors believe that the DNR is not contrary to Islamic rules. The study by Almoallem et al. shows that non-Saudi physicians conducting life-sustaining treatment or DNR decisions are more likely to consult ethics committees than Saudi physicians [36]. On the other hand, Saudi doctors who were educated and graduated abroad are confident in their knowledge of ethics in medical practice, but are less confident in making life-sustaining treatment decisions or DNR orders. They also suggest that additional educational programs would increase their competence in dealing with issues related to DNR discussions. One approach that has been proposed to improve knowledge is the establishment of a structured curriculum to teach skills relating to end-of-life issues, such as DNR orders in the Saudi medical system [5].

Essentially, physicians and nurses feel that the patient should be involved in the decision-making process and that each patient should receive advance directives [33–36]. A living will (advance directive) is a document in which a healthy person explains in writing what treatment one would accept or refuse at a critical moment when one may not be able to express one's wishes, i.e., in case of emergencies, incurable diseases and situations where they may not be able to make decisions. This document helps the attending physician to withhold or withdraw certain medical procedures and allows the patient to die naturally. In addition, Muslim patients, incompetent to make health care decisions, can approach an authorized representative to express their wishes and make treatment decisions on behalf of their best interests [2, 9, 22].

The most common limitation to meaningful DNR discussions is a lack of understanding of the patient's family, education level, and cultural background. The study by Abu Yahya et al. shows that most nurses want to be aware of a legal basis for DNR policy, and want to know more about patients' rights regarding end-of-life and the use of the DNR order [37]. The pattern reported by the nurses is similar to that seen in n = 203 pediatricians in the study by Aljethaily et al. Thus, most of the study sample could not correctly determine the DNR, the policies and procedures are unclear to them. While half of the participants believed that the DNR is a doctor's decision, only a few reported that they were comfortable discussing the DNR with parents [35]. Most believe that patients are entitled to intensive care, despite their incurable disease.

In contrast to this general knowledge of doctors, residents, and nurses about the DNR and its procedures, studies among medical students have found that most of them are familiar with the DNR order, and believe that there is a fatwa governing the DNR on an Islamic level [38]. Moreover, compared with information and knowledge about informed consent, students report that lectures at medical schools about the DNR are the main source of information. Similar to practicing doctors, Saudi medical students strongly agree that patients should be involved in DNR decision-making and suggest that misunderstanding patients and their families is one of the most important barriers to effective DNR discussions [36–38].

Data on the knowledge of the DNR order among the general public and patients show that while most populations in various studies can determine the DNR order to some extent, they require more in-depth knowledge. This is especially noticeable when participants' opinions regarding the compatibility of the DNR order, in terms of religion and ethics, are divided along ethical, religious, and medical grounds [5, 39, 40]. In fact, medical education, higher education, and knowledge of the DNR are associated with the acceptance of DNR. The most common reasons for the DNR's refusal are hope, cultural factors, and religious concerns, and the DNR's orders are thought to be a response to a reduction in the number of physicians providing clinical care. As with informed consent, the study by Al Ahmadi et al. shows that most participants choose the physicians responsible for the DNR decision [40]. The data synthesis can be expressed as follows: although patients can make informed judgments about end-of-life decisions, they also lack knowledge about health status, advance planning and life support, but are willing to participate in end-of-life care planning discussions with doctors.

As an extremely sensitive and controversial area that every doctor must deal with, the DNR remains an ethically elusive topic. In Saudi Arabia, the DNR is a legally binding order applicable only in the event of cardiopulmonary arrest, and does not cover the suspension or discontinuation of other supportive care. While this policy and fatwa are available to healthcare providers and the general Saudi public, the extensive evidence presented shows a significant degree of heterogeneity in knowledge and in the application of the law.

2. Summary

End-of-life care is the support and care provided in the period leading up to death. Some people may want to stay home when they die, while others prefer to be treated in a hospital or facility until the end. The truth is that everyone deserves to be allowed to maintain a sense of normality, despite death being the inevitable result. Everyone, regardless of age, culture, background, beliefs, or health condition, has the right to feel comfortable and pleased as their last day approaches.

The main goal of the healthcare system and providers is to cure the disease and alleviate symptoms and, in end-of-life care, the main goal is to improve the quality of life of patients facing complex problems associated with the disease and to provide psychological assistance to their families. While physicians have witness death many times, patients and their families need time to comprehend and understand the entire process and procedures of this unique and often devastating experience. Patients are primarily interested in discussing end-of-life care with their physicians. Therefore, clinicians should take responsibility for initiating a timely dialog to reduce patients' fear of pain, humiliation, abandonment, and fear of the unknown. Open and direct conversations with patients and their families can alleviate many of these fears and lessen the sense of isolation experienced by the dying person. Thus, providing quality end-of-life care requires understanding and empathetic communication through discussions in which most decisions are made comfortably and without disagreement.

Some of the core principles of end-of-life care in Saudi Arabia are respect for dignity of both the patient and caregiver; sensitivity to the wishes of the patient and family; management of pain or other symptoms; assessment and management of the psychological and social needs of the patient and family. However, despite this well-established evidence and these policies governing Saudi medical ethics, exploring the primary areas that define the basic needs for end-of-life care suggests that this domain is still in its infancy. What is even more alarming and thought-provoking is the lack of knowledge of physicians who are expected to educate patients and their families who are not always aware of all stages of treatment.

Healthcare professionals often neglect good clinical practice by failing to comply with informed consent. This insensibility leads to the reluctance of patients being aware of the procedures, although they have expressed an interest in decision-making. On the other hand, when treatment concerns children, doctors consider it their duty and obligation to present all stages to parents. This suggests that despite not being aware of certain fatwas or rules, Saudi physicians are aware of the importance of adherence to bioethics, which can be seen as another issue of selective application of medical ethics (e.g., children vs. adults).

In order to further develop end-of-life care services in this country and focus efforts on this vital sector, future research and education should aim to involve healthcare professionals, patients and their families in the decision-making process by providing knowledge on how to communicate openly and honestly, with empathy, dignity, and kindness. Moreover, multilateral cooperation is of great importance for enriching knowledge and improving the attitude of healthcare providers toward all areas of bioethics and their application in practice. This approach will help maintain transparency in care, better serve patients, and provide accountability for high-quality care and outcomes.

Author details

Alexander Woodman
University of Salford, Manchester, England

*Address all correspondence to: a.woodman1@edu.salford.ac.uk

References

[1] Düwell M. Bioethics: Methods, Theories, Domains. London: Routledge; 2012

[2] Al-Bar MA, Chamsi-Pasha H. Contemporary Bioethics: Islamic Perspective. London: Springer Nature; 2015

[3] Atighetchi D. Islamic Bioethics: Problems and Perspectives. Dordrecht: Springer; 2007

[4] Bukhari AA. Universal Principles of Bioethics and Patient Rights in Saudi Arabia. Pittsburgh, PA, the USA: Duquesne University; 2017

[5] Woodman A, Waheed KB, Rasheed M, Ahmad S. Current state of ethical challenges reported in Saudi Arabia: A systematic review & bibliometric analysis from 2010 to 2021. BMC Medical Ethics. 2022;**23**(1):1-36

[6] Huffman JL, Harmer B. End of Life Care. Treasure Island (FL): StatPearls Publishing

[7] Goold SD, Lipkin M Jr. The doctor–patient relationship: Challenges, opportunities, and strategies. Journal of General Internal Medicine. 1999 Jan;**14**(Suppl. 1):S26

[8] Morgan M. The Doctor-Patient Relationship: Sociology as Applied to Medicine. Edinburgh: Saunders Elsevier; 2008

[9] Hussein G, Alkabba A, Kasule O. Professionalism and Ethics Handbook for Residents (PEHR): A Practical Guide. Riyadh: Saudi Commission for Health Specialties; 2015

[10] Ministry of Health. Saudi Arabia. Available from: http://www.moh.gov.sa/ar/modules/news/print.php?storyid=281

[11] El-Sobkey SB, Almoajel AM, Al-Muammar MN. Knowledge and attitude of Saudi health professions' students regarding patient's bill of rights. International Journal of Health Policy and Management. 2014;**3**(3):117

[12] Alghanim SA. Assessing knowledge of the patient bill of rights in Central Saudi Arabia: A survey of primary health care providers and recipients. Annals of Saudi Medicine. 2012;**32**(2):151-155

[13] Saleh HA, Khereldeen MM. Physicians' perception towards patients' rights in two governmental hospitals in Mecca, KSA. International Journal of Pure and Applied Sciences and Technology. 2013;**17**(1):37

[14] Al Ali AA, Elzubair AG. Establishing rapport: Physicians' practice and attendees' satisfaction at a primary health care center, Dammam, Saudi Arabia, 2013. Journal of Family and Community Medicine. 2016;**23**(1):12

[15] Elagi AA, Jaber BA, Wassly AH, Ahmed RM, Bosily FA. Public's perception and satisfaction on the role and services provided by family physicians in Saudi Arabia: A cross-sectional study. Journal of Family Medicine and Primary Care. 2019;**8**(10):3282

[16] Aljaffary A, AlThumairi A, Almarhoon L, Alsaawi G. Measuring patient trust in public versus private physicians in the Kingdom of Saudi Arabia (KSA). Journal of Multidisciplinary Healthcare. 2021;**14**:151

[17] Fayez R, Nawwab A, Al-Jahdali H, Baharoon S, Binsalih S, Al SA. Negative ethical behaviors in Saudi hospitals: How prevalent are they perceived to be?—Statement agreement study. Avicenna Journal of Medicine. 2013;**3**(03):57-62

[18] Al-Zahrani BS, Al-Misfer MF, Al-Hazmi AM. Knowledge, attitude, practice and barriers of effective communication skills during medical consultation among general practitioners national guard primary health care center, Riyadh, Saudi Arabia. Middle East Journal of Family Medicine. 2015;**7**(10):4-17

[19] Banaser M, Stoddart K, Cunningham N. A qualitative study of patient satisfaction in oncology wards setting in Saudi Arabia. Research and Reviews: Journal of Nursing and Health Sciences. 2017;**3**(3):85-97

[20] Al-Yousefi NA. Observations of Muslim physicians regarding the influence of religion on health and their clinical approach. Journal of Religion and Health. 2012;**51**(2):269-280

[21] Leino-Kilpi H. Patient's Autonomy, Privacy and Informed Consent. The Netherlands: IOS Press; 2000

[22] Al-Amoudi SM, Al-Harbi AA, Al-Sayegh NY, Eldeek BS, Kafy SM, Al-Ahwal MS, et al. Health rights knowledge among medical school students at King Abdulaziz university, Jeddah, Saudi Arabia. PLoS One. 2017;**12**(5):e0176714

[23] Abolfotouh MA, Adlan AA. Quality of informed consent for invasive procedures in Central Saudi Arabia. International Journal of General Medicine. 2012;**5**:269

[24] Basharaheel H, Aidarous G, Halawani L, Bajeafer M, Al-Amoudi T, Al-Qurashi W, et al. Attitude and practice of surgical informed consent among the surgical team in a teaching center: A cross-sectional study. International Journal of Medical Research & Health Sciences. 2019;**8**(12):104-109

[25] Darwish MA, Sabra AA. Medical ethics: Knowledge about confidentiality among medical university students, Eastern province Saudi Arabia. Journal of American Science. 2012;**8**(6):299-304

[26] Alsaihati AM, Alotaibi AB, Alhawaj AM, Alabdulsalam AM, Alajmi NA, Boukhet MT, et al. Knowledge, opinions and attitude of surgeons in Saudi Arabia toward informed surgical consent. The Egyptian Journal of Hospital Medicine. 2017;**69**(4):2232-2237

[27] Al Qarny MA, Alsofiani AM, Garny AG. Medical Ethics Knowledge and Practice among Healthcare Workers at Prince Mansour Military Hospital. Taif, Saudi Arabia: PMMH; 2012

[28] Alahmad G, Al-Kamli H, Alzahrani H. Ethical challenges of pediatric cancer care: Interviews with nurses in Saudi Arabia. Cancer Control. 2020;**27**(1):1073274820917210

[29] Almohaimede K, Almogheer R, Alsubaie A, A-Turki T, Almuhanna A, Aljarallah JS. Informed consent for invasive procedures: A perspective from Saudi Arabia

[30] Hammami MM, Al-Gaai EA, Al-Jawarneh Y, Amer H, Hammami MB, Eissa A, et al. Patients' perceived purpose of clinical informed consent: Mill's individual autonomy model is preferred. BMC Medical Ethics. 2014;**15**(1):1-2

[31] Smith M, Saunders R, Stuckhardt L, McGinnis JM. Engaging patients, families, and communities. In: Best Care at Lower Cost: The Path to Continuously Learning Health Care in America. Washington (DC), the USA: National Academies Press (US); 2013

[32] Pasha HC, Albar MA. Do not resuscitate, brain death, and organ transplantation: Islamic perspective. Avicenna Journal of Medicine. 2017;**7**(02):35-45

[33] Amoudi AS, Albar MH, Bokhari AM, Yahya SH, Merdad AA. Perspectives of interns and residents toward do-not-resuscitate policies in Saudi Arabia. Advances in Medical Education and Practice. 2016;**7**:165

[34] Aljohaney A, Bawazir Y. Internal medicine residents' perspectives and practice about do not resuscitate orders: Survey analysis in the western region of Saudi Arabia. Advances in Medical Education and Practice. 2015;**6**:393

[35] Aljethaily A, Al-Mutairi T, Al-Harbi K, Al-Khonezan S, Aljethaily A, Al-HomaidhiHS.Pediatricians' perceptions toward do not resuscitate: A survey in Saudi Arabia and literature review. Advances in Medical Education and Practice. 2020;**11**:1

[36] Almoallem AM, Almudayfir MA, Al-Jahdail YH, Ahmed AE, Al-Shaikh A, Baharoon S, et al. Top ethical issues concerning healthcare providers working in Saudi Arabia. Journal of Epidemiology and Global Health. 2020;**10**(2):143

[37] AbuYahya O, Abuhammad S, Hamoudi B, Reuben R, Yaqub M. The do not resuscitate order (DNR) from the perspective of oncology nurses: A study in Saudi Arabia. International Journal of Clinical Practice. 2021;**75**(8):e14331

[38] Alsaati BA, Aljishi MN, Alshamakh SS, Banjar NS, Basharaheel HA, Alamri RS. The concept of do not resuscitate for students in King Abdulaziz University Hospital. Indian Journal of Palliative Care. 2019;**25**(4):544

[39] Al Sheef MA, Al Sharqi MS, Al Sharief LH, Takrouni TY, Mian AM. Awareness of do-not-resuscitate orders in the outpatient setting in Saudi Arabia: Perception and implications. Saudi Medical Journal. 2017;**38**(3):297

[40] Al Ahmadi JR, Aljehani SN, Bahakeem LM, Hijan BA, Mayet SA, Badahdah YA. Knowledge and attitude toward do-not-resuscitate among patients and their relatives visiting outpatient clinics at King Abdulaziz University Hospital, Jeddah, Saudi Arabia. Saudi Medical Journal. 2020;**41**(1):53

Chapter 8

Practice of Palliative Care at Home in Central Africa: Reflection and Lessons

Sah Tatsing Félix Désiré

Abstract

The importance of palliative care at home has been highlighted in the literature; however, the fact remains that its recent introduction in Central Africa faces a number of major challenges. These challenges form the backdrop of the reflection, which aims to lead to lessons to be learned of interest to the nine countries that make up the Central African zone (Angola, Cameroon, Congo, Gabon, Equatorial Guinea, Central African Republic, Democratic Republic of Congo, Sao Tome, and Principé, Chad) with which we associate Burundi and Rwanda because they share the same general health issues with regard to the palliative care of patients at home. The aim is to improve the quality of life of those who suffer and die at home due to lack of care.

Keywords: home-based palliative care, palliative care, life-limiting chronic diseases, quality of life, home care

1. Introduction

Palliative home care is a comprehensive package of care provided to patients and their families at home [1]. They include pain control and symptom management, psychosocial and spiritual care, and support with activities of daily living [2]. This healthcare model is most recently adopted in palliative care [3], and its development and practice over time varies from country to country [4]. In Central Africa, it is not always easy for a patient or his family to accept the transition from hospital to home [5], especially in a certain culture in which people are ashamed to die at home [6]. Perhaps this is why many poorly prepared and anxious patients die soon after returning home when unaccompanied.

To fill this gap, changes have taken place in health systems, in which there is an increasing emphasis on home care services to help families who want their loved ones to die at home [7]. This is a particular type of care that certainly fits into the paradigm of complexity [8] but which has proven itself in the countries that practice it. Today, with the resurgence of life-limiting chronic diseases such as HIV/AIDS, cancers, diabetes, and tuberculosis, to name but a few, the Central African countries that bear the heaviest burden are, therefore, the largest providers of palliative care at home. These countries, therefore, have an interest in breaking with the exclusivity of the very hospital-centered therapeutic model that they practice to the detriment of the home care model.

This new form of production of care and interdisciplinary practices is defined as a complete set of care provided at home to a patient suffering from a life-limiting illness and to his family [9]. In this case, the patient's and his family's place of residence becomes a specific care environment [9]. Hence, the purpose of this chapter is to reflect on this model of care in order to draw lessons for the countries of Central Africa.

2. Problematic situation of palliative home care in Central Africa

In Central Africa, the residential care of patients suffering from chronic diseases, 80 to 90% of whom arrive in hospitals at the advanced stage of the disease [10], is nowadays a major concern in palliative care. The question arises as to how to guarantee continuity of quality care to those who, after having stayed for days or even months in health facilities without recovery, are forced to be turned back to their homes because the structure cannot keep them longer. This decision-making happens in most cases when patients and their families are deprived of financial resources. In a context where almost all public hospitals have limited budgets for the management of these progressive diseases such as advanced-stage cancers or HIV/AIDS. What causes so much of a problem is sending these patients back to their living environments without any other means of follow-up [11] while simply waiting to watch them die, for lack of palliative care at home, training of caregivers in these kinds of interventions and of a relay organization for home care. In the absence of a proposal of choice, some patients refuse to leave the hospital, claiming that they are not yet cured. From this angle, care providers, and more generally physicians and nurses, are not always convinced that the care they provide to these types of patients is attentive, efficient, useful, and of high quality. A form of exclusion of those for whom the treatment of advanced chronic diseases is no longer the solution to cope with the burden of pathology [12].

Without any other alternative, these patients suffer enormous suffering that we could have limited, and we improved their quality of life by giving them early access to palliative care at home and by strengthening the skills of care workers. It is, therefore, a real public health problem. This problem affects many African countries which are permanently exposed to cancers, HIV/AIDS, pulmonary tuberculosis, and diseases of senescence. These diseases are the most dangerous and costly types, both in human and economic terms, for the health of Africans. According to the African Association for Palliative Care (2013), their rate will increase by 400% over the next 50 years in this part of the world. Moreover, the results of the study conducted by Sah Tatsing et al. [13] show that in these countries, 54.12% of patients suffering from life-limiting chronic diseases such as cancer wanted to receive their care at home so as not to be separated from family and friends. These results are similar to those of a study conducted in England, where 55% of people with cancer would prefer to die at home [14]. Unfortunately, during the same study, it emerged that very few health facilities in Central Africa provide home care. For those who do, this care is provided intuitively, without a repository, and is based much more on basic palliative care. Hospital structures that make efforts to provide palliative care favor the palliative model of hospital care, which focuses on the management of physical symptoms, psychosocial support, and ambulatory care for patients able to go to a health facility. They do not provide home care because of a lack of qualified staff and lack of financial means to meet travel costs. These shortcomings are in line with the observations noted by Clark et al. [15], who noted that the countries of Central Africa had a "localized provision" of palliative care, which boils down to a handful of services isolated from each other, with limited coverage.

Another observation made in these Central African countries concerns the insufficiency of teaching units on palliative care in the training programs of health personnel. This has resulted in a lack of knowledge and skills in palliative care at home.

Following this nonexhaustive list of shortcomings, it appears that palliative care at home in Central Africa is still not very present. Its expansion is a real requirement to the point where one could deduce that the patients who at home manage to survive for a few days are miracles of a hyper-hospital-centered system. Home palliative care in this part of Africa will fill the gap of continuous and integral care in order to meet the needs of the population and improve the efficiency of health systems. Indeed, the unavailability or inaccessibility of palliative care at home has many health and economic consequences.

In terms of health, the consequences are expressed in terms of inaccessibility and insufficient support for the care that patients may need, delay in the development of the practice of care actors in this area due to the fact that those – they are poorly prepared to deliver palliative care in general and palliative care at home in particular. Among other health consequences, there is the distress of patients and their relatives when people die in hospital when they would have preferred to die at home or when they have no medical reason to be hospitalized. In the absence of an organization that offers palliative care services at home, the data relating to this care, whether in an individual or collective home, remains poorly documented or disparate and constitutes an obstacle to their analysis in perspective [8].

On the economic level, there is an increase in the costs of care related to the prolonged care of patients in hospitals. This increase has an impact on the quality of care in health systems dominated by the absence of universal health coverage and the existence of selective health insurance.

In view of all the above, it appears that the challenge of palliative care with its model of home care is a worrying problem that interests decision-makers, NGOs, health professionals, and nonhealth professionals. These actors need more than ever contextual, targeted, and effective strategies to prevent and alleviate the suffering of patients and families who lack care in this context.

3. Reasons for choosing this therapeutic model

Many countries around the world practice palliative care at home [4]. In Central Africa, the method of admitting patients to these services differs from one country to another [4]. This can be continuity care after discharge from the hospital of a patient with a life-limiting illness [16] or simply the care provided to these types of patients, regardless of the stage of their illness [17], who express a desire to spend their last days at home [18] if circumstances permit. Other determinants of palliative care at home can be the absence of care [16], the unavailability or inaccessibility of hospitalization services [6], the high cost of medical care, technological innovation, such as home telemonitoring and teleconsultation [19], and the environment [20].

For Cordeiro et al. [16], there are three determinants of palliative home care: culture, economy, and health system. Costa et al. [20] add disease, the individual, and the environment. In the patient's home, care is centered on the patient, his expectations, his problems, and those of those around him [4] with the aim of controlling pain, as well as physical symptoms, providing psychosocial support and accompaniment, to improve their quality of life [21]. For Sun et al. [22], palliative home care brings together clinical services, nursing interventions, counseling, and social support.

4. Legal and juridical framework

In almost all Central African countries, there are no specific texts regulating the practice of palliative care at home. However, these practices are part of the intervention programs and agreements ratified by these countries. As such, the practice of palliative home care relies heavily on four guidelines.

The first relates to the integration of cancer care into primary care [23]. Primary health care as an approach centered on the needs of individuals emphasizes their well-being. This care ensures that low-income people receive palliative care as close as possible to their daily environment and therefore to their home. The "essential components of primary health care are therefore social justice, equity, universal access to care, community participation and multi and intersectoral approaches to health" [24].

The second guideline concerns the responsibility of healthcare actors to work toward the achievement of the Sustainable Development Goals adopted by the United Nations in 2015 to take over from the Millennium Development Goals (2000–2015), which places health at the heart of the third objective: "enable everyone to live in good health and promote well-being at all ages". From this perspective, palliative home care clearly has an essential role to play in achieving this objective.

Finally, the provisions of the National Strategic Plans for the Prevention and Control of Chronic Diseases in most Central African countries recognize the existence of palliative care with importance given to its home care model.

To this text should be added that of the WHO (2002) of which these countries are members, which invites them to:

> *"Develop, strengthen and implement, as appropriate, palliative care policies to support the overall strengthening of health systems with a view to integrating palliative care services into the continuum of care at all levels that are evidence-based, cost-effective and equitable, with an emphasis on primary, community and home-based care and universal coverage schemes".*

5. Procedure for palliative care at home: the specific case of Cameroon

In Cameroon, which is one of the countries of Central Africa, the team surrounding the patient is the same as in the hospital. In the first line, there is the family, the nurses, and the doctors and, in the second line, there can be the other members of the plural team of palliative care. When the hospital decides to send a patient home, the most likely scenario is that the nurse coordinating home care first goes to the patient's home to assess, with the help of the family, the adaptability of care at home and prepare for its installation. Once at home, the nurse coordinator calls on the general practitioner with whom she carries out the initial assessment of the patient before establishing a follow-up plan resulting from the scientific approach to care. This approach can be summed up in three essential phases: the identification of symptoms and patient needs, the implementation of multidisciplinary interventions, and their evaluation.

5.1 Identification of symptoms and patient needs

This phase is carried out by the nurse. After contact with the patient, she uses a hetero-questionnaire to evaluate the patient's condition to identify their socio-demographic and clinical aspects. The answers to these aspects can come directly from patients or their relatives and their medical records. This initial assessment follows the assessment of the symptoms (physical, psycho-sociological, and spiritual), the functional state, and the quality of life, before, during, and after the care interventions thanks to and with the same scales provided for this purpose. At the end of the initial assessment, the nurse coordinator establishes the baseline level of symptoms and needs that will be compared with those obtained during and after the interventions implemented.

5.2 Implementation of multi-professional interventions

Once the needs and symptoms of patients have been identified and measured, they are encouraged to follow the interventions set up by the multidisciplinary team. The interventions deployed come from the care protocol established beforehand. For issues requiring follow-up or special attention or even the opinion of the specialist, the coordinating nurse, with the permission of the patient and his family, contacts the specialist or the consensus team. For each patient, the caregiver draws up a multifaceted intervention plan including the care diagnosis(es), the care objective(s), and the interventions to be implemented.

5.3 Assessment

As in the phase of identification of symptoms and needs, the coordinating nurse also uses both the hetero-questionnaires and the self-questionnaires to regularly reassess the symptoms, the functional state, the interventions implemented, and the quality of life of the patients. Since the nursing staff is not always on-site, a 24-hour telephone service is available to patients and families in case of concerns. In the event of the patient's death at home, the nurse calls on the general practitioner to confirm the death. Afterward, the nurse and the family prepare the body for the destination of their choice. The nurse also helps them with the procedures for obtaining administrative documents such as the type of death certificate.

6. Benefits of palliative home care

Research findings show that palliative home care improves patient survival time and mood. They reduce hospital visits and patient travel time [1]. For these authors, this care reduces the duration of hospitalizations and the cost of medical care for patients with malignant neoplasms. For Morrison and Meier [25], palliative home care improves the efficiency and effectiveness of home care services. To this end, it has been shown that clinical procedures traditionally defined in hospitals can be carried out safely in the patient's home [26]. From this perspective, palliative home care is now considered one of the sectors toward which palliative interventions should be directed. But unfortunately, they present major challenges for practitioners.

7. Challenges to the development of palliative home care

In Central Africa, the home is full of symbols and memories. It is a place of tranquility, accommodated according to the patient's own wishes. The home is the best place that offers the patient a certain security when he is surrounded by the people dear to him, especially when crossing a new life induced by the fatal disease. It is a place where the patient finds his bearings, his life story which he needs to maintain the hope of living.

The carer must be able to keep in mind what makes home specific in African countries: "It is a place of life for the person and for their loved ones, which is part of a story, where questions of identity, intimacy and security are embodied in various forms" [27]. Care should be taken to ensure that the legitimate vision of broad access to palliative care at home is not accompanied by normative approaches or visions of this place, which refers first and foremost to the uniqueness of each life story [27]. From this point of view, far from being trivialized, palliative home care presents several challenges.

Indeed, the practice of palliative home care comes up against a number of obstacles. The first obstacle is his youthfulness [3]. It is perhaps for this reason that it is uncommon in Africa in general and relatively new in Central Africa [1]. In this part of the continent, palliative care at home is not recognized as a medical specialty, and it is not integrated into the diploma training of health personnel [1]. Waelli and Minvielle [28] add the lack of government support. In these countries, very little legislation governs the implementation of palliative care at home, as can be seen elsewhere. As a result, care pathways and appropriate symptom management interventions are underestimated or obsolete [1]. Linked to the person, one of the obstacles to the development of palliative care at home is the fear that the patient experiences, particularly with regard to the unfavorable opinion of his relatives and the ineffectiveness of the care he will receive at home compared to hospital care.

8. Conclusion

Home-based palliative care is defined as a comprehensive set of care provided at home to a patient suffering from a life-limiting illness and to their family [9]. The desire for this type of care originates from the observation that, in Central Africa, the suffering of patients is poorly taken into account in a good number of current programs for the treatment of chronic diseases, particularly those developed in countries with low income [1]. It is becoming urgent to carry out advocacy to make politicians and decision-makers listen to reason so that where palliative care at home does not exist, it can be instituted. Where it exists even in isolation, it can be strengthened.

Author details

Sah Tatsing Félix Désiré
Cameroon Ministry of Public Health – Yaounde, Cameroon

*Address all correspondence to: sahfelix@yahoo.fr

References

[1] Sah Tatsing FD, Bih SuH AM, Kimessouke OE. Plus-value des soins palliatifs à domicile pour les patients souffrant de cancers: une revue de littérature. Revue Internationale de Soins Palliatifs. 2021;**35**(4):189-195

[2] Bond C, Lavy V, Wooldridge R, Worldwide Palliative Care Alliance. Palliative Care Toolkit: Improving Care from the Roots Up in Resource-Limited Settings. London: Help the Hospices; 2008

[3] Wiencek C, Coyne P. Palliative care delivery models. Seminars in Oncology Nursing. 2014;**30**(4):227-233

[4] Boisserie-Lacroix L, Marquestaut O, de Stampa M. Patients en situation palliative en hospitalisation à domicile: trajectoires de soins et caractéristiques cliniques. Santé Publique. 2017;**29**(6):851

[5] Plummer S, Hearnshaw C. Reviewing a new model for delivering short-term specialist palliative care at home. International Journal of Palliative Nursing. 2006;**12**(4):183-188

[6] Campbell CS, Black MA. Dignity, death, and dilemmas: A study of Washington hospices and physician-assisted death. Journal of Pain and Symptom Management. 2014;**47**(1):137-153

[7] Cantwell P, Turco S, Brenneis C, Hanson J, Neumann CM, Bruera E. Predictors of home death in palliative care cancer patients. Journal of Palliative Care. 2000;**16**(1):23-28

[8] Daydé MC. Complexité, incertitude et interdisciplinarité : l'apport du travail en réseau. Médecine Palliat Soins Support – Accompagnement – Éthique. 2012;**11**(3):164-169

[9] Daydé MC. L'infirmière libérale et les soins palliatifs au domicile. Revue de l'Infirmière. 2017;**66**(235):36-38

[10] Kokka F, Bryant A, Brockbank E, Powell M, Oram D. Hysterectomy with radiotherapy or chemotherapy or both for women with locally advanced cervical cancer. Cochrane Database Systematic Review. 2015;**4**:CD010260

[11] Foucault C, Mongeau S. L'art de soigner en soins palliatifs: Perspectives infirmières. Presses de l'Université de Montréal; 2004. Available from: http://books.openedition.org/pum/10599

[12] Schüz J, Espina C, Wild CP. Primary prevention: A need for concerted action. Molecular Oncology. 2019;**13**(3):567-578

[13] Sah Tatsing FD, Bih SuH AM, Kimessouke OE. Vivre à domicile avec le cancer du col utérin et/ou du sein dans la région de l'Ouest-Cameroun: profil des patientes. Revue internationale de soins palliatifs. 2022;**36**(3):77-85

[14] Ward L, Fenton K, Maher L. The high impact actions for nursing and midwifery 6: Where to die when the time comes. Nursing Times. 2010;**106**(32):18-19

[15] Clark D. From margins to Centre: A review of the history of palliative care in cancer. Lancet Oncology. 2007;**8**(5):430-438

[16] Cordeiro FR, Kruse MHL, Carlin N. La sortie d'unités de soins palliatifs au Brésil et en France: expériences de patients atteints d'un cancer avancé et de leurs familles. Médecine Palliat. 2018;**17**(3):139-147

[17] Bookbinder M, Glajchen M, McHugh M, Higgins P, Budis J, Solomon N,

et al. Nurse practitioner-based models of specialist palliative care at home: Sustainability and evaluation of feasibility. Journal of Pain and Symptom Management. 2011;**41**(1):25-34

[18] Sneesby L. Home is where I want to die: Kelly's journey. Contemporary Nurse. 2014;**46**(2):251-253

[19] Ohannessian R, Guettier C, Lemaire A, Denis F, Ottavy F, Galateau Salle F, et al. L'utilisation de la télémédecine pour la prise en charge du cancer en France en 2016. European Research in Telemedicine / La Recherche Européenne en Télémédecine. 2017;**6**(1):44

[20] Costa V, Earle CC, Esplen MJ, Fowler R, Goldman R, Grossman D, et al. The determinants of home and nursing home death: a systematic review and meta-analysis. BMC Palliative Care. 2016;**15**(1). Available from: http://bmcpalliatcare.biomedcentral.com/articles/10.1186-1177

[21] Health Quality Ontario. Team-based models for end-of-life care: An evidence-based analysis. Ontology Health Technology Assessment Series. 2014;**14**(20):1-49

[22] Sun Z, Laporte A, Guerriere DN, Coyte PC. Utilisation of home-based physician, nurse and personal support worker services within a palliative care programme in Ontario, Canada: Trends over 2005-2015. Health & Social Care in the Community. 2017;**25**(3):1127-1138

[23] Sisler J, Chaput G, Sussman J, Ozokwelu E. Suivi après le traitement du cancer du sein. Canadian Family Physician. 2016;**62**(10):e578-e585

[24] Crismer A, Belche JL, Van der Vennet JL. Les soins de santé primaires, plus que des soins de première ligne. Santé Publique. 2016;**28**(3):375

[25] Morrison RS, Meier DE. The National Palliative Care Research Center and the Center to Advance Palliative Care: A partnership to improve care for persons with serious illness and their families. Journal of Pediatric Hematology/Oncology. 2011;**33**(Suppl. 2):S126-S131

[26] Peltzer K, Moetlo G, Pengpid S. An evaluation of the implementation of integrated community home-based care services in Vhembe District, South Africa. Indian Journal of Palliative Care. 2011;**17**(2):137

[27] Hirsch G. Soins palliatifs et accompagnement à domicile : quelles places respectives et quels liens entre les acteurs? Jusqu'à Mort Accompagner Vie. 2016;**127**(4):19

[28] Waelli M, Minvielle E. Facteurs clés pour une personnalisation du service rendu au patient: élaboration d'un cadre d'analyse. Journal de Gestion et D'économie Médicales. 2013;**31**(5):303

Chapter 9

Perspective Chapter: Palliative Care Experiences in Ethiopia – Call for Comprehensive Care Approach

Kalkidan Solomon, Yoseph Mamo Azmera and Mirgissa Kaba

Abstract

WHO estimated over 56 million people across the world require palliative care each year. Seventy-six percent of these are from low- and-middle-income countries. Due to the aging population, urbanization, and physical inactivity among others, chronic health problems are expanding. The number of individuals with such health problems is increasing. Even though access to palliative care is a patient's right and a duty of care provider, provision of comprehensive and integrated palliative care remains non-existent in Ethiopia. Within the health facilities where alleviation of pain and suffering is believed to improve quality of life, access to opioids is at best limited. Psychosocial needs and financial instability are primarily caused by persisting pain and diminishing livelihood. In Ethiopia, palliative care failed to pay attention to such components as social, economic, and spiritual support that are equally desirable to improve quality of life of those with chronic diseases. Coordinated care mechanisms are compromised with an inadequate understanding of the scope of palliative care, how to integrate different resources and lack of model that defines and guide provision of comprehensive palliative care.

Keywords: palliative care, comprehensive care, continuum of care, community-based care, Ethiopia

1. Introduction

World Health Organization (WHO) defines palliative care (PC) as an approach designed to be safe and effective to improve patients and their families' quality of life by preventing and relieving physical, psychological, social, and spiritual sufferings [1]. Through PC, individuals get relief from persistent pain while families cope with consequent challenges including bereavement to enhance the quality of life [2].

The development of palliative care is associated with movement of hospice centers with travelers where in ancient times sick travelers took rest. Such movement associated to sick travelers and dying patients have eventually developed into a center, which ultimately advanced into a formal palliative care service provided in conjunction with active treatment, and, as death nears [3]. It was in 1967 that Dr. Cicely Saunders, widely regarded as the founder of the modern hospice movement, opened the first team-based facility in the United Kingdom [4]. Palliative Medicine emerged as a medical specialty as a response to cancer and other chronic life-threatening illness. In the developing world, particularly sub-Saharan Africa, it had been the only available option for HIV/AIDS care before the era of antiretroviral drugs and remains relevant despite improved ART access [5].

Palliative care is an important agenda of the world health. In 2014, the World Health Assembly requested the Director General to ensure that PC is an integral component of all relevant global disease control and health system plans as well as consists into country and regional cooperation plans [6]. The resolution has clearly stated that it is the ethical duty of healthcare providers and the governmental organizations that support the delivery of healthcare to provide relief from pain, whether it is physical, psychological, or spiritual. This includes establishing appropriate local and national palliative care policies, supporting ongoing training and education on palliative care, providing budgetary support, ensuring appropriate access to necessary medications, supporting training programs, and ongoing education on palliative care [6].

Currently, PC is acknowledged as a necessary service in the Universal Health Coverage (UHC) package, which ensures that everyone has access to promotive, preventive, curative, rehabilitative, and palliative health services of adequate quality to be beneficial without putting the user in a financially difficult situation [7]. Whether a patient receives care in their own home, at community, at facility, at hospice inpatient unit, or at outpatient clinic holistic PC should be available wherever such care is needed [8]. Successful implementation of the PC program depends on how the different outlets are coordinated [9]. Studies revealed that patients and their caregivers prefer continued and comprehensive care service. Such continuity of care requires not only functional linkages between care outlets but also well-defined referral pathways and relevant capacities [10–13]. This chapter aims to describe the experience of palliative care in Ethiopia and discuss the importance to initiate a comprehensive care approach in consideration of what local culture offers.

2. Palliative care in Ethiopia

Globally, the use of traditional and complementary or alternative medicines are increasing in both developed and developing countries [14]. A sizeable number of people receiving modern medical care for chronic, incurable illnesses, use herbs and non-prescription drugs as well as communal prayers and holy water (Tsebel). There are initiatives in place to involve religious leaders in the treatment of critically ill patients [15].

In Ethiopia, a comprehensive palliative care movement has started in response to the HIV/AIDS epidemic. Inconsistencies between the number of patients, qualified caregivers and lack of adequate services and resources in the healthcare systems for people living with HIV/AIDS have led to the idea of providing healthcare services for this vulnerable population at home [16]. Nonetheless, such service is not standardized nor the component of it remains disintegrated.

Home-based care (HBC) focuses on comfort and the alleviation of suffering, similar to hospice care. Home-based care programs were developed with a view to assisting caregivers at family level in providing AIDS-related care yet such services could not cope with the increasing demand for treatment and care. Evidences reveal that such care is provided either by NGOs, government health clinics, or community groups with an additional role to improve adherence to antiretroviral therapy [17, 18]. Community members and minimally trained HBC volunteers filled the void by providing basic services, dispelling myths about HIV/AIDS, and reintegrating patients into the community [5, 19].

Home and community-based care (HCBC) is deeply ingrained in Ethiopian culture and has long predated the development of the contemporary medical system. When hospitals overflowed and sick people had to be sent home during the early stages of the HIV/AIDS epidemics, there was a significant shift. Thus, community members and minimally trained home care workers filled the void by providing basic services. Prior to antiretroviral treatment (ART), HIV had a rapid downward trajectory and care focused on comfort and alleviation of suffering similar to hospice care. There was no standardized training material and toolkit for patient care at the home level, and support from healthcare institutions was minimal. More organized initiatives in HCBC were introduced in the year 2000 when care and support services assessments were performed in the Oromia region of Jimma and Nekemte by The Organization for Social Services for AIDS (OSSA) and the Amhara region of Adama, Asela, Shashemene, and Zeway by the Family Guidance Association of Ethiopia (FGAE) [5]. Sensitization sessions on the fundamental ideas of HCBC, the roles and duties of different community groups, stakeholders, and the requirements for selecting volunteer caregivers were held in order to address the unmet needs of the patients, and caregivers, limitations of the organizational capabilities which include Non-Governmental Organizations (NGOs), Kebeles, (the smallest unit of Urban Dwellers) Self-Help Public Associations, and Idirs (community self-help associations) [5].

The Addis Ababa HCBC program was launched in September 2003 with the support of Family Health International (FHI), the Addis Ababa HIV/AIDS Prevention and Control Office (HAPCO), and Addis Ababa Health Bureau. The implementation of the program was started with 20 *idirs* and later expanded to 60 in the 10 sub-cities of Addis Ababa. FHI works with various local NGOs and provides HCBC both in Addis and several other regions of the country. People to People (P2P), a Diaspora healthcare professional organization has been providing HCBC in the Arada and Yeka sub-cities of Addis for several years. P2P has also provided training for 25 nurses and scores of auxiliary healthcare workers in HCBC, palliative care and hospice. Some organizations like the Mary Joy Development Association target the elderly, a clearly vulnerable group, in their care provision efforts [20].

According to assessments done in the beginning of 2000 by the African Palliative Care Association (APCA) and the World Health Organization (WHO), there were no institutions in Ethiopia that met the requirements for palliative care. Hospice Ethiopia was established in 2003 and offered the first multidisciplinary approach to healthcare, serving as a paradigm for future growth. Additional insights were gained from Ethiopia's early 2000 response to HIV/AIDS, which bolstered the country's overall healthcare delivery system. There are numerous additional groups involved in the Addis Ababa HCBC scene. Since 2003, Hospice Ethiopia has provided education and services [21].

In order to prepare guidelines for the standardization and implementation of PC, a technical working group (TWG) comprising stakeholders in the field was established in March 2011 under the direction of the Federal Ministry of Health (FMOH) of Ethiopia. Local morphine manufacture began in 2011, and the Ethiopian Public Health Association (EPHA) developed a pain training module in 2015, and PC was integrated into the public health system.

Over the last 10 years, the Federal Ministry of Health (FMOH) has created national palliative care standards, incorporated palliative care into the National Annual Plan, and integrated palliative care for the first time in the Ethiopian Hospital Services as part of the execution of policy of transformation guidelines. Palliative care was included in the Ethiopian Primary Health Care Clinical Guidelines. These recommendations were created using data from the Practical Approach to Care Kit (PACK), an integrated approach tool focused on symptoms that assist primary healthcare providers in making clinical decisions [22, 23].

FMOH has also been working on providing training for multi-disciplinary teams at hospitals, and some health centers both in Addis Ababa and the regions. FMOH has created a hub-and-spoke model for adult care, with the hospital serving as the hub and the hospital team connecting to community services and health centers. To create a multidisciplinary hospital team, in-service training for physicians, nurses, social workers, and pharmacists has been designed. The FMOH is working to increase the availability of drugs including morphine, as this is still a concern [22].

3. Disease dynamics and current state of palliative care in Ethiopia

The past century has shown a marked increase in life expectancy due to improved lifestyles, diagnostic facilities, and medical care as well as technological advances. Such an increase in life expectancy is not without cost. The vivid cost is complexities and burden of diseases that compromise the quality of life [24].

The WHO predicted an Epidemiological Transition due to a sharp increase in non-communicable diseases. While this may be the case in rich nations, many resource-constrained nations will likely experience a "triple epidemic," in which accidents, non-communicable diseases, and communicable diseases all have a significant impact. Among the 65 million annual deaths globally, 45 million are due to chronic illnesses, of these, 60% require palliative care. It is, therefore, crucial that we begin considering culturally competent and economically viable models of care for chronic illnesses as soon as possible rather than later [25].

As science has advanced and life expectancy has increased, PCs have become more and more important. The necessity of combining PC into routine care services is underscored by the rising prevalence of cancer, mental illness, chronic non-communicable diseases, and their related treatments [26]. There are different models of care being used for palliative care implementation including home-based, community-based, facility-based, and hospice-based care in Ethiopia [22]. Studies have shown that home-based palliative care is a preferred model by patients and family caregivers which is required to smoothen the continuum of palliative care from the facility level through the integration of the service to the current chain of health delivery system [27–29].

PC should be provided in the context of the continuum of care, yet studies showed that there are barriers ranging from structural to individual levels for adequate and continuum provision of PC [30]. Misconceptions about palliative care as under recognized specialty, lack of trained palliative care providers; late involvement of inpatient palliative care, lack of community hospice services, inadequate palliative care education and training, financial barriers, attitudes and beliefs around PC, and geographical barriers were commonly mentioned [30, 31].

Lack of access to basic and specialized palliative care training and education for healthcare workers, limited opioid availability, legal and regulatory restrictions on oral morphine and strong opioids, costs for transportation and healthcare services, turn-over of trained staff, overwhelmed health workers, physical inaccessibility, lack of holistic care model, lack of defined palliative care package, and the absence of established structure and care model for implementing palliative care continuity from facility to, community and home as key hindering provision of comprehensive palliative care service in Ethiopia [27, 28, 32].

Even though Ethiopia has a strong Primary Health Care (PHC) structure building from the community to specialized facility level with a very diverse and rich culture of community support groups such as "Idirs", Family kin system, Faith Based Organizations (FBOs), Civil Society Organization (CSOs), and Hospice centers, such resources are not translated to develop, and integrate PC services thereby contributing to meeting national and regional commitments to improve quality of life of chronically ill patients [22].

Ethiopians have long placed high value on their strong social fabric and sense of community responsibility for the sick. The culture of community support in Ethiopia is particularly strong since it takes into account the psycho-social aspects of a patient's illness in addition to their physical one. This approach is particularly relevant in palliative care where the emphasis is in addressing the "total pain" of patients and families. Stoicism is highly regarded in Ethiopian society, and expressing one's grief is seen as a sign of weakness or a lack of bravery. Pain management is therefore not given much thought. Ethiopia's low per capita opioid use suggests that even in established institutions, moderate-to-severe pain is not being adequately managed.

For their medical requirements, the majority of Ethiopians still turn to traditional healers, spiritual guidance, and home medicines. A considerable percentage of people seeking modern medical care for chronic, incurable illnesses also use herbal remedies, non-prescription medications, and/or religious practices like communal prayers and tebel (holy water). It is advised to make an effort to involve religious and community leaders in the care of patients with serious illnesses in order to allay their fears that pursuing modern treatment will conflict with the divine intervention required to recover [33].

Ensuring the continuity of care and attending to patient needs as they move through the referral routes between community, home, and facility-based treatments is a crucial aspect of PC service. Even though the majority of Ethiopians live in rural areas, PC is still mostly donor-dependent and concentrated in urban areas [34]. A study conducted in Addis Ababa and Sidama region reported that the majority of female cancer patients suffered from moderate to severe pain and there was an unmet need in psychosocial, spiritual, economic, and emotional support [28]. Another study done in rural part of Ethiopia reported that there are extensive unmet palliative care needs in Ethiopia.

Untreated pain and high costs of illness are the major contributors to psychosocial distress and financial crisis in the Ethiopian population [29, 35]. The majority of PC services in Ethiopia are focused on pain management, with little attention paid to other necessary components such as social, economic, and spiritual support. Coordinated care mechanisms has severely compromised, patient needs are not into consideration, and there is an inadequate translation of local resources to provide comprehensive care at various levels [22, 27].

4. A way of forward-call for comprehensive care approach

Evidence suggests that policymakers, medical professionals, and community members may not be fully aware of the comprehensive palliative care options available, which contributes to Ethiopia's poor palliative care practice. Lack of a comprehensive approach, poor stakeholder collaboration, and a dearth of funding and human resources all have an impact on the provision of palliative care. Thus, for millions of Ethiopians, access to comprehensive palliative care is either nonexistent or severely restricted [29].

Studies carried out in Ethiopia suggested additional studies on the underlying reasons for the dearth of integrated palliative care services and to design culturally relevant approaches. It is essential to have sincere discussions to raise awareness among decision-makers, healthcare professionals, and patient advocates about the importance of palliative care, shift tasks to primary care for improved access, and translate key terminologies and the concept of palliative care into working (official) language to support community ownership [27, 29, 35].

The Federal Ministry of Health's dedicated leadership and the active participation of all stakeholders, as well as the integration of palliative care into the continuum of care and preservice curriculums are also critical milestones which shall be in place. To the best of our knowledge, however, no comprehensive effort exists (**Figure 1**) that offers patients and caregivers ongoing support at the community level following the first course of treatment in the facilities.

Such comprehensive care approach could enhance the quality of life for those who are terminally, and chronically ill, as well as their families, and caregivers. Palliative care ought to be considered an integral aspect of healthcare, not limited to patients nearing the end of life. To guarantee sustainability and accessibility, palliative care ought to be developed within the framework of the current healthcare system, taking

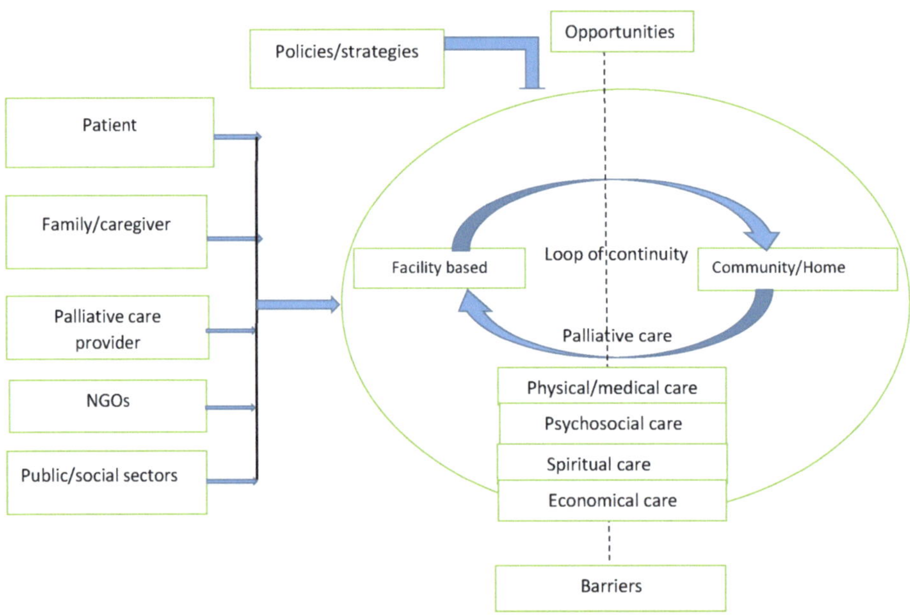

Figure 1.
Comprehensive palliative care model.

into account the cultural and social background as well as the requirements of patients and caregivers. Palliative care must begin early in order to be effective; as the disease progresses and the objectives of treatment shift, symptom-based care will become increasingly important and curative measures will become less common. Models that are both economically and culturally suitable have been developed and shown to work well in nations with limited resources, such Rwanda and Uganda. Because hospice and palliative care in these two nations support a long-lasting framework of community initiation and ownership, they can be used as a model for care in resource-constrained areas. It is the duty of national health systems to integrate PC with early detection, treatment, and prevention initiatives throughout the continuum of care.

5. Conclusion

Ethiopia has poor and fragmented palliative care services; the country's support systems are not well-coordinated nor do they have clear referral procedures or strategic guidelines to guarantee that palliative care is included in the country's overall healthcare strategy. Volunteers and other providers lack the tools and competencies needed to fulfill the expanding needs of palliative care. Patients' knowledge on what to do if they continue to demand care is remaining weak. Family and spiritual support as the most preferred services are generally accessible but should be reinforced. There is a fear associated with end-of-life planning, even though it has been shown to be rather effective. The palliative care continuum involves various stakeholders, including homes, health facilities, NGOs, and community structures, who should collaborate to improve quality of life.

Palliative care delivery mainly depends on NGOs based in urban settings, however, community volunteers had no chance to reach the hospitals to support patients besides primary healthcare units such as health centers, primary hospitals were missed in the process since palliative care provision is only provided in few specialized hospitals in Ethiopia. There is no responsible structure for the implementation of palliative care. Policy directions and guidance are missing as such in other departments like non-communicable disease, maternal, and child health.

Given Ethiopia's dearth of all-inclusive palliative care choices and the difficulties faced by participants and caregivers in programs, it is imperative that care professionals receive continual training and supervision within a well-defined organizational structure. The preference for home and community-based care in line with what is culturally acceptable necessitates the active participation of like-minded stakeholders in the community.

The continuum of care can be maintained by initiating a care model that holds the health system accountable to have a well-functioning system but also work in close collaboration with different stakeholders at the community level including a culturally established care system. Given Ethiopia is known to have multiple cultures, it is important to carry out studies to identify more robust local care system that could be developed to contribute to improved care to patients.

6. Recommendations

In response to the global call for comprehensive palliative care, the Ethiopian palliative care initiatives, competencies, and available resources at different level need to be studied and documented to inform the role of multiple sectors. It would be crucial for the nation to create a comprehensive care model that, on the one hand, outlines the responsibilities of various sectors and skills and, on the other hand, defines referral pathways with a continuum of care. Such an effort might raise people's quality of life and enhance Ethiopia's response to its commitment to universal health coverage.

Author details

Kalkidan Solomon[1], Yoseph Mamo Azmera[2] and Mirgissa Kaba[1*]

1 Department of Preventive Medicine, School of Public Health, College of Health Sciences, Addis Ababa University, Addis Ababa, Ethiopia

2 Hospice Ethiopia, Addis Ababa, Ethiopia

*Address all correspondence to: mirgissk@yahoo.com

References

[1] Organization WH. World Health Organization definition of palliative care. World Health Organization Website. 2014. Available from: http://www.whoint/cancer/palliative/definition/en

[2] WHO. Integrating Palliative Care and Symptom Relief into Paediatrics: A WHO Guide for Health-Care Planners, Implementers and Managers. Geneva: World Health Organization; 2018. Available from: https://creativecommons.org/licenses/by-nc-sa/3.0/igo

[3] Williams MA, Wheeler MS. Palliative care: What is it? Home Healthcare Now. 2001;**19**(9):550-556

[4] Twycross RG. Introducing Palliative Care. Radcliffe Publishing; 2003. Available from: Amazon.com

[5] World Health Organization. A community health approach to palliative care for HIV/AIDS and cancer patients in Sub-Saharan Africa. World Health Organization; 2004. Available from: https://iris.who.int/handle/10665/42919

[6] World Health Organization. Strengthening of palliative care as a component of integrated treatment throughout the life course. Journal of Pain and Palliative Care Pharmacotherapy. Jun 2014;**28**(2): 130-134. DOI: 10.3109/15360288.2014.911801. Epub 2014 Apr 29. PMID: 24779434

[7] Downing J, Rajagopal M, de Lima L, Knaul F. Universal Health coverage and serious health-related suffering: A case for children and young people. In: Downing J, editor. Children's Palliative Care: An International Case-Based Manual. Cham: Springer; 2020. pp. 13-23. DOI: 10.1007/978-3-030-27375-0_2

[8] Boston P, Bruce A, Schreiber R. Existential suffering in the palliative care setting: An integrated literature review. Journal of Pain and Symptom Management. 2011;**41**(3):604-618

[9] Graham F, Clark D. The changing model of palliative care. Medicine. 2008;**36**(2):64-66

[10] Bainbridge D, Brazil K, Krueger P, Ploeg J, Taniguchi A. A proposed systems approach to the evaluation of integrated palliative care. BMC Palliative Care. 2010;**9**(1):1-12

[11] Shamieh O, Hui D. A comprehensive palliative care program at a tertiary cancer center in Jordan. American Journal of Hospice and Palliative Medicine®. 2015;**32**(2):238-242

[12] Payne S, Eastham R, Hughes S, Varey S, Hasselaar J, Preston N. Enhancing integrated palliative care: What models are appropriate? A cross-case analysis. BMC Palliative Care. 2017;**16**(1):1-10

[13] Krakauer EL, Kane K, Kwete X, Afshan G, Bazzett-Matabele L, Ruthnie Bien-Aimé DD, et al. Essential package of palliative care for women with cervical cancer: Responding to the suffering of a highly vulnerable population. JCO Global Oncology. 2021;**7**:873-885

[14] Teshome-Bahire W. Initiation of healers in Ethiopia: A case study. Collegium Antropologicum. 2000;**24**(2):555-563

[15] Bishaw M. Promoting traditional medicine in Ethiopia: A brief historical

review of government policy. Social Science & Medicine. 1991;**33**(2):193-200

[16] Larki M, Roudsari RL. Home-based care, the missing link in caring of patients living with HIV/AIDS and their family members: A narrative review. International Journal of Community Based Nursing and Midwifery. 2020;**8**(3):190

[17] Uys L. Guest editorial: Longer-term aid to combat AIDS. Journal of Advanced Nursing. Oct 2003;**44**(1):1-2. DOI: 10.1046/j.1365-2648.2003.02787.x. PMID: 12956663

[18] Wood EM, Zani B, Esterhuizen TM, Young T. Nurse led home-based care for people with HIV/AIDS. BMC Health Services Research. 2018;**18**(1):1-13

[19] Gispen MEC. Human Rights and Drug Control: Access to Controlled Essential Medicines in Resource-Constrained Countries. Utrecht University Repository (Dissertation); 2017

[20] HIV/AIDS prevention and control Office annual report for 2011. HAPCO, Addis Ababa, Ethiopia (Un-published report)

[21] African Palliative Care Association (APCA). Standards for Providing Quality Palliative Care Across Africa. Kampala, Uganda: Elton John AIDS Foundation; 2010

[22] Mamo Y, Habte A, Abreha A, Ayers N, Abathun E, Reid E, et al. The evolution of hospice and palliative care in Ethiopia: From historic milestones to future directions. Ethiopian Journal of Health Development. 2020;**34**(4):310-312

[23] Cornick R, Picken S, Wattrus C, Awotiwon A, Carkeek E, Hannington J, et al. The practical approach to care kit (PACK) guide: Developing a clinical decision support tool to simplify, standardise and strengthen primary healthcare delivery. BMJ Global Health. 2018;**3**(Suppl. 5):e000962

[24] Crimmins EM. Lifespan and healthspan: Past, present, and promise. The Gerontologist. 2015;**55**(6):901-911

[25] Benziger CP, Roth GA, Moran AE. The global burden of disease study and the preventable burden of NCD. Global Heart. 2016;**11**(4):393-397

[26] Castro JA, Hannon B, Zimmermann C. Integrating palliative care into oncology care worldwide: The right Care in the Right Place at the right time. Current Treatment Options in Oncology. 2023;**24**(4):353-372

[27] Abate Y, Solomon K, Azmera YM, de Fouw M, Kaba M. Barrier analysis for continuity of palliative care from health facility to household among adult cancer patients in Addis Ababa, Ethiopia. BMC Palliative Care. 2023;**22**(1):1-9

[28] Kaba M, de Fouw M, Deribe KS, Abathun E, Peters AAW, Beltman JJ. Palliative care needs and preferences of female patients and their caregivers in Ethiopia: A rapid program evaluation in Addis Ababa and Sidama zone. PLoS One. 2021;**16**(4):e0248738

[29] Aregay A, O'Connor M, Stow J, et al. Palliative care in Ethiopia's rural and regional health care settings: A qualitative study of enabling factors and implementation challenges. BMC Palliat Care; 2023;**22**:156. DOI: 10.1186/s12904-023-01283-5

[30] Abu-Odah H, Molassiotis A, Liu J. Challenges on the provision of palliative care for patients with cancer in low-and middle-income countries: A systematic

review of reviews. BMC Palliative Care. 2020;**19**:1-16

[31] Cheng S-Y, Dy S, Hu W-Y, Chen C-Y, Chiu T-Y. Factors affecting the improvement of quality of dying of terminally ill patients with cancer through palliative care: A ten-year experience. Journal of Palliative Medicine. 2012;**15**(8):854-862

[32] Amare N, Gintamo B, Tukeni KN, Gebremichael EH, Abera EG. The prevalence of cancer patients requiring palliative care and its associated factors at St. Paul Hospital, Addis Ababa, Ethiopia: A cross-sectional study. Risk Management and Healthcare Policy. 28 Jun 2023;**16**:1203-1214. DOI: 10.2147/RMHP.S415532. PMID: 37404288; PMCID: PMC10315136

[33] Kassaye KD, Amberbir A, Getachew B, Mussema Y. A historical overview of traditional medicine practices and policy in Ethiopia. Ethiopian Journal of Health Development. 2006;**20**(2):127-134

[34] Reid E, Abathun E, Diribi J, Mamo Y, Hall P, Fallon M, et al. Rationale and study design: A randomized controlled trial of early palliative care in newly diagnosed cancer patients in Addis Ababa, Ethiopia. Contemporary Clinical Trials Communications. 2020;**18**:100564

[35] Aregay A, O'Connor M, Stow J, Ayers N, Lee S. Palliative care in Ethiopia's rural and regional health care settings: A qualitative study of enabling factors and implementation challenges. BMC Palliative Care. 2023;**22**(1):156

Section 3

Multidisciplinary Approaches and Clinical Practice

Chapter 10

Palliative Care in Advanced Chronic Obstructive Pulmonary Disease

Amon Banturaki

Abstract

There is a need to look at advanced chronic obstructive pulmonary disease in the eyes of palliative care. Many times, the eyes that are used may not reflect the objective of employing palliative care but rather an afterthought. It is, therefore, essential to look at how we can maximise professionalism in working as a team to provide palliative care. Palliative care should be built into the available professions and not introduced as separate care so that it improves the overall care but not replacing it. The chapter takes one through the commonly encountered problems facing a patient with advanced chronic obstructive pulmonary disease. It further raps this with the focus on a multi-disciplinary approach in a setting of shared decision-making.

Keywords: advanced chronic obstructive pulmonary disease, palliative care, multidisciplinary, shared decision making, patient-centred

1. Introduction

We introduce this chapter with a passage from a qualitative study published by palliative care experts. The authors summarised their findings with these statements, "In order to help patients to improve disease awareness, to accept their life situation and to improve their reduced quality of life, patients may benefit from the early integration of palliative care (PC), considering its multiprofessional patient-centred and team-centred approach" [1]. Palliative care means a lot to the patient with advanced chronic obstructive pulmonary disease (COPD). Since 2009, palliative care in Uganda has grown in volume, quality, and geographic reach. An important epidemiologic transition has occurred when non-communicable diseases have replaced HIV/AIDS as the leading diagnosis for patients receiving palliative care [2]. The challenges that these patients go through are worth accepting, targeting, and improving through the multidisciplinary care team offered in a palliative care setting.

Chronic obstructive pulmonary disease (COPD) has been defined by the Global Initiative for Chronic Obstructive Lung Disease (GOLD) as "a heterogeneous lung condition characterized by chronic respiratory symptoms (dyspnea, cough, sputum production) due to abnormalities of the airways (bronchitis, bronchiolitis) and/or alveoli (emphysema) that cause persistent, often progressive, airflow obstruction". It is diagnosed by performing spirometry, where a device measures the lung function.

IntechOpen

The forced expiratory volume in one second (FEV1) and forced vital capacity (FVC) ratio is calculated. A ratio less than 0.7 is indicative of an obstructive pattern. Spirometry measurements must persistently indicate obstruction, that is, consistent even after the patient is given an appropriate dose of a bronchodilator.

Palliative care is a multidisciplinary approach employed in health care. It has often been left to a few, but many who would have helped implement it mind other businesses [3]. The implementation gap must be sealed by showcasing the beauty of a multidisciplinary approach. Nonetheless, the typical current situation is the deception of fragmentation of care, being every day a 'hole in a doughnut' that the patients don't deserve. A team approach where patient-centred care is provided would be an outstanding achievement if persistently implemented. Palliative care avoids and alleviates the suffering of patients and their families by finding ways to care for their pain and other issues. The standard methods employed in palliative care include early detection of life-threatening illnesses, focusing on accurate diagnosis, and ensuring the use of effective treatments for the identified problems. The dimensions of the patients' issues in palliative care may be physical, psychosocial, or spiritual [4].

This chapter discusses the approach to handling palliative care among advanced COPD patients. Advanced COPD has been used in this chapter to refer to the COPD patients in Global Initiative for Chronic Obstructive Lung Disease (GOLD) grades III/IV as diagnosed by spirometry, and also the patients at "E" grading of the ADE GOLD classification, who are COPD patients with frequent exacerbations/hospitalisations in the previous one year at their time of presenting to the health care provider.

The sections of this chapter that follow will lightly explain the roles of the different players in the multidisciplinary approach in a palliative care team caring for a patient with advanced chronic obstructive pulmonary disease. The list presented in this chapter is not intended to show all needed members but instead gives a basis to start a functional team at a hospital. The chapter begins by mentioning the common symptoms or problems in palliative care for advanced COPD and concludes by explaining an active palliative care team for the advanced COPD patient.

2. Dyspnea management

One of the most distressing symptoms among Chronic Obstructive Lung Disease (COPD) patients is dyspnea. Dyspnea is an experience of abnormal, more significant effort required to breathe, the chest feeling heavy, air hunger, or gasping that COPD patients encounter [5]. This comes at any time and may be severe at some moments or consistently. The patients with dyspnea are at different severity levels.

The standard way to stratify the patients with dyspnea is using the Global Initiative for Chronic Obstructive Lung Disease (GOLD) classification. The classification considers the frequency of severe episodes of dyspnea and the associated disability in a patient's life.

This classification has been called the ADE classification [5]. The classification focuses on describing dyspnea in relation to forced expiratory volume in one second (FEV_1), the number of hospitalisations exacerbations in a year, and how the dyspnea affects their life.

The assessment of dyspnea is thus not only an issue of the presenting challenge but should involve having a good knowledge of the patient's past dyspnea experience for at least one year. The patient's experiences should then be categorised to make a treatment approach that will try to predict breathing challenges.

Having assessed the patient then, the treatment is prescribed depending on the individual patient's needs. The standard treatments include:

- Oxygen therapy usually prescribed for long-term use
- Bronchodilators, e.g. long-acting beta-agonist (LABA) like salmeterol, formoterol, and olodaterol; long-acting muscarinic receptor antagonists (LAMA) like tiotropium, aclidinium, umeclidinium, and glycopyrrolate
- Steroids, e.g. budesonide, beclomethasone, fluticasone

Other treatments target complications of COPD such as pulmonary embolism, e.g. use of anticoagulants; muscle weakness, e.g. pulmonary rehabilitation; stopping or getting alternatives to respiratory depressant drugs.

One of the key parts of the treatment of dyspnea in palliative care is patient empowerment. The patient needs to be empowered to benefit from the treatment. This may not apply to patients who are unconscious; thus, only their family members are empowered with knowledge in such instances. Patient empowerment starts with understanding the knowledge of the patient pertaining to the treatment prescribed. There is no need to teach a patient what they already know. Rather, effort should be focused on what they need to learn or understand better. An example of a knowledge gap may be how to use the medicine, such as the inhaler technique. The nurse or doctor thus goes ahead to teach the patient how best to use an inhaler. The earning process should be continuous rather than planned for counted times. This allows improvement throughout all interactions with the patient. Empowerment should be enhanced by using materials that the patient can access by themselves such recorded audio or video materials.

All patients who get exacerbations need to get reviewed by a respiratory physician or pulmonologist so that there is improved care for the added needs of the patient. In Uganda, we have a few internal medicine physicians who subspecialise in respiratory medicine (respiratory physicians). However, we often have general internal medicine physicians (with qualifications of master of medicine internal medicine) serving at various hospitals. Several have experience treating COPD patients and are thus a great resource. These usually prescribe guideline-directed treatments for COPD patients who get exacerbations. The patients are aware of their symptoms and are best at describing them to the physician. The patients are thus also experts in their illness. Dyspnea is most of the time chronic, and the patient needs to learn to also minimally adjust treatment to improve relief even before the pulmonologist sees them. The patient should be in control of up-titrating the bronchodilator and or/steroid doses. The patient empowerment sessions should guide the patient on safe practices for changing drug doses to relieve dyspnea as they wait to see their pulmonologist. This underscores the need to have repeated assessment and empowerment on how to use the prescribed treatment.

The use of morphine may be thought to be controversial among COPD patients. It has been used to treat refractory dyspnea [6]. The physician may not be willing to prescribe it for COPD patients due to its respiratory depression side effects. However, whenever prescribed, patient empowerment should be done so that the patient can identify the side effects and, if necessary, stop its use early. Morphine provides treatment for both dyspnea and pain in selected patients with advanced COPD, but this requires support from family members to be effectively utilised [7].

3. Role of pulmonary rehabilitation

COPD is a chronic disease. This allows for several processes to take place. Due to oxidative stress, genetics, hypercapnia, acidosis, metabolic problems, dietary irregularities, medicines, co-morbidities, and ageing, COPD reduces muscle mass. Common muscle remodeling leads to lower exercise capacity and impaired function.

The patient diagnosed with COPD usually needs extra assistance to be added to their physiological abilities. These assistances may come in to play when the health care team is multi-disciplinary. One of the relevant health care providers is a physiotherapist or at least the practice of physiotherapy, even if not by a registered physiotherapist.

The physiotherapist identifies the respiratory disabilities and plans how to administer the physiotherapy. The greatest challenge thus lies in the early identification of the physiotherapy needs of the patient. Delay in identifying the needs may result in wrongly diagnosing a patient to have a poor prognosis or sometimes wrong differential diagnoses.

There is, therefore, a need for the physiotherapist to be given adequate opportunities at ward rounds or outpatient respiratory clinics together with the physician to allow them understand the treatment options availed to the patient. This allows for the incorporation of pulmonary rehabilitation strategies. Pulmonary rehabilitation is a widely accepted comprehensive interdisciplinary exercise training technique.

Adherence to pulmonary rehabilitation is typically low, and obstacles include accessibility, financial constraints, a lack of enthusiasm, and the incapacity to participate in or carry out physical exercise [8].

The path to increase accessibility involves utilising the workforce that is already available. Underutilisation worsens the challenge of accessibility by preventing the availability of services. People can't adhere to services that have restricted access. It is also paramount that awareness of the need for pulmonary rehabilitation should increase.

Pulmonary rehabilitation improves the following aspects of palliative care [9]:

- Functional capacity
- Higher treatment of dyspnea
- Anxiety, and depression

Hospitalised advanced COPD patients may need practices such as those mentioned below for their improvement: [10]

- Humidification of respiratory gases
- Chest physical therapy
- Manual or ventilator pulmonary hyperinflation
    - Manual chest expiratory compressions
    - Mechanical in-exsufflation
    - High-frequency oscillations
- Muscle reconditioning

Although rehabilitation is important, it must be known that it does not help the patient, except other interventions are concurrently instituted. The patient under pulmonary rehabilitation equally require the help of all other specialists to have improvement in quality of life.

4. Social aspects

The approach discussed above of holistic approach in the palliative care is intended to include the social aspects of the patient. The COPD patient desires to live a satisfactory life, although it is at the end of their life. According to a study in 2021, patients with COPD who had more social support had a much decreased likelihood of experiencing depressed symptoms [11]. The involvement of peers and relatives in treating COPD patients is thus crucial to getting the best outcomes.

The holistic approach covers the social aspects, such as how the patient wishes to spend time if they were well. This means that the team caring for the patient gets to know the social life of the patient and then includes the social disabilities of the patient in the diagnosis. The common mistake is failure to include the social aspect in the diagnosis of the patient, resulting in not planning for palliative care needs for the social issues.

The diagnosis may thus have additional details such as:

- Sports, e.g. watching sports events
- Music and dancing, e.g. night clubbing
- Writing activities, e.g. authoring articles
- Eating for leisure, e.g. special meals
- Touring, e.g. places to visit before death
- People groups, e.g. people that one wishes to spend time with mostly

After the diagnosis then, the next step is to allocate the responsibility to one of the caring staff. This may mean having a very inclusive caring team that does not segregate social workers. This is important because most healthcare professionals do not get adequate training in handling issues that deal with social life. The staff that may be very helpful in managing the social aspects of the COPD patient conclude:

- Social workers
- Music trainers
- Tour/travel guides
- Journalists

The doctors and nurses should also use the opportunity to learn on the job by being present during the non-medical staff interview/therapy sessions. This helps to improve how they later interact with the patient knowledgeably. The presence of the health worker in the sessions helps to create a team and strengthen cooperation among the team members. Respect should be given to the non-health worker while they engage the patient. While the help of non-health workers is welcome, the confidentiality of information must be maintained since other professionals may not be trained in handling confidential data. There should be clear roles while working with team members, and none should feel embarrassed if reminded of the boundaries that should not be crossed. Such limitations include medical prescriptions which non-health workers should not be allowed to make. The involvement of family members is the usual inexpensive way to provide social palliative care. These can sing, help with sports, exercise, write, and play with the patients. This means that choosing an available and cheap method needs to be considered so that it is provided when it is never needed. The point to remember is that the family members may also be biased about certain sports activities or may even themselves be naïve about the interests of the patient, such as writing.

5. Home care and visits

In this section, we briefly discuss the care for a patient while at home. Many patients get to a time when all the needed services can be provided at their homes. This is usually a decision taken with the help of shared decision-making. The decision to care for the advanced COPD patient at home should be a collective choice with the inclusion of the patient. The caring team should look at the pros and cons of the decision. The patient will be visited by a team of palliative care providers at their home. The decision should guarantee that there will be uninterrupted communication through the sharing of telephone contacts between either parties and precisely locating the home. The home should be located by noting the details of the neighbourhood of the patient and road access with alternative routes. All these already exist in the patient register if the patient has been known to the hospital earlier. In case they aren't there need to document the data.

There should be caregivers with ability to respond to the daily immediate needs of the patient. This must be confirmed and the details taken so that responsibilities are clearly spelt out. The caregivers at home may be family members, friends, or those that the patient has entrusted such roles at a fee.

The palliative care team also equally identifies and gives specific roles to their hospital staff or volunteers to ensure that home visit are carried out. A system that involves periodic reports that are delivered to the hospital palliative care lead staff must be put in place. This ensures that support is continually given to the home visit staff or volunteers and quality improvement assured.

The common needs for home visits include the following but not limited to:

- Periodic assessment of palliative care problems since these change from time to time

- Offering a listening ear to share the challenging experiences

- Counselling sessions

- Bridging the gap between the staff at hospital and the team at home

- Delivering support to the patient such as medicines, e.g. nebulised bronchodilators, heart failure medicines, morphine, oxygen cylinders

- Delivering empowerment materials in any form, such as written, audio, or video

The care team should also plan for likely challenges while planning for home care. The commonly encountered problems include

- Poor adherence to the medicines and treatment prescribed.

- Meeting caregivers who don't usually stay with the patient. These may not provide relevant information during the home visit.

- Problems that the visiting team have never handled in their practice, e.g. homicide.

- Limited resources, e.g. due to reduced funding in the recent times of the COVID-19 pandemic.

- Change of physical address without notifying the visiting team.

- Inappropriate demands from family members, such as sexual harassment.

The health system may further complicate the challenges above in a given community. The laws governing patient care, as well as resources differ from country to country. In Uganda (where the author lives currently), the resources are usually centralised at health centres, and the district health care team may not be willing to extend the services to the patients at home. This may be eased by supporting non-governmental organisations where collaborations are feasible. Such organisations should be reached out to, and early engagement in patient care at hospitals before home visits would be a wise plan.

6. Role of multidisciplinary agreement and shared decision-making

The COPD patient is usually managed under the care of an internal medicine physician or pulmonologist. Depending on the set-up at the hospital, the patient's reviews will most of the time be scheduled by the above specialists. There is a tendency only to consult other specialists when the patient has requested or only when there is a new challenge to deal with. Such planning does not seem inclusive because it is limited and or/or depends on mainly the experience of the pulmonologist.

To improve the multidisciplinary team, the pulmonologist (who is the team lead) needs to treat the patient as a whole. Holistic management of the patient allows other specialists besides the pulmonologist to get involved in the treatment all through the care sessions.

With holistic treatment, the patients get scheduled reviews to identify the challenges that they may have in other organ systems besides the pulmonary system. Such reviews can be initiated by the pulmonologist initially seeking to involve the most common organ complication specialists.

These common complications experienced resulting from COPD that may need the involvement of other specialists include:

- Heart failure
- Depression
- Insomnia
- Weight loss
- Job loss

Specialists who may handle the above complications include

- Cardiologist
- Psychiatrist
- Nurse
- Nutritionist
- Social worker

Besides the attending pulmonologist, other specialists need to be given complete trust because of the need to have them on board all through the time the COPD patient gets hospital visits.

The role of the multidisciplinary team is to provide a comprehensive management plan. The complications of COPD may need palliative care that is beyond the capacity of the pulmonology department. An example is that of difficulty breathing. Difficulty breathing may initially be due to the severity of COPD but may at a time become a result of both the failing pulmonary system and heart failure. Such a patient may need treatments that are beyond what is usually prescribed for the dyspneic COPD patient under the care of a pulmonologist. Treatment of heart failure may be based on the ejection fraction of the patient (being reduced, mid-range or preserved ejection fraction). Optimising these treatments would be best done by teaming up with the cardiologist.

Patients who experience depression may be at risk of poor medicine adherence and may not live a satisfied life. The pulmonologist is responsible for involving the psychiatrist in the management of advanced COPD patients. Scheduling reviews or having discussions with the psychiatrist to enable both early detection and continued treatment of the depressed advanced COPD patient is crucial. Depression, if poorly managed, may result in difficulty in history taking, physical examination, and their associated failed shared decision-making. Caring for a patient who has lost hope, such as may be found among depressed patients, means caring for patients who have daily pain. Hope needs to be restored. This kind of approach that prioritises the challenges of the depressed advanced COPD patient can only be best handled while working with the psychiatrist.

Nutrition is vital for all advanced COPD patients. COPD is known to cause muscle wasting, and chronic inflammation has also been documented [12]. These issues require the adoption of nutritional care that emphasises the individual dietary needs of the patients since the needs vary. An appropriate assessment will require the involvement of a nutritionist not only a few times but always since COPD is chronic. The role of the nutritionist is to make a detailed assessment and design a long-term treatment plan for the patient. The treatment plans need to consider all other management plans that the patient has been given.

The health workers who spend the longest time with patients are usually nurses. These avail a credible place in knowing patient prognosis, adherence to therapy and reliable ways to detect patients' needs. These are not the only reasons they are important players in the palliative care of COPD patients but rather the more obvious reasons.

The nurse is usually equipped with both the patients' desires and the palliative care providers' desires. They thus play a great role in finding a balance between what care to give the patient. They often inform other care providers of the details they have observed while interacting with the patients, making the care patient-centred. Ignoring, delaying, or preventing the nursing team from providing their care view may result in not having patient-centred care.

Palliative care specialists are available in many countries nowadays. This has allowed many hospitals and clinics to offer specialised palliative care services. The patients are better managed with the involvement of these professionals. The professionals are at different levels of education, such as bachelor's, master's or even doctor of philosophy. Some professionals are medical doctors or nurses who have specialised to be palliative care specialists.

Their presence mainly acts as a guide in decision-making. They are custodians of best practices of palliative care and thus allow for improvement in care while mentoring other health care professionals regarding palliative care services. They improve early referral to better centres regarding palliative care. Early referral can be crucial in cases requiring dialysis or ventilator support. Some difficulties in decision-making, such as when to treat or not treat using specific therapies, are better reached with the help of palliative care specialists.

Other specialists have roles besides the pulmonologist's paths in caring for advanced COPD patients who need recognition, such as those mentioned above. There is, therefore, a need for the pulmonologist to think of making a team which is not permanent but varies depending on the individual patient's needs.

Although the patient is seeking help, their opinions in decision-making may not be at the forefront. Patients in palliative care wish to be involved in choices affecting their treatment [13]. Shared decision-making (SDM) has its role in palliative care because it helps patients understand better their illness and improve their adherence to therapy. The caring team also needs to understand the experiences of the patient. There is a challenge of presuming to understand even when deliberate processes are not engaged. This mistake is very likely to take place if one only trusts their opinion or professional decisions without remembering that care should be patient-centred. The way to make care patient-centred involves employing shared decision-making. Some health workers fear the outcomes of patients' opinions, thinking that it may result in poor prognoses or early death of the patient than expected. However, this is not true since the patient who seeks care already desires the best care.

7. Conclusions

Palliative care best operates at the peak of multidisciplinary teamwork. In caring for patients with advanced chronic obstructive pulmonary disease, all relevant discipline professionals need to liaise with each other, plan together, and apply interventions that are patient-centred. An approach that takes this form becomes easy to coordinate and allows time for decision-making. Patients with advanced COPD will realise better care when they receive palliative care services at all points whenever they meet healthcare professionals.

Acknowledgements

- Dr. Amandua Jacinto, MMED, MSc Palliative Care, Consultant Physician and Palliative Care Specialist, Kampala International University Teaching Hospital, Bushenyi, Uganda

- Caxton Bahemurwaki, BSc Palliative Care, Head of Palliative Care Services, Kabale Regional Referral Hospital, Kabale, Uganda

- Moureen Banturaki, Medical Clinical Officer, Bushenyi, Uganda

Conflict of interest

The authors declare no conflict of interest.

Author details

Amon Banturaki
Kampala International University Teaching Hospital, Bushenyi, Uganda

*Address all correspondence to: amon.banturaki@kiu.ac.ug

References

[1] Marx G, Nasse M, Stanze H, Boakye SO, Nauck F, Schneider N. Meaning of living with severe chronic obstructive lung disease: A qualitative study. BMJ Open. 2016;**6**(12):e011555. DOI: 10.1136/bmjopen-2016-011555

[2] Kagarmanova A, Mwesiga MD, Sisk ML, Kabagambe C, Nyakaisiki S, Marentette T, et al. Palliative care in Uganda: Quantitative descriptive study of key palliative care indicators 2018-2020. BMC Palliative Care. 2022;**21**:55. DOI: 10.1186/s12904-022-00930-7

[3] Kavalieratos D. Directing the narrative to define and present standardization in palliative care. Journal of Palliative Medicine. 2019;**22**(12):1486-1487. DOI: 10.1089/jpm.2019.0548

[4] WHO. Palliative care. 2020. Available from: https://www.who.int/news-room/fact-sheets/detail/palliative-care

[5] GOLD. 2023 GOLD Report. Global Initiative for Chronic Obstructive Lung Disease – GOLD. 2023. Available from: https://goldcopd.org/2023-gold-report-2/

[6] Verberkt CA, van den Beuken-van Everdingen MHJ, Schols JMGA, Hameleers N, Wouters EFM, Janssen DJA. Effect of sustained-release morphine for refractory breathlessness in chronic obstructive pulmonary disease on health status. JAMA Internal Medicine. 2020;**180**(10):1306-1314. DOI: 10.1001/jamainternmed.2020.3134

[7] Ferreira D, Kochovska S, Honson A, Phillips J, Currow D. Patients' and their caregivers' experiences with regular, low-dose, sustained-release morphine for chronic breathlessness associated with COPD: A qualitative study. BMJ Open Respiratory Research. 2022;**9**(1):e001210. DOI: 10.1136/bmjresp-2022-001210

[8] Kaasgaard M, Rasmussen DB, Andreasson KH, Hilberg O, Løkke A, Vuust P, et al. Use of singing for lung health as an alternative training modality within pulmonary rehabilitation for COPD: A randomised controlled trial. The European Respiratory Journal. 2022;**59**(5):2101142. DOI: 10.1183/13993003.01142-2021

[9] Neo H-Y, Yap C-W, Teo L-M, Lee L-T, Tan H-W, Xu H-Y, et al. Palliative rehabilitation improves health care utilization and function in frail older adults with chronic lung diseases. Journal of the American Medical Directors Association. 2021;**22**(12):2478-2485. DOI: 10.1016/j.jamda.2021.05.031

[10] Martí JD, McWilliams D, Gimeno-Santos E. Physical therapy and rehabilitation in chronic obstructive pulmonary disease patients admitted to the intensive care unit. Seminars in Respiratory and Critical Care Medicine. 2020;**41**(06):886-898. DOI: 10.1055/s-0040-1709139

[11] Turnier L, Eakin M, Woo H, Dransfield M, Parekh T, Krishnan JA, et al. The influence of social support on COPD outcomes mediated by depression. PLOS ONE. 2021;**16**(3):e0245478. DOI: 10.1371/journal.pone.0245478

[12] Bauer J, Morley JE, Schols AMWJ, Ferrucci L, Cruz-Jentoft AJ, Dent E, et al. Sarcopenia: A time for action. An SCWD Position Paper. Journal of Cachexia, Sarcopenia and Muscle. 2019;**10**(5):956-961. DOI: 10.1002/jcsm.12483

[13] Kuosmanen L, Hupli M, Ahtiluoto S, Haavisto E. Patient participation in shared decision-making in palliative care—An integrative review. Journal of Clinical Nursing. 2021;**30**(23-24):3415-3428. DOI: 10.1111/jocn.15866

Chapter 11

Kidney Palliative Care Metamorphose: Education, Ethics, and Quality Standard

Ana Mateus and Pedro Ponce

Abstract

This chapter addresses three main topics (subchapters): (i) acquisition of educational skills in palliative care that are relevant to all health professionals and ways to implement these skills in the field of nephrology; (ii) ethical considerations that are applicable and support clinical and specific decisions at different stages of chronic kidney disease, such as, respect for bioethical principles in decision making related to dialysis withdrawal, effective communication with the patient and family, end of life care; and (iii) implementation and definition of key performance indicators that ensure quality of care and are patient-centred. These three (interrelated) pillars will strongly contribute to the (positive and expected) changes in the field of kidney palliative care.

Keywords: kidney disease, palliative care, education, ethics, quality indicators

1. Introduction

Throughout history, dialysis has seen incredible technological advancements, from primitive cellophane tubing machines in the 1940s to today's modern hemodialysis and peritoneal dialysis procedures [1].

With dialysis becoming more widespread, however, patients and healthcare providers face new challenges.

On one hand, patients often suffer from more severe physical and psychological symptoms due to and comorbidity of the kidney patient population, and on the other hand, health systems face cost, access, and equity issues [2].

That's why updated palliative approach to renal care is becoming increasingly important.

Palliative care in general is focused on symptom management and improving the quality of life for seriously ill patients, namely those with advanced kidney disease [3].

To provide adequate palliative care nowadays, healthcare providers need advanced education and also training to deal with ethical dilemmas, which are inherent to extreme disease situations [4]. Education and ethics, as well as quality standards ensure that patients will receive compassionate, respectful, consistent, safe, effective, and equitable care. Thoughtful ethical decision-making is also essential to guarantee that care is consistent with the patient's values and goals [5].

The realm of kidney palliative care (KPC) has experienced significant advances in recent years due to progress in education, ethics, and quality standards, but still not enough to reach the level required to fulfill all the PC'goals [6].

In this chapter, we examine the crucial trends and progressions that are shaping the future of kidney palliative care (KPC) in the different areas. First, we explore how education and training of healthcare providers in KPC have developed over time. We then consider the ethical implications of managing end-stage kidney disease (ESKD), which is a multifaceted issue requiring careful consideration.

Regarding ethical issues, we believe that more efforts are still needed to establish ethical guidelines for decision-making, as well as education and training for professionals to support ethical practices in ESKD treatment. We also discuss the measures that need to be taken to achieve those objectives and any other unforeseen ethical challenge that may arise. Finally, we touch upon the future of quality standards in KPC. We discuss new frameworks for measuring and assessing the quality of care, such as patient-reported outcome measures, and underscore the importance of utilizing data systematically for continuous improvement.

Upon completion of this segment, readers will acquire a comprehensive understanding of how KPC has advanced and how it will likely continue to evolve in the future. Also, they will be well-equipped to navigate the rapidly changing landscape of kidney palliative care and will be able to provide high-quality, patient-centered care to patients with advanced kidney disease.

2. Palliative care education for nephrology team

2.1 Current situation of health-care professionals' education in Europe

The United Nations and the World Health Organization (WHO) have clearly stated that the provision of PC is a moral responsibility of health care systems, and it is the duty of health professionals to relieve pain and suffering, whether physical, psychosocial, or spiritual, regardless of whether the disease or condition can or not be cured. Indeed, end-of-life care is one of the most important components of PC [7].

The sustainable development goals call on member countries to "significantly improve health financing and the recruitment, development, and training, as well as retention of health workforce" [8].

To date, insufficient skills of health workers remain a significant problem limiting access to palliative care services worldwide [9, 10]. For that reason, enabling access to PC education must be addressed simultaneously at its various components to speed up the process [11].

The WHO palliative care roadmap introduces three levels of palliative care education: (i) basic education for primary care physicians, (ii) intermediate education for secondary care professionals, and (iii) tertiary education for specialists [12].

In 2013, the European Association for Palliative Care (EAPC) released a document with core competencies for palliative care addressed to physicians and other health professionals in Europe [13].

2.2 Competencies in palliative care in nephrology

So far, most of the studies regarding palliative care competencies were conducted in North America, but many of them are cross-cultural [14–18].

According to those studies, all nephrology care providers should have the following primary palliative care skills [19–22].

2.2.1 Understanding and communicating prognosis

The capability to prognosticate and communicate prognosis is crucial [23]. This can be a lengthy process that requires frequent repetition. In this matter, there is clearly a lack of studies enabling to translate prognostic factors into clinically useful prognostic tools, a topic scarcely addressed in the literature [24, 25].

2.2.2 Patient-centered decision-making

Ideally, patient-centered decision-making should be performed by a multidisciplinary team and be a family-oriented, as well as culturally appropriate process, in which the team and the patient agree on a course of action based on a shared understanding of the patient's treatment goals [26]. The benefits and harms of treatment and the likely outcomes should be considered. All possible options should be openly discussed. These should include all dialysis modalities, withholding or abandoning dialysis, and an "opt-out" option for the patient after a dialysis trial [26].

2.2.3 Symptom management in ESKD

Patients with advanced CKD suffer from numerous symptoms, contributing to a severe disease burden. Some guidelines have been compiled to assist healthcare providers in managing patients with symptoms associated with advanced CKD.

It is recommended that physical and emotional symptoms be routinely assessed at each consultation using validated tools, such as:

i. Integrated palliative care renal outcome scale-renal (IPOS-Renal) [27, 28]

ii. ESAS-r (Edmonton symptom assessment system-revised: Renal) [29]

iii. Brief pain inventory [30]

2.2.4 Communication

Compassionate and effective communication is key to develop a functioning and trusting relationship between patients, families, and healthcare professionals [31]. It requires knowing what, with whom, and when to have difficult conversations, while maintaining a positive, nonjudgmental attitude. These skills can be taught and must be practiced. Protocols, such as SPIKES (Breaking Bad News) and the serious illness conversations are examples of evidence-based communication approaches [32, 33]. All conversations about bad news, especially those related to refusal or discontinuation of dialysis, should be led by a senior clinician in the team [34].

All parties must convey the same message when communicating with patients and families to avoid raising false hopes or distrust. Difficult conversations should be clearly documented in patient records and should always be followed by reflection and, if necessary, debriefing. The moral distress of physicians involved in dialysis withdrawal or renunciation requires the collegial support of leaders and other health care providers.

There are many barriers to meaningful conversations with patients and family members [35]: (i) the patient and/or family may misunderstand the diagnosis and prognosis due to cultural differences, (ii) physicians' attitudes and beliefs about palliative care may not be adequately trained, and (iii) the time may be not sufficient to have difficult conversations. Those conversations should aim to manage conflict, acknowledge, and address all emotions, improve awareness of prognosis, and align care with patient and family expectations.

Essential conversations that should occur between health care professionals, patients, and families are: Breaking Bad News and Serious Illness Conversations [33].

Both types of conversations aim to offer a hopeful, achievable alternative with a carefully considered palliative care plan.

2.2.5 Advance care planning

Advance care planning (ACP) involves conversations with individuals about their preferences and wishes. They are best conducted when patients are relatively healthy, can communicate well, and are mentally capable of making independent decisions. Values, goals, and outcomes that are important to patients and their families should be addressed. The conversation should be ongoing and not a one-time event, with the opportunity for review as circumstances change. The plan helps the health care team make treatment recommendations that are consistent with the established values. This becomes increasingly important in preparation for the phase when the patient is no longer able to make or verbalize decisions independently [36].

Research shows that patients expect the physician to initiate those conversations. Experience shows that when conversations are done skillfully, they do not increase anxiety or hopelessness [37].

2.2.6 End-of-life care

Ethical and compassionate care is the primary goal in caring for a patient at the end of life [38]. This period can be defined as the "period of irreversible loss of function before death" [39]. Care plans must be adapted to provide patients with a "good death," in which distressing symptoms and suffering are managed competently and compassionately [38, 40].

The ethical framework underlying end-of-life care includes: [38, 40].

- Maintaining open communication with the patient and family.
- Providing appropriate relief of pain and other symptoms.
- Ensuring continuity of care for the patient.
- Not subjecting the dying patient to futile treatment that may only increase the level of suffering.
- Providing integrated bio-psycho-social and spiritual care.
- Supporting actively families during the time of their grief.

2.2.7 Withdrawal from dialysis

A periodic review of the decision to take dialysis should be included in the plan [41, 42]. The schedule for these reviews should be agreed upon at the initial consultation. For the following groups of patients, the American Renal Physicians Association suggests that it is reasonable to consider dialysis discontinuation (not starting or stopping dialysis), when: [43].

- A condition is present that precludes the technical process of dialysis (e.g., an uncooperative patient with advanced dementia), or the patient is medically unstable (e.g., suffers from severe hypotension).

- A terminal nonrenal disease (we recognize that some patients may see the benefit and choose dialysis).

- Refusal/discontinuation of dialysis in a patient who can make a decision and who is fully informed and makes a voluntary decision.

- Patients who are no longer capable of deciding and who have previously indicated in an advance directive that they refuse dialysis or whose legal representatives/representatives refuse dialysis or request its discontinuation.

- Patients with irreversible profound neurological impairments.

- Patients over 75 years of age with two or more of the following criteria for a poor prognosis:

    i. dependence on care from others due to increasing physical and/or emotional and/or mental health problems.

    ii. significant weight loss (> 10%);

    iii. high comorbidity score, e.g., modified Charlson comorbidity index of 8 or more;

    iv. significantly impaired functional status, for example, Karnofsky score < 40 with limited reversibility;

    v. Patient requests palliative care or chooses to reduce, discontinue, or not receive treatment.

3. Ethical challenges, strategies and legal considerations faced by the kidney palliative care movement

And so, he'd live another day.
To bleed and cough and waste away.
The family, they were not impressed,
And wanted dad to get all the best.

Ryon D 1996.

In this section, we will address the most relevant aspects of medical ethics in the field of palliative care, applied to ESKD.

3.1 Ethical framework in renal palliative care

It is fair to state that, in general, treatment of end-stage kidney disease (ESKD) with dialysis is associated with a significant patient survival advantage, but this advantage is dramatically reduced for older people (mostly above 75 years) with major comorbidities (mainly coronary artery disease), or poor functional status, and may be lost if we consider hospital free survival and health-related quality of life (HRQOL) [44, 45].

In patients older than 85 years of age, receiving the highest intensity of care, the median duration of survival after dialysis initiation is typically less than 6 months, with more than a third of that time spent in the hospital [46].

Kurella and coworkers [47] showed that of all ESKD patients nursing home residents in the United States (U.S.), within the first year after initiation of dialysis, 58% had died and 29% had a decrease in functional status, maintained in only 13%.

Most elderly patients accept dialysis treatment but do not choose it [48]. A recent survey [49] showed 61% of dialysis patients sampled reported that they regretted beginning dialysis. Over half of these indicated that they started dialysis because of the urging of their nephrologists, and in 14% it was their family wish.

Therefore, for aged and frail patients, conservative medical treatment (CMT) without dialysis should be discussed not as a last resort, but as a clear treatment option that may be most effective in promoting patient goals [50].

Nephrologists are responsible for presenting relevant information as unbiased and easily as possible, sharing the decision process with patients/families, to support and implementing the treatment decisions reached by all stakeholders without ever closing the door to an opinion change by the patient or his family in favor of life-prolonging [49, 51].

Despite the urgency of a new approach to this selected group of patients, well known to all working in the field of chronic dialysis, we must be cautious, as age and frailty may be used as targets for cost-containment policies and resource rationing, disguising a hidden agenda of saving family resources, reducing costs on behalf of the community or the health system, that cynically perverts the movements for patient's autonomy and "death with dignity" [52].

3.2 Communicating information and informed consent

The initiation of dialysis presumes the appropriate provision of informed consent. Ideally, informed consent begins as part of advance care planning (ACP) long before a person decides about renal replacement treatment (RRT).

The importance of ACP is underscored by the high rates of withdrawal from dialysis, which is second only to cardiovascular disease as a cause of death and accounts for one-quarter of dialysis patient deaths [53].

Informed consent is the modern clinical ritual of trust. It is more than simply getting a patient to sign a written consent form.

A physician obtaining consent from a patient or family does not have to present all treatment options available; his professional responsibility, according to the shared decision-making guideline, is to exercise clinical judgment and guide the patient/family only through medically indicated options and not present choices that are not real choices [54].

Nephrologists in dialysis units have an ethical obligation to provide their patients with information on their policies about advance directives and to offer the patient an opportunity to complete an advance directive. We are equally obliged to participate in shared decision-making with patients and families. A large part of a physician's role in that process is providing the information patients and families require to make informed decisions [40].

Because the quality of our patients′ lives changes, so do their goals for care and treatment.

Because these potential patients′ representatives performed no better than chance, we must allow our patients to express their will timely while competent to do it and that we educate their designated surrogates.

Advance directives (AD) are part of the ACP and include the issue of a living will (LW), written evidence of an individual's wishes concerning future care in the event (and only then) he becomes incompetent.

Also, part of it and, in the authors' opinion, extremely relevant is the appointment of a health care proxy, an agent (surrogate) to act on the patient's behalf should he become incompetent. This is the most effective way to guarantee that patient autonomy will be protected, even in cases not mentioned or predicted in the LW. Coaching surrogates on why dialysis is no longer an appropriate and useful treatment for a certain patient is key to helping them represent the patient [40].

3.3 Shared decision-making

The Renal Physicians Association (RPA) and the American Society of Nephrology (ASN), following the Institutes of Medicine's (IOM) recommendation [42], published the shared decision-making guideline, whose goal was to provide clinicians, patients, and families with the most current evidence about the benefits and burdens of dialysis for patients with diverse conditions, followed in 2010 by the second edition of this guideline, enriched by new evidence on outcomes of dialysis in different patient populations.

The shared decision-making guideline also proposes a structured approach to identifying, analyzing, and resolving ethical issues in clinical medicine. The four topics approach includes (a) Medical indications, (b) Patient preferences, (c) Quality of life, and (d) Contextual features. This approach incorporates in intricate relationships the ethical principles of (i) respect for patient autonomy, (ii) beneficence, (iii) nonmaleficence, (iv) distributive justice, and (v) professional integrity. These principles, not rarely, may conflict among them in individual cases [55].

Medical indications imply the consideration of the patient's diagnosis, disease progression, predictable prognosis, and treatment alternatives that interact with the ethical principles of beneficence, nonmaleficence, and professional integrity, this last one requiring the physician to refrain from providing dialysis when it is not medically indicated, that is. whenever the burdens of treatment substantially outweigh the benefits.

Regarding *patient preferences*, it is important to raise some key questions: What are the patient's goals? Did he receive sufficient information? Does he comprehend that information? If the patient lacks decision-making capacity, the nephrologist must decide who has the authority to decide on behalf of that patient. This point reflects the ethical principle of autonomy and how to protect it for those unable to exert it. There are high rates of disagreement among surveyed nephrologists about the management of incompetent patients without clear advance directives [56].

3.4 Respecting without enforcing autonomy

According to Singer and coworkers, what patients want at the end of life is: (i) receiving adequate pain and symptom management, (ii) avoiding inappropriate prolongation of dying, (iii) a feeling of control over their lives and decisions, (iv) not becoming a burden to their family, and (v) getting closer to their loved ones [57].

Modern medical ethics reflects the erosion of trust in the doctor-patient relationship because, in our clinical decisions, the autonomy model is replaced by the beneficence model. However, the irony is that these efforts to safeguard patient autonomy and offer protection against possible abuse have failed to reestablish trust [58–60].

Public trust in medicine has faltered despite successes, efforts to respect persons and their rights, and regulations to protect them. Why? The short answer is: contracts (such as informed consent) cannot be a substitute for beneficence and the trust accompanying it.

Unfortunately, in the large majority of scenarios, where we desperately need to share decisions with our patients, they have no capacity to exert their rights.

A patient's inability to complete a written advance directive or make an end-of-life decision does not alter the standards his healthcare provider must hold his surrogates to when making decisions on his behalf. Those standards include the patient's wishes, substituted judgment, and best interests.

So, the question stands. How to give autonomy to those who cannot use it? Moreover, never impose it on those who want to forgo their right. The answer to the first question is ACP/living wills/health care proxy, but unless formerly designated and properly coached, surrogate decision-makers are quite imperfect to represent patient's wishes. On the other hand, not every patient, or family member wants to participate in difficult decisions. In ICUs in France, more than 50% prefer to forgo autonomy [61].

To make things more difficult, patient preferences are not stable, rather evolve, as they get sicker and elder, so does their preference for a higher level of care [62].

3.5 Withholding and withdrawing dialysis

Dialysis can sustain life, but dialysis may also be viewed as merely a forestalling of death, a prolongation without progress for patients suffering many indignities. This dilemma highlights the need to emphasize clinically meaningful outcomes, the focus of which may be quality of life rather than quantity of survival. Technical success and availability of kidney replacement therapy (KRT) have blurred the distinction between the opportunity to extend life and the obligation to do so [63].

In its practice guidelines, the RPA identified some conditions in which it is ethical to withhold or withdraw dialysis, many of which were later incorporated in the KDIGO 2015 conference on supportive care in CKD [26].

Regarding withdrawal from dialysis, KDIGO states that this "is ethically and clinically acceptable after a process of shared decision making," however, not before all potentially remediable factors contributing to that decision, such as depression, pain, or other kind of suffering, as well as reversible social factors have been excluded, or properly addressed [26].

3.6 Legal implications of our ethical decisions

The definition of a competent patient has key legal implications in assessing our ethically guided decisions. The competent patient must fully understand: (i) the relevant clinical information provided, (ii) the possible consequences and outcomes of his clinical situation, (iii) and tell apart the different diagnostic and therapeutic options presented and also be able to communicate his decisions and choices [64].

Patients have the right to decline medical treatment after receiving a full explanation of the diagnosis, prognosis, and all appropriate treatment options for their case, or even to refuse to receive distressing clinical information or participate in shared decision-making [60].

According to the RPA guidelines, an explanation of treatment options should include: (i) available dialysis modalities, (ii) not starting dialysis and proceeding with conservative management, including palliative care, (iii) a time-limited trial of dialysis, and (iv) discontinuation of dialysis and receiving end-of-life care.

A time-limited trial is "an agreement between clinicians and patient/surrogate decision-makers to use medical therapies such as mechanical ventilation, enteral feeding, or dialysis over a defined period to determine if the patient improves or deteriorates according to predefined clinical outcomes" [65].

It is important to highlight that most published policy and research in the field of medical ethics in the end-of-life in dialysis patients has been conducted in the U.S. and other Anglo-Saxon countries [66–70]. In many other places, withdrawing has not always had the same legal value as withholding dialysis. The legal system and medical profession do not always recognize ACP and living wills, and local religion and culture may constitute important hurdles to modern ethics, as depicted in this chapter.

4. Quality standards for kidney care

4.1 The current model of kidney care

The current healthcare model for advanced chronic kidney disease (CKD) and end-stage kidney disease (ESKD) is primarily focused on optimizing dialysis care. That model, however, fails to support complex treatment decisions, such as starting or stopping dialysis, and it also overlooks the emotional and existential challenges faced by patients with advanced illnesses [2, 71]. Many patients with severe CKD and ESKD display unmet care needs, namely distressing symptoms and functional limitations [27]. Despite receiving costly and highly intensive end-of-life care, the quality of care in many cases is considered insufficient by their families [49].

To meet the needs of those gravely ill patients, it is proposed to integrate palliative care into their care plans [72, 73]. Kidney palliative care (KPC) is an interdisciplinary model of person-centered medicine that seeks to optimize health-related quality of life (HRQoL) and preserve human dignity through strategies. Among them are: (i) dedicated communication with patient and family, (ii) shared decision making, (iii) planning future health care/treatment, and (iii) management of pain as well as (iv) biopsychosocial and spiritual problems, including grief and proper end-of-life care [26].

In recent years, reimbursement models have incorporated incentives based on healthcare quality indicators (QI), which are based on international best practice guidelines [74–76]. Compensating healthcare units upon meeting specific QI values may be among those incentives.

In the United States and in some Europe healthcare systems, a range of QI have been used to integrate patient data related to kidney disease [77, 78].

Outcome measures (mortality, hospital readmission, and patient experience of care), intermediate outcome measures (dialysis adequacy and vascular access), process measures (blood transfusion), and safety measures (bloodstream infections and hypercalcemia) are examples of quality indicators suitable to aggregate patient data [79].

However, those metrics, according to Hayward, fail to offer a comprehensive evaluation of quality [80]. Intermediate outcomes can only provide useful measurements if they are directly linked to clinically outcomes.

Regarding palliative and end-of-life care, Holloway and Quill explore the significance of mortality as a QI. They argue that while mortality can be a suitable indicator for people with acute illnesses, who are not expected to survive, it is inadequate for those approaching end of their lives, suffering from several chronic illnesses [81].

Mortality may provide a reliable quality indicator for many people, but not for chronically ill people. This raises a critical question regarding quality measurements: "*Could some measures be adequate for some patients but not for others?*" Indeed, each patient initiating therapy has his own goals, and many issues may affect the ways patients make decisions about health care, even when the diseases are similar. They include age, frailty, genetics, life experiences, psychosocial anatomy, and differences intrinsic to each person, which are difficult to describe or measure. This leads to the questions "*In in a patient-centered care, should not the decisions and the patient's characteristics tell us what kind of care he wants?" and "Should quality measures be based on the patient individual characteristics?*" For example, a patient who initiates dialysis as part of a plan for end-of-life palliative care has goals different than others who begin the same treatment to extend his life.

Special attention should be paid to end-of-life care as the current care models for critically ill patients with advanced CKD and ESKD are still inadequate [82, 83]. The hospice care model, which is the most recognized palliative care model in Europe, Canada, and the United States, needs revision to meet the needs of those end-of-life patients [6, 84, 85].

Hospice care is primarily intended for terminally ill patients who choose to forgo curative treatment. However, eligibility criteria for hospice care restrict access for ESKD patients unless they discontinue dialysis or display a terminal condition unrelated to ESKD, which allows concurrent hospice and dialysis care [86]. Furthermore, the reimbursement structure s dialysis care over ambulatory palliative care, creating a financial incentive to initiate dialysis rather than choosing interdisciplinary palliative care [87, 88].

The lack of coordinated and meaningful advance care planning highlights the absence of a patient-centered care paradigm for patients with advanced CKD and ESKD. For that reason, few patients are engaged in advance care planning. The current emphasis on dialysis overlooks the opportunity to explore patient goals as part of the advanced care planning process [89]. In this way, the separation between dialysis decision-making and advance care planning can result in care misaligned with the patient preferences. Patients are left with limited choices or unaware of the different options available.

Additionally, dialysis patients rarely receive advance care planning, which leads to high use of intensive treatment in the phase nearing death [90].

To summarize, with the current ESKD quality and performance incentive structure the result is that health care in many cases is misaligned with patient-centered care [91].

Given the heterogeneity of the dialysis population, it becomes clear that one-size-fits-all should not be suitable. However, it is difficult to incentivize palliative care provision under the quality payment programe due to the lack of appropriate and individualized quality measures [92].

4.2 Toward more meaningful and sustainable kidney care models

During the past few years, a notable shift toward a healthcare model that emphasizes patient-centered approaches has occurred [93].

However, clinical guidelines are based solely on the evidenced-based paradigm, where populations are the primary focus rather than individuals [94]. Nevertheless, there is a growing awareness of the need to better align patient-valued quality metrics with clinical guidelines and with this purpose several strategies have been put forward, namely: (i) establishing quality measures that correspond to the priorities and preferences of the patients, (ii) strengthening access to palliative care, and (iii) incorporating routinely advanced care planning [72, 94–96].

4.2.1 Establishing quality measures that correspond to the priorities and preferences of patients

Incorporating patient-reported outcomes (PROs) and patient-centered care approaches that match patients' priorities and preferences is essential [97, 98]. This can be accomplished by developing and utilizing standard assessment tools that capture the unique needs, values, and goals of patients undergoing kidney palliative care. Involving patients in shared decision-making and care-planning processes guarantees that their priorities and preferences are properly valued [97].

Recently, it has been attempted to include patient-reported outcomes in the quality incentive program (QIP), such as pain and depression [83]. Although studies have highlighted the importance of integrating patient perspectives into palliative care quality measures, a debate about that topic is still missing [72, 83]. In assessing symptom burden and quality of life in patients receiving palliative care for advanced kidney disease, Davison S et al. identified the value of patient-reported outcomes [99].

4.2.2 Strengthening access to palliative care

Access to palliative care can be enhanced by using several approaches. Those include improving healthcare professionals' knowledge and skills in palliative care through education and training programs, implementing early identification and referral processes to ensure timely access, integrating palliative care into standard kidney care pathways, and addressing barriers such as misconceptions and limited resources.

Several studies have shown the effectiveness of those strategies in improving access to palliative care for kidney patients. For example, in the study by Wachterman et al. with patients displaying end-stage kidney disease, it was found that increased palliative care should be associated with higher likelihood of receiving hospice care and lower intensive care unit utilization rates [100]. Another study by *Davison et al.*

demonstrated that implementing a palliative care pathway for patients with advanced chronic kidney disease improved their access to supportive care services and led to better symptom management and patient satisfaction [26].

4.2.3 Integrating advance care planning

Advance care planning and the existence of advanced directives are crucial quality measures in kidney palliative care, facilitating patient-centered decision-making and honoring patients' end-of-life preferences [37].

Sudore et al. and Wright et al. have demonstrated that advance care planning and the use of advanced directives result in improved patient satisfaction, enhanced communication between patients and healthcare providers, and a higher likelihood of receiving care consistent with patients' wishes, leading to better end-of-life outcomes in the context of kidney disease [36].

5. Conclusions

In kidney care, it is critical to take a multifaceted approach to address the needs of patients and their families, especially in palliative care. Healthcare providers must have the education and training to provide appropriate care while addressing ethical issues, such as end-of-life decisions and cultural and spiritual considerations. Quality indicators are important and is equally important to understand what quality renal palliative care really incorporates. By addressing education, ethics, and quality measurements, a comprehensive approach can be developed for KPC that responds to the unique needs of this patient population. Collaboration and communication among healthcare providers, patients, families, and stakeholders are crucial to ensure that kidney palliative care is evidence-based, patient-centered, and of the highest quality.

Author details

Ana Mateus[1*] and Pedro Ponce[2]

1 Hospital Cruz Vermelha, Lisboa, Portugal

2 NephroCare Portugal, Portugal

*Address all correspondence to: anaamateus@yahoo.com

References

[1] Wańkowicz Z. The role of technological progress vs. accidental discoveries and clinical experience in the evolution of dialysis. Medical Science Monitor. 2013;**19**:984-992. DOI: 10.12659/MSM.889710

[2] Luyckx VA, Tonelli M, Stanifer JW. The global burden of kidney disease and the sustainable development goals. Bulletin of the World Health Organization. 2018;**96**(6):414-422C. DOI: 10.2471/BLT.17.206441

[3] Gelfand SL, Schell J, Eneanya ND. Palliative care in nephrology: The work and the workforce. Advances in Chronic Kidney Disease. Jul 2020;**27**(4):350-355. e1. DOI: 10.1053/j.ackd.2020.02.007

[4] Connor S. Global Atlas of Palliative Care. 2nd ed. 2020

[5] Connor S, Sepulveda C. The Global Atlas of Palliative Care at the End of Life. 2014

[6] Lam DY, Scherer JS, Brown M, Grubbs V, Schell JO. A conceptual framework of palliative care across the continuum of advanced kidney disease. Clinical Journal of the American Society of Nephrology. 2019;**14**(4):635-641. DOI: 10.2215/CJN.09330818

[7] Davison SN, Jassal SV. Supportive care: Integration of patient-centered kidney care to manage symptoms and geriatric syndromes. Clinical Journal of the American Society of Nephrology. 2016;**11**(10):1882-1891. DOI: 10.2215/CJN.01050116

[8] Powell RA, Mwangi-Powell FN, Radbruch L, et al. Putting palliative care on the global health agenda. The Lancet Oncology. 2015;**16**(2):131-133. DOI: 10.1016/S1470-2045(15)70002-1

[9] Centeno C, Garralda E, Carrasco JM, et al. The palliative care challenge: Analysis of barriers and opportunities to integrate palliative care in Europe in the view of national associations. Journal of Palliative Medicine. 2017;**20**(11):1195-1204. DOI: 10.1089/jpm.2017.0039

[10] Hawley P. Barriers to access to palliative care. Palliative Care: Research and Treatment. 1 Jan 2017;**10**:117822421668888. DOI: 10.1177/1178224216688887

[11] Elsner F, Centeno C, Ellershaw JE. Early integration needs early education. Palliative Medicine. 2016;**30**(9):805-806. DOI: 10.1177/0269216316664455

[12] Callaway MV, Connor SR, Foley KM. World Health Organization public health model: A roadmap for palliative care development. Journal of Pain and Symptom Management. 2018;**55**(2):S6-S13. DOI: 10.1016/j.jpainsymman.2017.03.030

[13] Gamondi C, Larkin P, Payne S. Core competencies in palliative care: An EAPC white paper on palliative care education - Part 1. European Journal of Palliative Care. 2013;**20**:86-91

[14] Rawlinson F, Finlay I. Assessing education in palliative medicine: Development of a tool based on the Association for Palliative Medicine core curriculum. Palliative Medicine. 2002;**16**(1):51-55. DOI: 10.1191/0269216302pm508oa

[15] Moss AH, Armistead NC. Improving end-of-life care for ESRD patients: An initiative for professionals. Nephrology News & Issues. 2013;**27**(10):30-32

[16] Holley JL, Davison SN, Moss AH. Nephrologists' changing practices in

reported end-of-life decision-making. Clinical Journal of the American Society of Nephrology. 2007;**2**(1):107-111. DOI: 10.2215/CJN.03080906

[17] Davison SN, Jhangri GS, Holley JL, Moss AH. Nephrologists' reported preparedness for end-of-life decision-making. Clinical Journal of the American Society of Nephrology. 2006;**1**(6):1256-1262. DOI: 10.2215/CJN.02040606

[18] Cohen LM, Moss AH, Weisbord SD, Germain MJ. Renal palliative care. Journal of Palliative Medicine. 2006;**9**(4):977-992. DOI: 10.1089/jpm.2006.9.977

[19] Gutmann A. Safeguarding children—Pediatric research on medical countermeasures. New England Journal of Medicine. 2013;**368**(13):1171-1173. DOI: 10.1056/nejmp1302093

[20] Carroll T, Weisbrod N, O'Connor A, Quill T. Primary palliative care education: A pilot survey. American Journal of Hospice and Palliative Medicine. 2018;**35**(4):565-569. DOI: 10.1177/1049909117723618

[21] Quérin S, Clermont MJ, Dupré-Goudable C, Dalmon P. Physician-patient communication in nephrology. Nephrologie et Therapeutique. 2011;**7**(4):201-206. DOI: 10.1016/j.nephro.2011.01.009

[22] Moss AH, Holley JL, Davison SN, et al. Palliative care. American Journal of Kidney Diseases. 2004;**43**(1):172-185. DOI: 10.1053/j.ajkd.2003.12.009

[23] Wachterman MW, Marcantonio ER, Davis RB, et al. Relationship between the prognostic expectations of seriously ill patients undergoing hemodialysis and their nephrologists. JAMA Internal Medicine. 2013;**173**(13):1206-1214. DOI: 10.1001/jamainternmed.2013.6036

[24] Cohen LM, Ruthazer R, Moss AH, Germain MJ. Predicting six-month mortality for patients who are on maintenance hemodialysis. Clinical Journal of the American Society of Nephrology. 2010;**5**(1):72-79. DOI: 10.2215/CJN.03860609

[25] Couchoud C, Labeeuw M, Moranne O, et al. A clinical score to predict 6-month prognosis in elderly patients starting dialysis for end-stage renal disease. Nephrology Dialysis Transplantation. 2009;**24**(5):1553-1561. DOI: 10.1093/ndt/gfn698

[26] Davison S, Levin A, Moss A, Jha V, Brown E, Brennan F, et al. Executive summary of the KDIGO Controversies Conference on Supportive Care in Chronic Kidney Disease: Developing a roadmap to improving quality care. Kidney International. 2015;**88**. DOI: 10.1038/ki.2015.110

[27] Murphy EL, Murtagh FEM, Carey I, Sheerin NS. Understanding symptoms in patients with advanced chronic kidney disease managed without dialysis: Use of a short patient-completed assessment tool. Nephron. Clinical Practice. 2009;**111**(1):c74-c80. DOI: 10.1159/000183177

[28] Raj R, Ahuja K, Frandsen M, Murtagh FEM, Jose M. Validation of the IPOS-renal symptom survey in advanced kidney disease: A cross-sectional study. Journal of Pain and Symptom Management. 2018;**56**(2):281-287. DOI: 10.1016/j.jpainsymman.2018.04.006

[29] Davison SN, Jhangri GS, Johnson JA. Longitudinal validation of a modified Edmonton symptom assessment system (ESAS) in haemodialysis patients. Nephrology Dialysis Transplantation. 2006;**21**(11):3189-3195. DOI: 10.1093/ndt/gfl380

[30] Tan G, Jensen MP, Thornby JI, Shanti BF. Validation of the brief pain inventory for chronic nonmalignant pain. Journal of Pain. 2004;**5**(2):133-137. DOI: 10.1016/j.jpain.2003.12.005

[31] Kwame A, Petrucka PM. A literature-based study of patient-centered care and communication in nurse-patient interactions: Barriers, facilitators, and the way forward. BMC Nursing. 2021;**20**(1):158. DOI: 10.1186/s12912-021-00684-2

[32] Baile WF, Buckman R, Lenzi R, Glober G, Beale EA, Kudelka AP. SPIKES—A six-step protocol for delivering bad news: Application to the patient with cancer. The Oncologist. 2000;**5**(4):302-311. DOI: 10.1634/theoncologist.5-4-302

[33] Bernacki RE, Block SD. Communication about serious illness care goals: A review and synthesis of best practices. JAMA Internal Medicine. 2014;**174**(12):1994-2003. DOI: 10.1001/jamainternmed.2014.5271

[34] Holley JL, Carmody SS, Moss AH, et al. The need for end-of-life care training in nephrology: National survey results of nephrology fellows. American Journal of Kidney Diseases. 2003;**42**(4):813-820. DOI: 10.1016/s0272-6386(03)00868-0

[35] Russell JSC, Oliverio A, Paulus A. Barriers to conservative management conversations: Perceptions of nephrologists and fellows-in-training. Journal of Palliative Medicine. 2021;**24**(10):1497-1504. DOI: 10.1089/jpm.2020.0690

[36] Sudore RL, Lum HD, You JJ, et al. Defining advance care planning for adults: A consensus definition from a multidisciplinary Delphi panel. Journal of Pain and Symptom Management. 2017;**53**(5):821-832.e1. DOI: 10.1016/j.jpainsymman.2016.12.331

[37] O'Halloran P, Noble H, Norwood K, et al. Advance care planning with patients who have end-stage kidney disease: A systematic realist review. Journal of Pain and Symptom Management. 2018;**56**(5):795-807.e18. DOI: 10.1016/j.jpainsymman.2018.07.008

[38] Akdeniz M, Yardımcı B, Kavukcu E. Ethical considerations at the end-of-life care. SAGE Open Medicine. Jan 2021;**9**:205031212110009. DOI: 10.1177/20503121211000918

[39] Hui D, Nooruddin Z, Didwaniya N, et al. Concepts and definitions for "actively dying," "end of life," "terminally ill," "terminal care," and "transition of care": A systematic review. Journal of Pain and Symptom Management. 2014;**47**(1):77-89. DOI: 10.1016/j.jpainsymman.2013.02.021

[40] Green R. Ethical Considerations. 2014. DOI: 10.1016/B978-0-12-409503-8.00040-8

[41] Yu X, Nakayama M, Wu MS, et al. Shared decision-making for a dialysis modality. Kidney International Reports. 2022;**7**(1):15-27. DOI: 10.1016/j.ekir.2021.10.019

[42] Renal Physicians Association. Shared Decision-Making in the Appropriate Initiation of and Withdrawal from Dialysis. Rockville, Maryland, USA: Renal Physicians Association; 2010. Available from: www.renalmd.org

[43] Galla JH. Clinical practice guideline on shared decision-making in the appropriate initiation of and withdrawal from dialysis. Journal of the American Society of Nephrology. July 2000;**11**(7):1340-1342. DOI: 10.1681/asn.v1171340

[44] Murtagh FEM, Burns A, Moranne O, Morton RL, Naicker S. Supportive care: Comprehensive conservative care in

end-stage kidney disease. Clinical Journal of the American Society of Nephrology. 2016;**11**(10):1909-1914. DOI: 10.2215/CJN.04840516

[45] Carson RC, Juszczak M, Davenport A, Burns A. Is maximum conservative management an equivalent treatment option to dialysis for elderly patients with significant comorbid disease? Clinical Journal of the American Society of Nephrology. 2009;**4**(10):1611-1619. DOI: 10.2215/CJN.00510109

[46] Wong SPY, Kreuter W, O'Hare AM. Healthcare intensity at initiation of chronic dialysis among older adults. Journal of the American Society of Nephrology. 2014;**25**(1):143-149. DOI: 10.1681/ASN.2013050491

[47] Kurella Tamura M, Covinsky KE, Chertow GM, Yaffe K, Seth Landefeld C, McCulloch CE. Functional status of elderly adults before and after initiation of dialysis. The New England Journal of Medicine. 2009;**61**(16):1539-1547

[48] Russ AJ, Kaufman SR. Discernment rather than decision-making among elderly dialysis patients. Seminars in Dialysis. 2012;**25**(1):31-32. DOI: 10.1111/j.1525-139X.2011.01047.x

[49] Davison SN. End-of-life care preferences and needs: Perceptions of patients with chronic kidney disease. Clinical Journal of the American Society of Nephrology. 2010;5(2):195-204. DOI: 10.2215/CJN.05960809

[50] Arnold RM, Zeidel ML. Dialysis in frail elders—A role for palliative care. The New England Journal of Medicine. 2009;**16**:1597-1598

[51] Moss AH, Hozayen O, King K, Holley JL, Schmidt RJ. Attitudes of patients toward cardiopulmonary resuscitation in the dialysis unit. American Journal of Kidney Diseases. 2001;**38**(4):847-852. DOI: 10.1053/ajkd.2001.27705

[52] Levinsky NG. Age as a criterion for rationing health care. New England Journal of Medicine. 21 Jun 1990;**322**(25):1813-1816. DOI: 10.1056/nejm199006213222512

[53] USRDS 2006 ADR: Chronic kidney disease. American Journal of Kidney Diseases. Jan 2007;**49**:S47-S66. DOI: 10.1053/j.ajkd.2006.11.006

[54] Post LF, Blustein J. Handbook for Health Care Ethics Committees. JHU Press; 30 Jun 2015

[55] Jonsen AR, Siegler M, Winslade WJ. Clinical Ethics: A Practical Approach to Ethical Decisions in Clinical Medicine, 9th Ed. McGraw Hill Professional. 17 Dec 2021

[56] Singer PA, Thiel EC, David Naylor C, et al. Life-sustaining treatment preferences of hemodialysis patients: Implications for advance directives. Journal of the American Society of Nephrology. 1995;**6**:1410-1417. Available from: http://journals.lww.com/jasn

[57] Singer PA, Martin DK, Kelner M. Quality end-of-life care patients' perspectives. JAMA. 1999;**281**:163-168. Available from: www.jama.com

[58] Pellegrino ED, Thomasma DC. The conflict between autonomy and beneficence in medical the conflict between autonomy and beneficence in medical ethics: Proposal for a resolution ethics: Proposal for a resolution. The Journal of Contemporary Health Law and Policy. 1985;**3**:23-46. Available from: https://scholarship.law.edu/jchlp/vol3/iss1/7

[59] Dardis A, Gefter WI, Manahan WD, McIntyre RL, Pellegrino ED, Wolfson EA.

Medical ethics: Plain talk about ethics in practice. Patient Care. 1978;**12**(5):186-188, 190, 192+

[60] Varkey B. Principles of clinical ethics and their application to practice. Medical Principles and Practice. 2021;**30**(1):17-28. DOI: 10.1159/000509119

[61] Azoulay É, Pochard F, Chevret S, et al. Half the family members of intensive care unit patients do not want to share in the decision-making process: A study in 78 French intensive care units. Critical Care Medicine. 2004;**32**(9):1832-1838. DOI: 10.1097/01.CCM.0000139693.88931.59

[62] Ostermann M. Cardiac arrests in hemodialysis patients: An ongoing challenge. Kidney International. 2008;**73**(8):907-908. DOI: 10.1038/ki.2008.40

[63] Schmidt RJ. Informing our elders about dialysis: Is an age-attuned approach warranted? Clinical Journal of the American Society of Nephrology. 2012;**7**(1):185-191. DOI: 10.2215/CJN.10401011

[64] Ganzini L, Volicer L, Nelson WA, Fox E, Derse AR. Ten myths about decision-making capacity. Journal of the American Medical Directors Association. 2005;**6**(3):S100-S104. DOI: 10.1016/j.jamda.2005.03.021

[65] Chung GS, Lawrence RE, Curlin FA, Arora V, Meltzer DO. Predictors of hospitalised patients' preferences for physician-directed medical decision-making. Journal of Medical Ethics. 2012;**38**(2):77-82. DOI: 10.1136/jme.2010.040618

[66] Luyckx VA, Martin DE, Moosa MR, et al. Developing the ethical framework of end-stage kidney disease care: From practice to policy. Kidney International Supplements (2011). 2020;**10**(1):e72-e77. DOI: 10.1016/j.kisu.2019.11.003

[67] Canadian Medical Association. Code of ethics: CMA policy summary. CMAJ. 1987;**137**(8):760A-760D

[68] Chamber of Physicians (Poland). The code of medical ethics. Kennedy Institute of Ethics Journal. 1992;**2**(4):371-384. DOI: 10.1353/ken.0.0058

[69] Feely MA, Albright RC, Thorsteinsdottir B, Moss AH, Swetz KM. Ethical challenges with hemodialysis patients who lack decision-making capacity: Behavioral issues, surrogate decision-makers, and end-of-life situations. Kidney International. 2014;**86**(3):475-480. DOI: 10.1038/ki.2014.231

[70] Murtagh FEM, Marsh JE, Donohoe P, Ekbal NJ, Sheerin NS, Harris FE. Dialysis or not? A comparative survival study of patients over 75 years with chronic kidney disease stage 5. Nephrology Dialysis Transplantation. 2007;**22**(7):1955-1962. DOI: 10.1093/ndt/gfm153

[71] Bristowe K, Horsley HL, Shepherd K, et al. Thinking ahead-the need for early advance care planning for people on haemodialysis: A qualitative interview study. Palliative Medicine. 2015;**29**(5):443-450. DOI: 10.1177/0269216314560209

[72] Kurella Tamura M, Meier DE. Five policies to promote palliative care for patients with ESRD. Clinical Journal of the American Society of Nephrology. 2013;**8**(10):1783-1790. DOI: 10.2215/CJN.02180213

[73] O'Hare AM, Armistead N, Funk Schrag WL, Diamond L, Moss AH. Patient-centered care: An opportunity to accomplish the "three aims" of the national

quality strategy in the medicare ESRD program. Clinical Journal of the American Society of Nephrology. 2014;**9**(12):2189-2194. DOI: 10.2215/CJN.01930214

[74] Hogan M. ESRD quality incentive program a cautious first pass at pay-for-performance. Nephrology Times. Jan 2011;**4**(1):1. DOI: 10.1097/01.nep.0000394216.40483.60

[75] Coelho AP, Sá HO, Diniz JA, Dussault G. The integrated management for renal replacement therapy in Portugal. Hemodialysis International. 2014;**18**(1):175-184. DOI: 10.1111/hdi.12064

[76] Finalized PY 2018 Clinical Measure Kt/V Dialysis Adequacy Measure Topic: Peritoneal Dialysis Peritoneal Dialysis Adequacy Clinical Performance Measure III-Delivered Dose of Peritoneal Dialysis Above Minimum Higher Rate Desired Measure Description

[77] Mendes A. The KDIGO roadmap to improving care in chronic kidney disease. Journal of Kidney Care. 2 Nov 2016;**1**(4):205-205. DOI: 10.12968/jokc.2016.1.4.205

[78] National Kidney Foundation. K/DOQI clinical practice guidelines for chronic kidney disease: Evaluation, classification, and stratification. American Journal of Kidney Diseases: The Official Journal of the National Kidney Foundation. 2002;**39**(2 Suppl 1):S1-S266

[79] Kliger AS. Quality measures for dialysis. Clinical Journal of the American Society of Nephrology. Feb 2016;**11**(2):363-368. DOI: 10.2215/cjn.06010615

[80] Smith KA, Hayward RA. Performance measurement in chronic kidney disease. Journal of the American Society of Nephrology. 2011;**22**(2):225-234. DOI: 10.1681/ASN.2010111152

[81] Holloway RG, Quill TE. Mortality as a measure of quality implications for palliative and end-of-life care. JAMA. 2007;**298**(7):802-804. Available from: http://www.nhpco.org/files/public/2005-facts-and-figures.pdf

[82] Chen SS, Unruh M, Williams M. In quality we trust; but quality of life or quality of care? Seminars in Dialysis. 2016;**29**(2):103-110. DOI: 10.1111/sdi.12470

[83] Moss AH, Davison SN. How the ESRD quality incentive program could potentially improve quality of life for patients on dialysis. Clinical Journal of the American Society of Nephrology. 2015;**10**(5):888-893. DOI: 10.2215/CJN.07410714

[84] Mathews J, Hannon B, Zimmermann C. Models of integration of specialized palliative care with oncology. Current Treatment Options in Oncology. 2021;**22**(5):44. DOI: 10.1007/s11864-021-00836-1

[85] Grubbs V, Moss AH, Cohen LM, et al. A palliative approach to dialysis care: A patient-centered transition to the end of life. Clinical Journal of the American Society of Nephrology. 2014;**9**(12):2203-2209. DOI: 10.2215/CJN.00650114

[86] Schell JO, Johnson DS. Challenges with providing hospice care for patients undergoing longterm dialysis. Clinical Journal of the American Society of Nephrology. 2021;**16**(3):473-475. DOI: 10.2215/CJN.10710720

[87] Grubbs V, Tuot DS, Powe NR, O'Donoghue D, Chesla CA. System-level barriers and facilitators for foregoing or withdrawing dialysis: A qualitative study of nephrologists in the United States and England. American Journal of Kidney Diseases. 2017;**70**(5):602-610. DOI: 10.1053/j.ajkd.2016.12.015

[88] Tamura MK, Montez-Rath ME, Hall YN, Katz R, O'Hare AM. Advance directives and end-of-life care among nursing home residents receiving maintenance dialysis. Clinical Journal of the American Society of Nephrology. 2017;**12**(3):435-442. DOI: 10.2215/CJN.07510716

[89] Song MK, Lin FC, Gilet CA, Arnold RM, Bridgman JC, Ward SE. Patient perspectives on informed decision-making surrounding dialysis initiation. Nephrology Dialysis Transplantation. 2013;**28**(11):2815-2823. DOI: 10.1093/ndt/gft238

[90] Eneanya ND, Hailpern SM, O'Hare AM, et al. Trends in receipt of intensive procedures at the end of life among patients treated with maintenance dialysis. American Journal of Kidney Diseases. 2017;**69**(1):60-68. DOI: 10.1053/j.ajkd.2016.07.028

[91] Kliger AS. Quality measures for dialysis: Time for a balanced scorecard. Clinical Journal of the American Society of Nephrology. 2016;**11**(2):363-368. DOI: 10.2215/CJN.06010615

[92] Evangelidis N, Tong A, Manns B, et al. Developing a set of Core outcomes for trials in hemodialysis: An international Delphi survey. American Journal of Kidney Diseases. 2017;**70**(4):464-475. DOI: 10.1053/j.ajkd.2016.11.029

[93] Mead N, Bower P. Patient-centredness: A conceptual framework and review of the empirical literature. Social Science & Medicine. 2000;**51**(7):1087-1110. Available from: www.elsevier.com/locate/socscimed

[94] O'Hare AM, Rodriguez RA, Bowling CB. Caring for patients with kidney disease: Shifting the paradigm from evidence-based medicine to patient-centered care. Nephrology Dialysis Transplantation. 2016;**31**(3):368-375. DOI: 10.1093/ndt/gfv003

[95] Tamura MK, Goldstein MK, Pérez-Stable EJ. Preferences for dialysis withdrawal and engagement in advance care planning within a diverse sample of dialysis patients. Nephrology Dialysis Transplantation. 2010;**25**(1):237-242. DOI: 10.1093/ndt/gfp430

[96] O'Hare AM, Song MK, Kurella Tamura M, Moss AH. Research priorities for palliative care for older adults with advanced chronic kidney disease. Journal of Palliative Medicine. 2017;**20**(5):453-460. DOI: 10.1089/jpm.2016.0571

[97] Umeukeje EM, Nair D, Fissell RB, Cavanaugh KL. Incorporating patient-reported outcomes (PROs) into dialysis policy: Current initiatives, challenges, and opportunities. Seminars in Dialysis. 2020;**33**(1):18-25. DOI: 10.1111/sdi.12854

[98] Lavallee DC, Chenok KE, Love RM, Petersen C, Holve E, Segal CD, et al. Incorporating patient-reported outcomes into health care to engage patients and enhance care. Health Affairs. Apr 2016;**35**(4):575-582. DOI: 10.1377/hlthaff.2015.1362

[99] Davison SN, Klarenbach S, Manns B, et al. Patient-reported outcome measures in the care of in-centre hemodialysis patients. Journal of Patient-Reported Outcomes. 2021;**5**:93. DOI: 10.1186/s41687-021-00365-3

[100] Wachterman MW, Hailpern SM, Keating NL, Tamura MK, O'Hare AM. Association between hospice length of stay, health care utilization, and medicare costs at the end of life among patients who received maintenance hemodialysis. JAMA Internal Medicine. 2018;**178**(6):792-799. DOI: 10.1001/jamainternmed.2018.0256

Chapter 12

Comprehensive Insights into Palliative Nephrology: A Chapter in Contemporary Renal Medicine

Asad Merchant and Adel Moideen

Abstract

Chronic Kidney disease (CKD) is a global epidemic, affecting more than 800 million people worldwide. Advanced CKD patients experience a substantial symptom burden, compromising their Health-Related Quality of Life. It is crucial for healthcare practitioners to understand the palliative needs of CKD patients, and participate in Advance Care Planning (ACP) and shared decision-making, aligning medical care with patients' preferences and values. Prognostication tools can help identify those unsuitable for dialysis, leading to consideration of conservative kidney management (CKM), prioritizing supportive care over invasive interventions. Early palliative care referral improves symptom control, patient satisfaction, and goal-concordant care. Symptom management is an important consideration and requires careful consideration of drug dosing and toxicities due to impaired renal function. Dialysis, while extending life, may exacerbate patient suffering; optimizing comfort-oriented therapy can enhance quality of life. End-of-life care, including dialysis withdrawal and hospice care, is a key feature of palliative nephrology, but ethical dilemmas and cultural context must be carefully considered. With an aging CKD population, nephrologists will need to integrate palliative care principles into routine kidney care. This will include improving confidence and competence in providing palliative renal care, and implementing system-level changes to remove barriers to effective palliation and end-of-life care.

Keywords: palliative nephrology, chronic kidney disease (CKD), conservative kidney management (CKM), symptom management, end-of-life care

1. Introduction

Chronic kidney disease (CKD) has become a global epidemic, affecting more than 800 million people [1]. More than 2 million people worldwide receive dialysis [2], with incidence of dialysis disproportionately higher in the older age groups [3, 4]. While advances in medical therapies has improved outcomes related to CKD, having renal disease confers significant morbidity and mortality. In the past few decades, CKD has emerged as a leading cause of death worldwide [5]. Patients on dialysis have mortality rates approximately 6–8 times higher than that of the general population [6]. The overall prognosis for stage 5 CKD (Estimated Glomerular Filtration

Rate (eGFR) less than 15 ml/min/1.73 m^2) can be worse than that for patients with acquired immunodeficiency syndrome (AIDS) or cancer [7].

Patients with advanced CKD have heavy symptom burdens, including uremic symptoms, as well as those related to metabolic bone disease, cardiovascular disease, heart failure, polypharmacy, and the dialysis treatments themselves [8]. Comorbid conditions have powerful deleterious impacts on patients' health-related quality of life (HRQoL) [9]. It is important for health care practitioners to develop knowledge of the palliative needs of CKD patients, including advance care planning (ACP), prognosis of CKD, risks and benefits of proposed treatments such as dialysis and end- of- life (EOL) care.

2. Conservative kidney management

2.1 Trajectory of CKD

Kidney disease progression occurs asymptomatically, only evident by eGFR decline. The eGFR is an important prognostic marker of risk of developing end stage kidney disease (ESKD), as well as risk of death and morbidity [10], however it loses some of its predictive ability in older patients[11], who are at most risk of increased frailty, multi-morbidity, and being exposed to aggressive therapies with limited benefit. Sicker patients may experience more rapid deterioration of GFR, with more frequent hospitalizations [11]. Each acute event experienced increases the risk of functional decline, and may eventually lead to transformation into frailty trajectory with need for institutionalization, and a switch towards palliative care philosophy [12]. The risk of developing ESKD may be highest around this transition, and may require important and difficult conversations with patients and their families about the benefits and risks of renal replacement therapies. The converse is also true; transitioning to ESKD can cause marked frailty. Tamura *et al* demonstrated a sharp decline in functional independence in elderly patients starting dialysis [13]. Only 13% of the sampled cohort maintained their functional status after 1 year. Similarly Jassal *et al* demonstrated marked loss of independence in patients starting dialysis after the age of 80 [14]. Acute illness events can serve as triggers for ACP conversations: a patient's evolving experience of illness may be leveraged to align their expressed goals of care to the realities of their CKD. Without such experiences, patients and families are left in an unenviable situation of having to choose from abstract therapies with limited context. Regardless of whether patients choose to pursue renal replacement therapy, or a conservative (non dialytic) kidney management (CKM), there is usually an inflection point towards the end of their life at which point patients will experience an inexorable worsening of health unmitigated by disease specific therapies [15].

2.2 Conservative care pathways for CKD

Conservative Kidney Management (CKM) is a treatment approach for stage 5 CKD (estimated glomerular filtration rate (eGFR) below 15 mL/min/1.73 m^2), aimed at delivering kidney supportive care to manage renal disease symptoms and complications without pursuing dialysis or transplantation. While CKD is associated with tremendous mortality risk, treatment with renal replacement therapy (e.g. dialysis) can be of limited benefit, especially in older patients with multiple co-morbidities and high baseline frailty [16]. Such patients may have median survival of no greater than 2–3 years after initiation of dialysis, and much of that may be spent hospitalized. Patients may experience increased functional dependence, institutionalization, and cognitive decline and a decrease in quality of life after reaching ESKD [13]. In older patients with multiple co-morbid conditions, there is little if any survival advantage to choosing a dialytic pathway [13, 17].

Conservative non-dialytic kidney management is, thus, a viable option for certain patients whose goals of care do not align with aggressive life sustaining measures such as dialysis. It is important that health care providers in nephrology participate discuss goals of care with patients, and educate patients about the risks and benefits of the different options available to patients upon reaching ESKD, including renal replacement therapy (RRT) and CKM [18]. Patients should have a complete understanding of what life on dialysis entails, in terms of not only survival, but also its effect on their quality of life. On the other hand, patients, for whom CKM is recommended, should know that their overall survival may be impacted by foregoing dialysis, and what end of life care entails.

Patients that are well educated about end stage kidney disease and are invited to share in the decision making with their families and the nephrology team are more less likely to have decisional regret and have a stronger relationship with the medical team [19].

Patients who choose CKM do not always end up foregoing dialysis; reasons for decisional switch include family influences, worsening symptoms including fluid overload that are refractory to medical management, or decisional regret. For some patients it may be a consequence of poor communication about CKM early on in the education process [20]. It is also possible that some may not be able to foresee the implications of their decision and may conflate CKM with the expression of their desire to avoid dialysis. In other cases, deferring the decision of choosing a RRT modality may be a maladaptive coping mechanism to deal with their progressive chronic kidney disease diagnosis. There is a paucity of literature to help understand the reasons for changing decisions, but there may be an increased rate of acute hospital-based dialysis starts in this population, which the literature has shown leads to poorer outcomes [21]. CKM patients tend to spend less time in the hospital compared to those on dialysis [22, 23]. CKM offers opportunities for more effective symptom management, palliative care, and hospice services.

2.3 Shared decision making and advanced care planning (ACP)

Shared decision-making is the cornerstone of kidney supportive care; it involves information giving, discussing prognosis, and advanced care planning (ACP). The care plan must be attuned to the patient's needs and perspective, accommodating their lifestyle, family, community, and cultural beliefs. This involves allowing patients to prioritize medical care components most important to them, balancing symptom management and quality of life with long-term survival [24, 25]. ACP involves understanding and sharing personal values, life goals, and medical care preferences It is imperative that these discussions happen in a sensitive manner; for patients, the idea of losing their kidney function is naturally distressing [26]. Using a framework for communication that helps to prepare patients for receiving bad news can be helpful, and it is important to ensure that the patient is well supported [27]. There is ample evidence that patients wish to be well informed about the trajectory and prognosis of their condition [28]; nephrologists will need to be prepared to be able to accurately prognosticate, and incorporate objective and subjective measures of the individual in front of them to provide an estimation of the survival and HRQoL impacts. ACP should be integrated into routine kidney care, and ideally readdressed as the illness progresses, normalizing the process.

One particular tool may be the use of the best-case/ worst-case scenario framework, which is increasing being used in the surgical and palliative fields [29]. Patients are provided with the best-case scenario, the worst-case scenario and the most likely scenarios of starting dialysis or not; this helps provide a spectrum of possible outcomes, giving the patients a deeper understanding of what life with or without dialysis entails instead of an abstract picture.

Unfortunately, many dialysis providers do not feel comfortable addressing end of life issues [30]. This is counter to the evidence that dialysis patients have clear preferences about end of life care [31]. Similarly, many nephrologists do not feel comfortable discussing conservative models of kidney care where dialysis may be deferred in those with limited life expectancy, poor functional status (frail, institutionalized), or those whose preferred goals of care do not include renal replacement therapy [32].

2.4 Prognostication

Prognostication is a key element in the shared decision-making process and advanced care planning. Having knowledge of the trajectory of disease in CKD and the factors that predict poor outcomes in CKD or ESKD allow nephrologists to identify those individuals who may benefit from a palliative approach to CKD. With the help of prognostic tools, the nephrologist can provide realistic expectations to the patients allowing them and their families to make a more informed decision about their plans. Patients with a likelihood of limited survival would also benefit from a more timely referral to palliative care services. Prognostication tools can be useful in identifying those who would not necessarily benefit from dialysis. Studies have shown that patients over 75 with eGFR <15 $ml/min/1.73m^2$ and with multiple comorbidities who have chosen to dialysis if they reach ESKD do not fare much better than those who opt for a conservative care pathway [17, 33].

Certain risk factors such as age, serum albumin, functional status, and co-morbidities predict poor outcomes on dialysis [34]. The Charlson comorbidity index (CCI) has also been shown to have some predictive ability, with a score of ≥ 8 signifying an approximately 50% one year mortality rate [35, 36].

One relatively simple yet effective tool that is used extensively by palliative specialists is the "surprise question (SQ)": "Would you be surprised if this patient were to die in the next 12 months?" It has been validated and prevents overestimation of survival prognosis [37]. The SQ has been shown to identify dialysis patients with lower functional status scores, higher co-morbidity scores and who are 3.5x more likely to die in the next year [37]. Cohen *et al* combined more traditional risk factors with the surprise question to create an integrated prognostic tool, this includes age, serum albumin, PVD, dementia and the surprise question to predict one year mortality in maintenance hemodialysis patients [38]. More investigations are required to determine its predictive accuracy, and its performance in peritoneal dialysis patients is uncertain [38].

Using the French Renal Epidemiology and Information Network (REIN) database, Couchoud *et al* developed a model for incident dialysis patients [39]. It integrated measures of function (dependence for transfers), nutritional metrics

(BMI) and comorbidities to predict 6-month mortality rates. There are similar tools developed for patients with CKD IV and V that estimate 6 month and 12-month mortality. One such calculator was developed by Schmidt *et al* (2019) that uses a modified Karnofsky scale as a measure of functionality, as well as the SQ and age [40]. The authors found that subjective measures were more discriminating than objective values like albumin, although bias from potential variability in how providers assessed patients could not be excluded. The data set for developing the model was also limited; important variables such as albuminuria could not be captured [40].

2.5 Role of palliative care in nephrology

Palliative care addresses physical, psychological, social, spiritual, and existential needs of serious illness patients, aiming to enhance quality of life by alleviating suffering and managing symptoms [41]. A palliative philosophy of kidney care places equal emphasis on both symptom management and life extension, and it can be instrumental in providing holistic patient centered care. In order to provide such care optimally, this philosophy needs to be integrated within the overall structure of nephrology practice. The key components of kidney palliative care include Advanced care planning, pain and symptoms management, end of life care and bereavement support [42]. A palliative philosophy is not exclusive to CKM patients, but also relevant in patients whose goals of care include dialysis.

Partnerships with palliative care services help bridge the transition to end of life care without acute crises. Early or timely referral to palliative care may be the best way to facilitate a smooth transition from CKD stage V to ESKD without inflicting emotional or physical suffering on the patient (usually via unnecessary hospitalizations, and aggressive medical interventions such as surgical procedures in acute settings) [43]. This is associated with higher patient satisfaction, and improved control of symptoms with overall more goal concordant care [43]. It may also provide support to the patients with respect to existential dread and grief as they approach end of life.

Including palliative care experts in goals of care conversations can be very important, and helpful in exploring advanced care planning and end of life transitions. Creating a plan and aligning patients' expectations with illness progression can ensure seamless transitions, avoiding unnecessary hospitalizations and other end of life crises [44].

3. Symptom management

3.1 The burden of symptoms in CKD

Patients with advanced CKD approaching ESKD bear a substantial symptom burden. This necessitates continuous attention throughout their illness journey, with particular focus as they approach the end of life. In a study involving 472 patients with advanced CKD, where imminent death was anticipated, pain emerged as the most prevalent symptom (69%), followed by respiratory secretions (46%), anxiety (41%), confusion (30%), dyspnea (22 percent), and nausea (17%) [45].

CKD patients have a multitude of pain syndromes including arthritis, neuropathic pain from diabetes or inflammatory diseases [46, 47]. Among patients with ESKD, a notable 63.1% reported musculoskeletal-related pain as the predominant issue, while 13.6% experienced pain linked to the dialysis procedure [47].

Uremic neuropathy was common in the past; this was due to thiamine deficiency from the B1 vitamin being easily dialyzable but now patients are supplemented with renal vitamins. Dialysis related amyloidosis related to B2 microglobulin can cause various musculoskeletal ailments, including carpal tunnel syndrome and osteoarthropathies. Renal osteodystrophy related to dysregulation of the calcium – phosphate axis can also lead to severe bone disease including pathologic fractures, osteolytic lesions, brown tumors (osteitis fibrosa cystica), Calcific uremic arteriolopathy (calciphylaxis), muscle weakness and pain. Ischemia to the gut during dialysis in vasculopathic patients may lead to severe abdominal pain, GI bleeding, and nausea/ vomiting. Peritoneal dialysis patients may experience GI discomfort from the presence of peritoneal fluid, pain from drainage, increased pill burden from reduced efficiency, and in rare cases encapsulating peritoneal sclerosis leading to bowel adhesions, and obstruction. Access related complications are a concern in both modalities of dialysis. Gout can also be quite debilitating in the CKD population.

Unfortunately, the ability of dialysis to treat uremia related symptoms may also be limited and may be outweighed by unintended adverse effects of dialysis precipitating symptoms that worsen quality of life and cause a significant burden of suffering. Patients on dialysis may experience symptoms related either to undertreated uremia, intradialytic symptoms, or due to other co-morbid conditions exacerbated by ESKD. 40% of hemodialysis sessions are associated with symptomatic hypotension, nausea, cramping and/ or vomiting [48]. Dialysis patients often experience pruritus, either due to poor clearance of their toxins, or as a reaction to dialyzers or other products used during the treatment (e.g. chlorhexidine). Patients may also have chest pain, difficulty with cognition during the treatment, and difficulty sleeping after. Many patients complain of a "washed out" feeling after dialysis that may not improve until close to their next session.

3.2 Symptom assessment

A study comparing symptoms and quality of life in patients with cancer and those with end-stage renal disease found that advanced CKD patients experience a symptom burden and quality of life impairment akin to terminal malignancy patients [49]. CKM patients also experience a similar number and severity of symptoms as those on dialysis. Understanding the physical and emotional symptom burdens in all chronic kidney disease patients, whether on dialysis or receiving conservative management, is pivotal for enhancing their health-related quality of life.

Clinicians may find it useful to employ established assessment tools such as The Edmonton Symptom Assessment System modified for nephrology care– developed in Canada (ESAS-r:Renal) [50], the Integrated Palliative Care Outcome Scale (IPOS-renal) or the Kidney Disease Quality of Life (KDQOL-36) [51]. These tools can help identify patients with large burden of uremia, and monitor the effectiveness of treatment. The Brief Pain Inventory can be used to evaluate pain management [52].

3.3 Managing symptoms

The goal of symptom management is to alleviate symptoms without causing drug toxicity. Administering medications in advanced CKD is complex due to its impact on renal excreted drug pharmacokinetics. For those undergoing dialysis, the influence of dialysis on the drug must also be considered.

3.4 Pain

Addressing pain requires a careful evaluation of the source, and nature of the pain and a nuanced multimodal approach. Integral to chronic pain management are non-pharmacologic therapies, which can serve as standalone treatments or complement pharmacologic approaches. These can include physiotherapy, massage, chiropractic adjustments, ice/heat applications and meditation.

Pharmacologic treatments work best when targeted to the causal factors, and the pathologic mechanisms (e.g. nociceptive vs. neuropathic pain). The classic approach to pain control is that of a stepwise careful escalation of analgesia, aligning with the World Health Organization's (WHO) guidelines [53]. The WHO ladder approach advocates starting with non-opioids with or without adjuvants, and then adding opioids of increasing potencies as needed. Although this strategy is often successful, there are some important departures, the most notable of which is the contraindication of NSAID use in CKD. Occasionally, short-course NSAIDs might be prescribed, assuming a calculated risk, particularly in patients without residual renal function or nearing the end of life. Topical NSAIDs have fewer adverse effects, although there may be some increased systemic absorption in patients with lower muscle mass [54].

Neuropathic pain is common in CKD and ESKD. In cases of conservative kidney management, the frontline approach to neuropathic pain involves calcium channel-α 2δ-ligands like gabapentinoids [55]. These do accumulate in CKD, and can cause drowsiness and increased risk of falls [55]. They should be started at low doses, and slowly titrated up. Atypical antidepressants such as duloxetine, and anti-epileptics may also treat neuropathic pain.

If pain is not well controlled, opioid use may be necessary. The initiation of opioids should involve low doses, careful adverse effects monitoring, and gradual titration. Most opioids undergo liver metabolism into either active or inactive metabolites, with the kidneys being the typical excretion route for these compounds, including some unchanged opioids [56]. If a substantial portion of unchanged opioid is excreted via the kidneys and the metabolites remain active, the opioid is likely to induce toxicity when eGFR drops below 30 ml/min/m^2 [56]. Opting for short-acting preparations over longer-acting ones is strongly recommended, especially if patient is opioid naïve [46]. Hydromorphone may be preferred over morphine, whose metabolites are more likely to accumulate in kidney disease causing risk of over-narcotization [46].

Constipation is a common side effect of opioid use. Medications like sennosides, stool softeners (bisacodyl), lactulose or polyethylene glycol (PEG) can be safe and effective laxatives. However, laxatives containing magnesium, citrate, or phosphate should be avoided in ESKD [57].

3.5 Pruritus

The etiology of uremic pruritus remains intricate and not fully understood. Factors like uremic neuropathy, chronic systemic inflammation triggering skin or nerve inflammation [58], and heightened μ-opioid receptor activity are all implicated contributors. Due to the complexity of pruritus in CKD, managing this symptom can be challenging, with various treatments proposed, each offering only modest effectiveness.

Initiating management begins with optimizing renal care. Addressing elevated phosphate levels and hyperparathyroidism, which could contribute to pruritus, is important, involving dietary adjustments and the use of phosphate binders. Preventive measures like nail care and maintaining a cool environment through lightweight clothing and tepid baths are also beneficial. Emollients and other topical analgesics (e.g. camphor and/ or menthol) constitute the primary treatment for uremic pruritus, especially for dry skin.

Navigating pharmacological interventions can be challenging due to a lack of clear evidence favoring one approach over another. While some evidence supports use of UVB light therapy, its accessibility may be limited[77]. A recent systematic review highlighted the effectiveness of low-dose gabapentin or pregabalin for uremic pruritus, although evidence for other interventions remains limited [59]. Antihistamines are not recommended as first line, given that uremic pruritus operates through a non-histaminergic itch pathway Mirtazapine, with adjusted dosing for renal impairment, also demonstrates some efficacy [60].

3.6 Nausea and vomiting

Nausea and vomiting often have multifactorial origins. Uremia may cause unremitting nausea, and sensitive gag reflex. In CKM patients, treatments include dietary changes such as decreased protein intake, and smaller meals may help. Other factors such as gastroparesis, and medication side effects should be excluded or treated. Symptoms like bloating, epigastric fullness, flatulence, hiccups, or heartburn may accompany this condition. Gastritis-related nausea often coincides with heartburn, dyspepsia, or epigastric pain. Constipation can exacerbate nausea and vomiting.

Antipsychotics such as olanzapine in low doses are effective in treating uremic nausea. Haloperidol can also be effective, but can cause extrapyramidal symptoms, and are often reserved for nausea in end-of-life patients. 5HT3 antagonists such as ondansetron may be effective as well. Prolonged QTc may limit usage of all these compounds [61].

3.7 Restless legs syndrome (RLS)

Restless legs syndrome (RLS) manifests as an urge to move the legs accompanied by discomfort, exacerbated during rest, particularly at night. RLS's precise cause remains uncertain, with factors like dopaminergic system dysfunction, and iron deficiency, and uremia. Effective management involves addressing these factors and minimizing exacerbating agents like caffeine, alcohol, nicotine, and certain drugs. Gabapentin or pregabalin, often effective for dialysis patients, are often first line options [62]. Dopamine agonists like pramipexole are also effective, but can cause side effects like nausea, dreams, and nightmares.

3.8 Palliative dialysis

Renal replacement therapies include intermittent hemodialysis, peritoneal dialysis and kidney transplantation, as well as CKM. Hemodialysis can be offered both at home as a self-administered therapy or in monitored facilities (hospitals or clinics) by nurses or technicians, while peritoneal dialysis is exclusively a home-based therapy, with or without the help of a trained nurse. Dialysis is purported to have two major benefits – prolongation of life in the context of ESKD, and to treat uremic symptoms (dyspnea, peripheral edema, nausea, anorexia, dysgeusia, pruritus, cramping, etc.). Dialysis does have a role in palliating symptoms of uremia, although this benefit is not always realized in all patients. Dialysis can be quite effective in controlling volume overload in patients, and may treat severe nausea, and vomiting, however other symptoms mentioned above are inconsistently treated. Many patients on dialysis continue to complain of pruritus, fatigue, insomnia and cramping, especially older, frail patients with comorbid illnesses [63]. Paradoxically, dialysis therapy can precipitate the very same symptoms that it is supposed to treat and may cause or exacerbate other symptoms such as pain, weakness and worsened cognition [64]. The latter is often due to dialysis related hypotension, or due to its effects on cardiac function and cerebral perfusion [65]. Symptom burden accounts for 29% of the impairment in physical HRQoL, and 39% of the impairment in mental HRQoL in ESKD [50].

Despite the poor performance of extracorporeal renal replacement therapy in quality of life and survival metrics, especially in older patients, many patients approaching ESKD will not eschew the therapy, often due to existential angst or having goals they wish to achieve before death [66].

For patients who desire to continue dialysis despite poor survival prognosis, an attempt should be made to tailor their treatments to optimizing symptom control, while minimizing the associated adverse effects. This concept is known as palliative or "comfort" dialysis. Rather than a "one- size- fits- all" style of dialysis, focused on conventional disease-oriented treatment, the approach of palliative dialysis is that it should align with the specific needs, values and goals of the patient, thus fitting with the principles of palliative care; it should provide relief from pain and other symptoms, regardless of life expectancy and prognosis, prioritizing comfort [66, 67].

Palliative dialysis may entail a de-emphasizing of clearance adequacy targets; rather than tailoring frequency and length of dialysis to achieve lowered urea levels, symptom control is the end goal. Older patients may require less dialysis time if they have lower metabolic needs, and thus lower uremic toxin production. Lower blood flow rates and dialysis flow rates may theoretically allow better tolerance of dialysis with increased fluid removal. Patients with residual urine output may not require as much ultrafiltration permitting them to dialyse less frequently. Reduction of dialysis may help reduce the burden of travel to and waiting at the dialysis unit, which can be substantial. Sitting in uncomfortable postures for 4 hours maximum may be a source of pain and suffering for patients.

On the other hand, palliative dialysis does not automatically equate to less dialysis. Some ESKD patients may benefit from increased length or frequency of dialysis to control uremic symptoms or improve their bone mineral metabolism parameters. Nocturnal (in-center or home) hemodialysis may help achieve those results. Patients that find it difficult to sit for the requisite 4 hours, but still benefit from additional clearance, may prefer shorter but more frequent sessions, if they do not find the travel to a dialysis center cumbersome. Some patients who suffer from isolation may enjoy the socialization that a communal dialysis unit offers.

Home dialysis with assisted PD or assisted home hemodialysis may be ways to get adequate clearances with less discomfort [68]. More clearance may also allow patients to liberalize their diet, and optimize nutrition, leading to less weakness, fatigue, overall better health and HRQoL. Access issues are also a major consideration in palliative dialysis approaches. Older patients with poor vasculature and limited life expectancy may not necessarily require a permanent AV access; instead, a CVC may be reasonable, with less concern of pain and bruising related to needling of a fistula or graft [67]. In frail patients, graft and fistulas may not be as successful with respect to creation and may have higher rates of steal syndromes leading to pain and weakness in the involved arm and hand [69].

Medications such as anti-hypertensives, phosphate binders may not need to be aggressively prescribed, and management of traditional CKD and ESKD parameters should be balanced with potential negative impacts on their quality of life. Using erythropoietin-stimulating agents to target higher hemoglobin levels in patients with severe fatigue may outweigh the potential risks of hypertension and thrombosis that have been seen with hemoglobin levels over 115 g/L. While studies did not show a significant HRQoL benefit of targeting higher hemoglobin levels, there were few older individuals in such studies [67], and the results may not be applicable to patients with limited life expectancy undergoing palliative dialysis. There may be a potential trade-off between survival and comfort with any of these strategies; nephrologists should discuss these issues with their patients to ensure that all parties have a good understanding of the risks and benefits of palliative dialysis in order to make an informed choice that reduces regret. Involving palliative care physicians to help with identifying areas of suffering in ESKD patients may help formulate palliative strategies.

There are certain barriers to providing palliative dialysis – Physicians face pressures to achieve certain adequacy and quality targets that are based on metrics like clearance; these can be tied to remuneration policies [66]. Dialysis staff and facility schedules are predicated on patients having a fixed schedule with limited changes on a day to day or week to week basis [66].

4. End of life care

End-of-life care is a critical aspect of kidney palliative care; and is required for patients with CKM who approach ESKD, or who withdraw from dialysis Patients with advanced kidney disease experience a high symptom burden and require intensive care at the end of life [70]. The disease continuum for patients with kidney disease is characterized by psychological distress, high physical symptom needs, and increased medicalization that escalates at the end of life [70]. Anuric patients survive a median of 7 days without dialysis, depending on their nutritional intake and activity [71]. Those individuals that have residual urine output despite exceedingly low GFR have an uncertain survival prognosis without dialysis; an individual with less than 5 – 7 ml/min/1.73m^2 of GFR would likely have a life expectancy of less than 6 months [72]. In conservatively managed patients, symptoms tend to remain stable until the final 2 months before death. However, in a study of such patients, the last 2 months were marked by an escalation in symptoms, including fatigue, pruritus, drowsiness, dyspnea, agitation, and pain. Patients and caregivers also experienced elevated levels of psychological concerns and practical issues [73]. Addressing challenging symptoms or conflicting care objectives can be aided by the involvement of an interdisciplinary palliative care team, and patients undergoing CKM and their caregivers may benefit from hospice services.

Common end-of-life symptoms include dyspnea from volume overload, fatigue, respiratory secretions, cramping, nausea and pruritus [74]. Patients with urine output may benefit from high dose diuretics. Oxygen use may provide comfort. Strategies such as the use of a fan to blow air on one's face may help to alleviate feelings of breathlessness. Low doses of opioids, like hydromorphone, can alleviate dyspnea, initiating with lower doses due to reduced renal excretion of active metabolites [74]. Hydromorphone 0.5 mg S.C / P.O every 1–2 hours prn can be effective without causing delirium or severe constipation. However, if the patient has pain, higher doses may be required. If the patient has both pain and anxiety along with breathlessness, a small dose of a benzodiazepine like midazolam (1 mg PRN) or lorazepam may be helpful [75]. Pain management can also include fentanyl, buprenorphine, methadone, or morphine, depending on the patient's condition. Fentanyl has the advantage that it has no active metabolites with minimal renal excretion. Haloperidol is recommended for restlessness or agitation due to its safety profile and parenteral route of administration [76]. Nausea can be treated with antipsychotics such as olanzapine or haloperidol [61]. Emollients, topical steroids, gabapentinoids, and mirtazapine may be effective for uremic pruritus. In addition to targeted symptom management, it is imperative to emphasize general supportive care for terminally ill patients. This includes interventions to ensure comfort, such as the use of lip balm, mouth swabs, proper positioning, back rubs, fans, and reduction of blood draws and dietary restrictions.

Bereavement support is the final pillar of palliative care. This includes communicating with the family, providing privacy and support, and honoring cultural requests. Conscientious and comprehensive bereavement support can mitigate complex grief reactions in families.

5. Dialysis withdrawal

The decision to withdraw from dialysis can be a difficult one for patients, fraught with emotion. Globally, dialysis withdrawal is a major cause of death in ESKD patients and is becoming more common. In 2020, it became the second leading cause of death among US ESKD patients [77]. About 17% of hemodialysis and 16% of peritoneal dialysis patients in the US stopped dialysis before death in 2020 [77].

Withdrawal of dialysis is suitable in cases where the patients have decision-making capacity but who choose to withdraw. It can also be considered in ESKD patients with severe anguish and suffering, hospitalized patients with multiple organ failure, those with irreversible mental incapacity, and limited life expectancy due to conditions unresponsive to dialysis [78]. Factors such as pain and depression, if amenable to treatment, should be addressed by the care team. It is imperative that mental health issues be treated, especially psychosis. Complex cases may benefit from an evaluation by psychiatric and palliative care specialists. The involvement of family members and caregivers in a patient's decision to withdraw from dialysis is not mandatory but is strongly encouraged [79].

Palliative care should be made available to all patients who choose this path, with an emphasis on educating patients and families about post-dialysis care, symptom management, and end-of-life care locations. Emotional, spiritual, and social support services should be provided, and access to palliative or hospice care should be offered as needed [80]. On average, patients typically survive for 7 to 10 days after discontinuing dialysis, with longer survival rates noted in those retaining residual urine output. Barriers to dialysis withdrawal include policy limitations, conflicting cultural expectations, inadequate training, societal norms, and differing opinions among nephrologists [81]. Overcoming these barriers requires concerted efforts, including education, awareness campaigns, promotion of advanced directives, and facilitation of multidisciplinary discussions, all supported by close collaboration between nephrology and palliative care teams and guided by national bodies.

5.1 Barriers to effective palliation and end of life care

Patients with ESKD are less likely to receive hospice care than patients with other types of terminal illness [5]. Only 20% of patients with ESKD in the US utilize hospice compared with 55% of patients with cancer, and 39% with congestive heart failure [4]. The main barriers to appropriate end of life care in CKD patients include access, as well as patient and practitioner attitudinal factors [67]. Knowledge gaps and competing priorities are other challenges[111].

The current model of renal care in most centers is poorly equipped to help patients and their families address the emotional and existential challenges of navigating their advanced CKD and the complex treatment decisions required, such as whether to start dialysis, or stopping dialysis when it becomes burdensome. Access to specialized palliative care for patients with ESKD on maintenance dialysis is limited, despite dialysis providers identifying it as the second highest priority to improve palliative care for their patients [82]. Palliative care services can be limited geographically and available only in tertiary care centers [83]. Patients that are ill but not hospitalized or imminently dying may be precluded from such care. Workforce shortages are also a major barrier; the specialty of palliative care has certainly grown rapidly; however, the existing demand still outpaces the available number of trained palliative care physicians. The burden thus falls on the primary nephrologist; however, there is limited training in palliative care in nephrology curricula. Trainees graduating fellowship programs have identified palliative care in nephrology as a major unmet learning need [84].

The hospice model is insufficient to meet the needs of seriously ill patients with CKD and ESKD. In the US Medicare beneficiaries are only eligible for hospice care if they agree to forgo or withdraw from dialysis therapy unless they have another terminal illness unrelated to their renal disease [83]. Outpatient palliative care programs suffer from lack of parity in reimbursement; there may be an incentive to initiate dialysis therapy than to manage conservatively in an interdisciplinary palliative care program.

Patient attitudes towards palliative and end of life care can create a barrier in itself. Many patients on dialysis express a desire for life prolongation even at the cost of increased suffering. This is borne out in so far that nearly half of dialysed patients die in hospital compared with 35% of all Medicare beneficiaries with other severe illnesses [85]. However, a Canadian study did show that patients were willing to forgo 7 months of life expectancy to reduce the number of visits to hospital, and up to 15 months to increase their ability to travel [86].

5.2 Ethical and legal issues

There are many ethical issues around the care of dialysis patients. One question that many nephrologists grapple with is that of the appropriateness of withholding or withdrawing dialysis. This dilemma presents itself particularly when goals and expectations are not congruent between the provider, the patient, and their families. Certainly, patients have the autonomy to refuse, or stop dialysis; they have an ethical and legal right of self-determination. Physicians also can determine if dialysis will not offer a reasonable expectation of medical benefit on the basis principle of beneficence and non-maleficence. However, it is difficult to determine that risk benefit trade-off in ESKD where trajectory of disease progression can be unpredictable as can be a patient's response to, and tolerance of dialysis [87]. Many Nephrologists would elect to provide dialysis at the behest of the legal agent, against their reservations. In one study, 17% of nephrologists surveyed reported they would start dialysis at the family's request for a permanently unconscious patient despite being deeply conflicted [88]. The reasons for doing so include fear of litigation, uncertainty of the law, and their own unqualified valuation for the preservation of life [88].

To guide renal physicians through these complex issues, the Renal Physician's Association and American society of nephrology developed a clinical practice guideline about the appropriate initiation and withdrawal from dialysis [87]. The key emphasis was on the importance of communication, education and shared decision making [88]. The guidelines recommended that it was reasonable not to initiate dialysis in patients with terminal illnesses or medical conditions that would preclude the technical process of dialysis, or in those with profound neurological impairment. A systematic approach to conflict resolution was recommended in all cases of disagreement. Conflicts often rise due to miscommunication or misunderstanding about the nature of disease progression and the prognosis, or due to a misalignment of values. There was a provision that a time limited trial be considered in those patients with uncertain prognosis, or where there was no consensus about the utility of dialysis.

6. Future directions

Nephrologists are beginning to face the reality of an older CKD population with increased frailty and burden of comorbidity. It is becoming imperative that the tenets of renal palliative care become commonplace in renal programs and clinics. To accomplish this goal of enveloping a palliative philosophy into routine kidney care, there will need to be concerted effort to increase confidence and competence in nephrologists and trainees in palliative renal care. There already exist several professional development programs such as NephroTalk that can help teach nephrology specific communication skills [89]. Developing relationships with palliative care will also be helpful to develop these skills.

More research into conservative care is necessary for the nephrology community. To improve clinical practice and policy making, there needs to be a consensus on conservative kidney management. The research priorities should include understanding of disease progression for those managed conservatively, evaluating the health-related quality of life symptoms and functional status of patients receiving CKM, and comparing the cost-effectiveness of different models of conservative care across various health systems (**Table 1**).

Finally, system level changes will be needed to remove barriers to effective palliation and end of life care for patients with CKD. Development of programs with proficiency in managing kidney disease conservatively will help reduce dialysis starts in patients whose goals may not be congruent with aggressive dialytic management. Stakeholder engagement with nurses, management and physicians would be

Symptom	Nonpharmacologic	Pharmacologic
Restless leg syndrome, Cramps [24, 62].	Address iron deficiency avoid antidepressants and dopamine antagonists. Abstinence from stimulants like alcohol, caffeine, and nicotine. Incorporate regular exercise.	First-line treatment: gabapentin, 50 to 300 mg nightly, or pregabalin, 25 to 75 mg nightly Second-line: non-ergot-derived dopamine agonists e.g. pramipexole, which can be taken orally at doses of 0.125 to 0.25 mg three times daily as needed Consider low-dose magnesium supplementation.,
Uremic pruritus [24, 59].	Skin care and moisturizing. Avoid hot showers/ baths, aqueous emollients. Choose gentle soaps without fragrances or additives. Maintain a cool environment. Resist the urge to scratch. Keep fingernails short and smooth, consider gentle massages, and use gloves at night if necessary.	Topical treatments like camphor and menthol-based compounds, low-potency steroids, capsaicin-based creams/ointments (0.025% or 0.03%), and pramoxine 1%. Low doses of gabapentin and SSRIs (Paroxetine or mirtazapine). Use antihistamines cautiously, but hydroxyzine (10 mg twice daily) is an option if needed. Ultraviolet-B therapy can be considered, limited evidence.
Nausea and vomiting [24, 61].	Address constipation. Avoid triggers such as large meals and strong odors. Avoid alcohol and greasy, spicy, or overly sweet foods. Encourage a relaxed, upright position after eating. Wear loose-fitting clothes. Consider complementary therapies like relaxation techniques, acupressure, and using ginger.	First line: atypical antipsychotics like olanzapine at 2.5 mg every 8 hours PRN or low-dose haloperidol at 0.5 mg every 8 hours PRN. Second line: Use ondansetron at 4–8 mg every 8 hours PRN. Third line: Consider metoclopramide at 2.5 mg every 4 hours PRN.
Dyspnea [90].	Restrict salt and fluid intake. Optimize anemia treatment. Try pursed lip breathing. Use supplemental oxygen, if needed. Explore complementary methods like relaxation techniques and music.	Higher furosemide dose if patient urinates and volume overloaded. Use low-dose opioids, hydromorphone (e.g., 0.5 mg PO or 0.2 mg S/C) Oxygen by nasal prongs
Fatigue [24, 91].	Improve nutrition. Optimize anemia treatment. Ensure proper cardiac function and diuretic dosages. Evaluate reducing β-blocker doses. Explore exercise programs. Employ cognitive and psychological approaches like relaxation therapy. Use energy-saving techniques.	
Sleep disturbance [92].	Incorporate exercise. Decrease caffeine and restrict evening fluid intake. Administer diuretics earlier in the day (e.g., the second dose of furosemide no later than 2 pm). Address benign prostatic hyperplasia if relevant. Treat pain, restless leg syndrome, and pruritus.	melatonin 2–5 mg at night. mirtazapine 7.5 – 15 mg, Trazadone 25 – 100 mg nightly
Depression [24].	Manage contributing symptoms like pain, insomnia, and pruritus. Enhance social support. Explore cognitive-behavioral therapy and exercise.	Dose-adjusted antidepressants such as mirtazapine, sertraline or escitalopram may be effective.

Symptom	Nonpharmacologic	Pharmacologic
Pain [46, 55].	Utilize physical therapies like physiotherapy, aerobic exercise, massage, acupressure, and acupuncture. Consider behavioral therapies, such as cognitive-behavioral therapy (the most commonly used), biofeedback, relaxation techniques, and psychotherapy in individual or group counseling. Explore interventional and surgical options, including ablative techniques, nerve blocks, and trigger point injections.	Begin with nonopioid analgesics, like acetaminophen (up to 3 g daily) and topical NSAIDs for localized pain. Neuropathic agents like gabapentin (start with 100 mg orally daily) can be considered but monitor for falls. hydromorphone (starting at 0.5 to 1 mg orally every 4–6 hours), if needed. Limited evidence exists for cannabinoid use in CKD.

Table 1.
Summary of symptom management guidelines for patients receiving CKM.

necessary. Similarly, engaging dialysis unit leadership to promote palliative dialysis for certain patients would help to usher in a new paradigm of dialysis care. Changes in how we measure quality delivery of dialysis care will be important; remuneration indices will need to be shifted from laboratory measure of adequacy and aligned more with patient goals and satisfaction [66].

Author details

Asad Merchant and Adel Moideen*
Division of Nephrology, Department of Medicine, University Health Network, University of Toronto, Toronto, Ontario, Canada

*Address all correspondence to: adel.moideen@gmail.com

References

[1] Kovesdy CP. Epidemiology of chronic kidney disease: An update 2022. Kidney International Supplement. 2022;**12**(1): 7-11. DOI: 10.1016/j.kisu.2021.11.003

[2] Couser WG, Remuzzi G, Mendis S, Tonelli M. The contribution of chronic kidney disease to the global burden of major noncommunicable diseases. Kidney International. 2011;**80**(12):1258-1270. DOI: 10.1038/ki.2011.368

[3] Kurella Tamura M. Incidence, management, and outcomes of end-stage renal disease in the elderly. Current Opinion in Nephrology and Hypertension. 2009;**18**(3):252-257. DOI: 10.1097/mnh.0b013e328326f3ac

[4] U.S. Renal Data System. USRDS Annual Data Report: Epidemiology of kidney disease in the United States. National Institutes of Health, National Institute of Diabetes and Digestive and Kidney Diseases, Bethesda, MD. 2022. Available from: https://usrds-adr.niddk.nih.gov/2022/end-stage-renal-disease/1-incidence-prevalence-patient-characteristics-and-treatment-modalities [Accessed: September 11, 2023]

[5] Sturgill D, Bear A. Unique palliative care needs of patients with advanced chronic kidney disease—The scope of the problem and several solutions. Clinical medicine (London, England). 2019;**19**(1):26-29. DOI: 10.7861/clinmedicine.19-1-26

[6] Collins AJ et al. US Renal Data System 2012 Annual Data Report. American Journal of Kidney Diseases. 2013;**61**(1 Suppl. 1):A7, e1-476. DOI: 10.1053/j.ajkd.2012.11.031

[7] Jha V et al. Chronic kidney disease: Global dimension and perspectives. Lancet. 2013;**382**(9888):260-272. DOI: 10.1016/S0140-6736(13)60687-X

[8] Brown EA, Chambers EJ, Eggeling C. Palliative care in nephrology. Nephrology, Dialysis, Transplantation: Official Publication of the European Dialysis and Transplant Association – European Renal Association. 2008;**23**(3):789-791. DOI: 10.1093/ndt/gfm874

[9] Brown EA. Epidemiology of renal palliative care. Journal of Palliative Medicine. 2007;**10**(6):1248-1252. DOI: 10.1089/jpm.2007.0033

[10] Al-Aly Z et al. Rate of kidney function decline associates with mortality. Journal of the American Society of Nephrology. 2010;**21**(11):1961-1969. DOI: 10.1681/ASN.2009121210

[11] Al-Aly Z, Balasubramanian S, McDonald JR, Scherrer JF, O'Hare AM. Greater variability in kidney function is associated with an increased risk of death. Kidney International. 2012;**82**(11):1208-1214. DOI: 10.1038/ki.2012.276

[12] Schell JO, O'Hare AM. Illness trajectories and their relevance to the care of adults with kidney disease. Current Opinion in Nephrology and Hypertension. 2013;**22**(3):316-324. DOI: 10.1097/MNH.0b013e32835ffaaf

[13] Kurella Tamura M, Covinsky KE, Chertow GM, Yaffe K, Landefeld CS, McCulloch CE. Functional status of elderly adults before and after initiation of dialysis. The New England Journal of Medicine. 2009;**361**(16):1539-1547. DOI: 10.1056/NEJMoa0904655

[14] Jassal SV, Chiu E, Hladunewich M. Loss of independence in patients starting dialysis at 80 years of age or older. The New England Journal of Medicine. 2009;**361**(16):1612-1613. DOI: 10.1056/NEJMc0905289

[15] Murtagh FEM, Sheerin NS, Addington-Hall J, Higginson IJ. Trajectories of illness in stage 5 chronic kidney disease: A longitudinal study of patient symptoms and concerns in the last year of life. Clinical Journal of the American Society of Nephrology. 2011;**6**(7):1580-1590. DOI: 10.2215/CJN.09021010

[16] Naylor KL, Kim SJ, McArthur E, Garg AX, McCallum MK, Knoll GA. Mortality in incident maintenance dialysis patients versus incident solid organ cancer patients: A population-based cohort. American Journal of Kidney Diseases. 2019;**73**(6):765-776. DOI: 10.1053/j.ajkd.2018.12.011

[17] Murtagh FEM, Marsh JE, Donohoe P, Ekbal NJ, Sheerin NS, Harris FE. Dialysis or not? A comparative survival study of patients over 75 years with chronic kidney disease stage 5. Nephrology, Dialysis, Transplantation: Official Publication of the European Dialysis and Transplant Association – European Renal Association. 2007;**22**(7):1955-1962. DOI: 10.1093/ndt/gfm153

[18] Koncicki HM, Swidler MA. Decision making in elderly patients with advanced kidney disease. Clinics in Geriatric Medicine. 2013;**29**(3):641-655. DOI: 10.1016/j.cger.2013.05.004

[19] Saeed F, Ladwig SA, Epstein RM, Monk RD, Duberstein PR. Dialysis regret: Prevalence and correlates. Clinical Journal of the American Society of Nephrology. 2020;**15**(7):957-963. DOI: 10.2215/CJN.13781119

[20] Low J et al. The experiences of close persons caring for people with chronic kidney disease stage 5 on conservative kidney management: Contested discourses of ageing. Health (London, England : 1997). 2014;**18**(6):613-630. DOI: 10.1177/1363459314524805

[21] Roy D, Chowdhury AR, Pande S, Kam JW. Evaluation of unplanned dialysis as a predictor of mortality in elderly dialysis patients: A retrospective data analysis. BMC Nephrology. 2017;**18**(1):364. DOI: 10.1186/s12882-017-0778-0

[22] Wong SPY, Yu MK, Green PK, Liu C-F, Hebert PL, O'Hare AM. End-of-life Care for Patients with Advanced Kidney Disease in the US veterans affairs health care system, 2000-2011. American Journal of Kidney Diseases. 2018;**72**(1):42-49. DOI: 10.1053/j.ajkd.2017.11.007

[23] Tam-Tham H et al. Association of Initiation of dialysis with hospital length of stay and intensity of Care in Older Adults with Kidney Failure. JAMA Network Open. 2020;**3**(2):e200222. DOI: 10.1001/jamanetworkopen.2020.0222

[24] Davison SN, Jassal SV. Supportive care: Integration of patient-centered kidney care to manage symptoms and geriatric syndromes. Clinical Journal of the American Society of Nephrology. 2016;**11**(10):1882-1891. DOI: 10.2215/CJN.01050116

[25] Brown EA, Bekker HL, Davison SN, Koffman J, Schell JO. Supportive care: Communication strategies to improve cultural competence in shared decision making. Clinical Journal of the American Society of Nephrology. 2016;**11**(10):1902-1908. DOI: 10.2215/CJN.13661215

[26] Barnes S et al. Enhancing patient-professional communication about end-of-life issues in life-limiting conditions: A critical review of the literature. Journal of Pain and Symptom Management. 2012;**44**(6):866-879. DOI: 10.1016/j.jpainsymman.2011.11.009

[27] Schell JO, Cohen RA. A communication framework for dialysis

decision-making for frail elderly patients. Clinical Journal of the American Society of Nephrology. 2014;**9**(11):2014-2021. DOI: 10.2215/CJN.02190314

[28] Fine A, Fontaine B, Kraushar MM, Rich BR. Nephrologists should voluntarily divulge survival data to potential dialysis patients: A questionnaire study. Peritoneal Dialysis International. 2005;**25**(3):269-273

[29] Kruser JM et al. 'Best case/worst case': Qualitative evaluation of a novel communication tool for difficult in-the-moment surgical decisions. Journal of the American Geriatrics Society. 2015;**63**(9):1805-1811. DOI: 10.1111/jgs.13615

[30] Davison SN, Jhangri GS, Holley JL, Moss AH. Nephrologists' reported preparedness for end-of-life decision-making. Clinical Journal of the American Society of Nephrology. 2006;**1**(6):1256-1262. DOI: 10.2215/CJN.02040606

[31] Davison SN. End-of-life care preferences and needs: Perceptions of patients with chronic kidney disease. Clinical Journal of the American Society of Nephrology. 2010;**5**(2):195. DOI: 10.2215/CJN.05960809

[32] Parvez S, Abdel-Kader K, Pankratz VS, Song M-K, Unruh M. Provider knowledge, attitudes, and practices surrounding conservative Management for Patients with advanced CKD. Clinical Journal of the American Society of Nephrology. 2016;**11**(5):812-820. DOI: 10.2215/CJN.07180715

[33] Chandna SM, Da Silva-Gane M, Marshall C, Warwicker P, Greenwood RN, Farrington K. Survival of elderly patients with stage 5 CKD: Comparison of conservative management and renal replacement therapy. Nephrology, Dialysis, Transplantation: Official Publication of the European Dialysis and Transplant Association – European Renal Association. 2011;**26**(5):1608-1614. DOI: 10.1093/ndt/gfq630

[34] Cohen LM, Moss AH, Weisbord SD, Germain MJ. Renal palliative care. Journal of Palliative Medicine. 2006;**9**(4):977-992. DOI: 10.1089/jpm.2006.9.977

[35] Beddhu S, Bruns FJ, Saul M, Seddon P, Zeidel ML. A simple comorbidity scale predicts clinical outcomes and costs in dialysis patients. The American Journal of Medicine. 2000;**108**(8):609-613. DOI: 10.1016/s0002-9343(00)00371-5

[36] Hemmelgarn BR, Manns BJ, Quan H, Ghali WA. Adapting the Charlson comorbidity index for use in patients with ESRD. American Journal of Kidney Diseases. 2003;**42**(1):125-132. DOI: 10.1016/s0272-6386(03)00415-3

[37] Moss AH et al. Utility of the 'surprise' question to identify dialysis patients with high mortality. Clinical Journal of the American Society of Nephrology. 2008;**3**(5):1379-1384. DOI: 10.2215/CJN.00940208

[38] Cohen LM, Ruthazer R, Moss AH, Germain MJ. Predicting six-month mortality for patients who are on maintenance hemodialysis. Clinical Journal of the American Society of Nephrology. 2010;**5**(1):72-79. DOI: 10.2215/CJN.03860609

[39] Couchoud C et al. A clinical score to predict 6-month prognosis in elderly patients starting dialysis for end-stage renal disease. Nephrology, Dialysis, Transplantation: Official Publication of the European Dialysis and Transplant Association – European Renal Association. 2009;**24**(5):1553-1561. DOI: 10.1093/ndt/gfn698

[40] Schmidt RJ et al. Derivation and validation of a prognostic model to predict mortality in patients with advanced chronic kidney disease. Nephrology, Dialysis, Transplantation: Official Publication of the European Dialysis and Transplant Association – European Renal Association. 2019;**34**(9):1517-1525. DOI: 10.1093/ndt/gfy305

[41] Task Force on Palliative Care, Last Acts Campaign, and Robert Wood Johnson Foundation. Precepts of palliative care. Journal of Palliative Medicine. 1998;**1**(2):109-112. DOI: 10.1089/jpm.1998.1.109

[42] Levy JB, Chambers EJ, Brown EA. Supportive care for the renal patient. Nephrology, Dialysis, Transplantation: Official Publication of the European Dialysis and Transplant Association – European Renal Association. 2004;**19**(6):1357-1360. DOI: 10.1093/ndt/gfh178

[43] Eneanya ND, Paasche-Orlow MK, Volandes A. Palliative and end-of-life care in nephrology: Moving from observations to interventions. Current Opinion in Nephrology and Hypertension. 2017;**26**(4):327-334. DOI: 10.1097/MNH.0000000000000337

[44] Combs SA, Davison SN. Palliative and end-of-life care issues in chronic kidney disease. Current Opinion in Supportive and Palliative Care. 2015;**9**(1):14-19. DOI: 10.1097/SPC.0000000000000110

[45] Axelsson L et al. Unmet palliative care needs among patients with end-stage kidney disease: A National Registry Study about the last week of life. Journal of Pain and Symptom Management. 2018;**55**(2):236-244. DOI: 10.1016/j.jpainsymman.2017.09.015

[46] Davison SN, Koncicki H, Brennan F. Pain in chronic kidney disease: A scoping review. Seminars in Dialysis. 2014;**27**(2):188-204. DOI: 10.1111/sdi.12196

[47] Davison SN. Pain in hemodialysis patients: Prevalence, cause, severity, and management. American Journal of Kidney Diseases. 2003;**42**(6):1239-1247. DOI: 10.1053/j.ajkd.2003.08.025

[48] Brown E, Chambers EJ, Germain M. *Supportive Care for the Renal Patient*. Second ed, Supportive Care. Oxford, New York: Oxford University Press; 2010

[49] Saini T, Murtagh FEM, Dupont PJ, McKinnon PM, Hatfield P, Saunders Y. Comparative pilot study of symptoms and quality of life in cancer patients and patients with end stage renal disease. Palliative Medicine. 2006;**20**(6):631-636. DOI: 10.1177/0269216306070236

[50] Davison SN, Jhangri GS, Johnson JA. Cross-sectional validity of a modified Edmonton symptom assessment system in dialysis patients: A simple assessment of symptom burden. Kidney International. 2006;**69**(9):1621-1625. DOI: 10.1038/sj.ki.5000184

[51] Hays RD, Kallich JD, Mapes DL, Coons SJ, Carter WB. Development of the kidney disease quality of life (KDQOL) instrument. Quality of Life Research. 1994;**3**(5):329-338. DOI: 10.1007/BF00451725

[52] Daut RL, Cleeland CS, Flanery RC. Development of the Wisconsin brief pain questionnaire to assess pain in cancer and other diseases. Pain. 1983;**17**(2):197-210. DOI: 10.1016/0304-3959(83)90143-4

[53] Ventafridda V, Saita L, Ripamonti C, De Conno F. WHO guidelines for the use of analgesics in cancer pain. International Journal of Tissue Reactions. 1985;**7**(1):93-96

[54] Andrews P. Topical non-steroidal drugs are systemically absorbed and may cause renal disease. Nephrology, Dialysis, Transplantation. 1999;**14**(1):187-189. DOI: 10.1093/ndt/14.1.187

[55] Atalay H, Solak Y, Biyik Z, Gaipov A, Guney F, Turk S. Cross-over, open-label trial of the effects of gabapentin versus pregabalin on painful peripheral neuropathy and health-related quality of life in haemodialysis patients. Clinical Drug Investigation. 2013;**33**(6):401-408. DOI: 10.1007/s40261-013-0080-2

[56] Davies G, Kingswood C, Street M. Pharmacokinetics of opioids in renal dysfunction. Clinical Pharmacokinetics. 1996;**31**(6):410-422. DOI: 10.2165/00003088-199631060-00002

[57] Xing JH, Soffer EE. Adverse effects of laxatives. Diseases of the Colon and Rectum. 2001;**44**(8):1201-1209. DOI: 10.1007/BF02234645

[58] Kimmel M et al. The role of micro-inflammation in the pathogenesis of uraemic pruritus in haemodialysis patients. Nephrology, Dialysis, Transplantation: Official Publication of the European Dialysis and Transplant Association – European Renal Association. 2006;**21**(3):749-755. DOI: 10.1093/ndt/gfi204

[59] Simonsen E et al. Treatment of uremic pruritus: A systematic review. American Journal of Kidney Diseases. 2017;**70**(5):638-655. DOI: 10.1053/j.ajkd.2017.05.018

[60] Davis MP, Frandsen JL, Walsh D, Andresen S, Taylor S. Mirtazapine for pruritus. Journal of Pain and Symptom Management. 2003;**25**(3):288-291. DOI: 10.1016/s0885-3924(02)00645-0

[61] Leach C. Nausea and vomiting in palliative care. Clinical Medicine. London. Jul 2019;**19**(4):299-301. DOI: 10.7861/clinmedicine.19-4-299. PMID: 31308107; PMCID: PMC6752233

[62] Gopaluni S, Sherif M, Ahmadouk NA. Interventions for chronic kidney disease-associated restless legs syndrome. Cochrane Database of Systematic Reviews. 2016;**11**(11):CD010690. DOI: 10.1002/14651858.CD010690.pub2

[63] Jablonski A. The multidimensional characteristics of symptoms reported by patients on hemodialysis. Nephrology Nursing Journal: Journal of the American Nephrology Nurses' Association. 2007;**34**(1):29-37; quiz 38

[64] Kurella Tamura M et al. Effect of more frequent hemodialysis on cognitive function in the frequent hemodialysis network trials. American Journal of Kidney Diseases. 2013;**61**(2):228-237. DOI: 10.1053/j.ajkd.2012.09.009

[65] Weiner DE et al. Cardiovascular disease and cognitive function in maintenance hemodialysis patients. American Journal of Kidney Diseases. 2011;**58**(5):773-781. DOI: 10.1053/j.ajkd.2011.03.034

[66] Grubbs V et al. A palliative approach to dialysis care: A patient-centered transition to the end of life. Clinical Journal of the American Society of Nephrology. 2014;**9**(12):2203-2209. DOI: 10.2215/CJN.00650114

[67] Tentori F, Hunt A, Nissenson AR. Palliative dialysis: Addressing the need for alternative dialysis delivery modes. Seminars in Dialysis. 2019;**32**(5):391-395. DOI: 10.1111/sdi.12820

[68] Harris SAC, Lamping DL, Brown EA, Constantinovici N, North Thames Dialysis Study (NTDS) Group. Clinical outcomes and quality of life in elderly

patients on peritoneal dialysis versus hemodialysis. Peritoneal Dialysis International. 2002;**22**(4):463-470

[69] Moist LM et al. Optimal hemodialysis vascular access in the elderly patient. Seminars in Dialysis. 2012;**25**(6):640-648. DOI: 10.1111/sdi.12037

[70] Lam DY, Scherer JS, Brown M, Grubbs V, Schell JO. A conceptual framework of palliative care across the continuum of advanced kidney disease. Clinical Journal of the American Society of Nephrology. 2019;**14**(4):635-641. DOI: 10.2215/CJN.09330818

[71] Chen JC-Y et al. End of life, withdrawal, and palliative care utilization among patients receiving maintenance hemodialysis therapy. Clinical Journal of the American Society of Nephrology. 2018;**13**(8):1172-1179. DOI: 10.2215/CJN.00590118

[72] Chou A, Li KC, Brown MA. Survival of older patients with advanced CKD managed without dialysis: A narrative review. Kidney Medicine. 2022;**4**(5):100447. DOI: 10.1016/j.xkme.2022.100447

[73] Murtagh FE et al. Symptoms in the month before death for stage 5 chronic kidney disease patients managed without dialysis. Journal of Pain and Symptom Management. 2010;**40**(3):342-352. DOI: 10.1016/j.jpainsymman.2010.01.021

[74] Murtagh FEM. End-stage kidney disease. In: Cherny NI, Fallon MT, Kaasa S, Portenoy RK, Currow DC, Cherny NI, Fallon MT, Kaasa S, Portenoy RK, Currow DC, editors. *Oxford Textbook of Palliative Medicine*. Eds: Oxford University Press; 2021. p. 0. DOI: 10.1093/med/9780198821328.003.0095

[75] Douglas CA. Palliative care for patients with advance chronic kidney disease. The Journal of the Royal College of Physicians of Edinburgh. 2014;**44**(3):224-231. DOI: 10.4997/JRCPE.2014.309

[76] Yasui-Furukori N et al. Delirium in hemodialysis predicts mortality: A single-center, long-term observational study. Neuropsychiatric Disease and Treatment. 2017;**13**:3011-3016. DOI: 10.2147/NDT.S152355

[77] United States Renal Data System. 2022 USRDS Annual Data Report: Epidemiology of Kidney Disease in the United States. Bethesda, MD: National Institutes of Health, National Institute of Diabetes and Digestive and Kidney Diseases; 2022

[78] Lambie M et al. Starting and withdrawing haemodialysis—Associations between nephrologists' opinions, patient characteristics and practice patterns (data from the dialysis outcomes and practice patterns study). Nephrology, Dialysis, Transplantation: Official Publication of the European Dialysis and Transplant Association – European Renal Association. 2006;**21**(10):2814-2820. DOI: 10.1093/ndt/gfl339

[79] Hines SC, Glover JJ, Holley JL, Babrow AS, Badzek LA, Moss AH. Dialysis patients' preferences for family-based advance care planning. Annals of Internal Medicine. 1999;**130**(10):825-828. DOI: 10.7326/0003-4819-130-10-199905180-00016

[80] Davison SN et al. Executive summary of the KDIGO controversies conference on supportive Care in Chronic Kidney Disease: Developing a roadmap to improving quality care. Kidney International. 2015;**88**(3):447-459. DOI: 10.1038/ki.2015.110

[81] Holley JL, Foulks CJ, Moss AH. Nephrologists' reported attitudes about

factors influencing recommendations to initiate or withdraw dialysis. Journal of the American Society of Nephrology. 1991;**1**(12):1284-1288. DOI: 10.1681/ASN.V1121284

[82] Culp S, Lupu D, Arenella C, Armistead N, Moss AH. Unmet supportive care needs in U.S. dialysis centers and lack of knowledge of available resources to address them. Journal of Pain and Symptom Management. 2016;**51**(4):756-761.e2. DOI: 10.1016/j.jpainsymman.2015.11.017

[83] Tamura MK, O'Hare AM, Lin E, Holdsworth LM, Malcolm E, Moss AH. Palliative care disincentives in CKD: Changing policy to improve CKD care. American Journal of Kidney Diseases. 2018;**71**(6):866-873. DOI: 10.1053/j.ajkd.2017.12.017

[84] Holley JL et al. The need for end-of-life care training in nephrology: National survey results of nephrology fellows. American Journal of Kidney Diseases. 2003;**42**(4):813-820. DOI: 10.1016/s0272-6386(03)00868-0

[85] Wong SPY, Kreuter W, O'Hare AM. Treatment intensity at the end of life in older adults receiving long-term dialysis. Archives of Internal Medicine. 2012;**172**(8):661-663; discussion 663-664,. DOI: 10.1001/archinternmed.2012.268

[86] Morton RL et al. Factors influencing patient choice of dialysis versus conservative care to treat end-stage kidney disease. Canadian Medical Association Journal. 2012;**184**(5):E277-E283. DOI: 10.1503/cmaj.111355

[87] Galla JH. Clinical practice guideline on shared decision-making in the appropriate initiation of and withdrawal from dialysis. The renal physicians association and the American Society of Nephrology. Journal of the American Society of Nephrology. 2000;**11**(7):1340-1342. DOI: 10.1681/ASN.V1171340

[88] Moss AH, Stocking CB, Sachs GA, Siegler M. Variation in the attitudes of dialysis unit medical directors toward decisions to withhold and withdraw dialysis. Journal of the American Society of Nephrology. 1993;**4**(2):229-234. DOI: 10.1681/ASN.V42229

[89] Schell JO et al. NephroTalk: Evaluation of a palliative care communication curriculum for nephrology fellows. Journal of Pain and Symptom Management. 2018;**56**(5):767-773.e2. DOI: 10.1016/j.jpainsymman.2018.08.002

[90] Barnes H, McDonald J, Smallwood N, Manser R. Opioids for the palliation of refractory breathlessness in adults with advanced disease and terminal illness. Cochrane Database of Systematic Reviews. 2016;**3**(3):CD011008. DOI: 10.1002/14651858.CD011008.pub2

[91] Yennurajalingam S, Bruera E. Palliative management of fatigue at the close of life: 'It feels like my body is just worn out'. JAMA. 2007;**297**(3):295-304. DOI: 10.1001/jama.297.3.295

[92] Furey SA, Hull SG, Leibowitz MT, Jayawardena S, Roth T. A randomized, double-blind, placebo-controlled, multicenter, 28-day, polysomnographic study of gabapentin in transient insomnia induced by sleep phase advance. Journal of Clinical Sleep Medicine : JCSM : Official Publication of the American Academy of Sleep Medicine. 2014;**10**(10):1101-1109. DOI: 10.5664/jcsm.4110

Chapter 13

Oncopediatric Palliative Care

Mariuska Forteza Sáez and Marìa del Carmen Llantà

Abstract

Palliative Care in children and adolescents with cancer has become a great challenge in current times, not only because of the mortality and morbidity statistics, but also because of the great experience of suffering that it can lead to for patients, their parents and relatives, as well as for the staff that provide health services. The adequate preparation for professional performance within the framework of a humanized medicine constitutes a challenge; Lack of competencies are recognized for their intervention by the work teams. The objectives of this chapter are to describe some barriers and challenges of this care in Latin American countries, as well as to frame the main functions and areas of intervention with the aim of minimizing experiences of suffering, adequate control of symptoms, and preserving or potentiating Health-Related Quality of Life from a bioethical approach.

Keywords: pediatric palliative care, pediatric oncology, pediatric cancer, quality of life, death

1. Introduction

Cancer is one of the leading causes of death for children and adolescents worldwide, and approximately 280,000 children aged 0–19 are diagnosed with cancer each year. In Latin America and the Caribbean, it is estimated that at least 29,000 children and adolescents under 19 years of age will be affected by cancer each year. Of these, about 10,000 will die from this disease. In high-income countries, more than 80% of children with cancer are cured, but in many low- and middle-income countries, the cure rate is only 20% [1].

Although major improvements have been achieved in pediatric cancer treatment over the last decades, about 4 million children with oncological diseases worldwide require palliative care due to the nature of their condition [2–4].

The WHO in 2002 defines palliative care: "Comprehensive active care of patients whose disease does not respond to active therapies. Its foundation is the relief of pain and other accompanying symptoms and the consideration of psychological, social and spiritual problems. Your goal should be to achieve the highest possible quality of life for the patient and his family. Many aspects are also applicable in previous phases of the disease [5]. "In 2004 "...they seek to improve the quality of life of patients and their families when facing problems associated with life-threatening diseases, thanks to the prevention and relief of suffering from through early identification, assessment, and impeccable treatment of pain and other physical, psychosocial, and spiritual problems [6].

The WHO defines pediatric palliative care (PPC) as the prevention and relief of suffering in patients with life-threatening or life-limiting disease, as well as for their families [7]. To this definition, the American Academy of Pediatrics adds that this care must be offered comprehensively from the moment of diagnosis and throughout the entire disease, whatever the final outcome: cure or death of the child [8].

PPC relies on the comprehensive and multidisciplinary management of the child and the family's physical, psychological, spiritual, and social needs. Importantly, PPC begins at a diagnosis of incurability or supposed incurability, and continues regardless of whether the patient receives any oncological treatment [9]. As such, PPC is a general approach continuing over the entire disease trajectory, which includes, but is not limited to, end-of-life (EoL) care [9–11].

It is widely accepted that the implementation of PPC in pediatric oncology improves the quality of life (QoL) of the child and family, helps reduce symptom burden, diminishes costs of care and access to intensive care units at EoL, and makes dying at home more frequent [12–14]. Of note, PPC implementation is not associated with shorter survival of the patient [15]. Despite the wide availability of dedicated literature and the numerous advantages of PPC implementation in the management of pediatric patients, PPC is still poorly implemented in oncology practice [16].

Indeed, 56% of children with cancer do not have access to PPC before death, and 44.2% of children with advanced cancer are referred to PPC only at EoL [17, 18]. Moreover, only 5% of pediatric oncologists and the child's family discuss palliative advanced care planning [19]. Some barriers persist and prevent a standardized approach to PPC in settings with limited resources and high-income countries [20–22]. These barriers include poor access to essential analgesic drugs in many countries, lack of services and providers dedicated to PPC, scant allocation of resources, limited development of care models, and non-specific educational curricula for healthcare providers [23–26]. Furthermore, PPC is often misperceived as a mutually exclusive service from pediatric oncologists by healthcare providers, patients, and families, and is often associated only with EoL care [9]. Due to all of these barriers, it is not surprising that PPC integration in pediatric oncological practice remains suboptimal. Of note, evidence in the literature suggests that most pediatric oncologists feel that PPC should be consulted more frequently than currently. Thus, further research exploring these specific barriers is necessary to understand the disconnection between oncologists' attitudes and PPC consultation [22].

A comprehensive assessment is required that has an ethical impact on the actions of professionals who work with diseases that can have a fatal course. Pediatric palliative care is the best option for a patient with advanced cancer since people make contact with health institutions. Promoting palliative care does not imply renouncing life in pursuit of its fullness or quality as many may interpret, it only means reconsidering the meaning of clinical measures and concentrating on aspects such as pain and suffering, hope, death management, etc. so that they contribute -above all- to preserving what we have called quality of life or fullness of life. Ramón Bayés [27] a well-known Spanish psycho-oncologist, expressed: "Palliative care is not only the last resort for a group of "biological losers" whom medicine cannot save; they are something to which all human beings have the right to aspire".

Both the WHO and the American Academy of Pediatrics (AAP) and the EAPC (European Association for Palliative Care) [7, 28] establish that the moments in which onco-pediatric palliative care should ideally be started are:

- At the time of diagnosis of a life-limiting disease, to ensure treatment focused on quality of life and symptom relief.

- In cancer patients at the time of diagnosis, regardless of their prognosis.

During the trajectory of the disease, not all pediatric palliative patients are cared for by units specialized in pediatric palliative care; this care is adapted to the needs of each patient at each moment of their life. Depending on the degree of complexity of the pediatric palliative patient, three different levels of care are established [29]:

1. Palliative approach: the pediatrician accepts the irreversibility of the patient's process and the possibility of death as a natural event, without depriving the patient of what they need to be Any health professional with basic knowledge in palliative care can facilitate the palliative approach of the disease.

2. General palliative care: it consists of optimizing symptom control, improving decision-making and caring for the family in order to facilitate their adaptation to grief. It requires intermediate knowledge to manage the most common problems in these patients, and must be administered by professionals who have received at least intermediate training in pediatric palliative care.

3. Specific palliative care: offered by units with specific training and exclusive dedication to palliative care. They cover the needs of a palliative approach and general palliative care and also give control to difficult symptoms, collaborate in making complex decisions taking into account the interest superior of the child, his needs and problems; and in accompanying the family during the life and after the death of the child.

Children are special patients, they do not understand death and pain in the same way as adults. To this fact adds the ethical problems that arise about who should make such tough decisions. Therefore it is important to adequately inform the family and the patient to avoid suffering and uncertainty, and also accompanying them properly.

2. Materials and methods

A bibliographic search was carried out to date in PubMed. The search strategy used the following keywords: palliative care, pediatrics, and their combination, end of life care, pain relief, terminal care, pediatric oncology, quality life. Only articles available in English or Spanish were included. The search has focused on the last 10 years, and if publications of interest do not appear in that period, an attempt has been made to find the most recent and best quality experiences. Articles containing information exclusively on adults or whose results could not be extrapolated were excluded. Children from 0 to 19 years of age have been taken as a reference for pediatric patients, which is the classification that the WHO follows in palliative care.

2.1 Pediatric palliative care (PPC) in oncology

To better understand the basic principles of PPC in oncology, it is of the utmost importance to consider the wide variability in the prognosis and disease trajectory across different types of pediatric cancer. Indeed, cancer rates in children and adolescents have been steadily increasing since 1975, with leukemia and brain tumors being the most frequently diagnosed [30]. This increase is paralleled by a marked increase in survival rates at 5 years, from 58% in the 1970 to >80% nowadays [31, 32]. Prognosis was also varied: in the 1970s, the poorest surviving rates were found in leukemia's; nowadays, despite the general improvement in survival, solid tumors, and particularly rhabdomyosarcoma, bone tumors, central nervous system tumors, and neuroblastoma, are associated with the worst prognosis [33]. Moreover, advances in therapeutic approaches have led to a dramatic change in cancer trajectory, which is reflected not only in the above-mentioned improvement in survivorship, but also in a transition of cancer from an acute disease to a chronic condition that includes complex medical needs and medical device dependence [34, 35]. The clinical and natural history is different according to the type of cancer. Hematological malignancies in younger children with acute onset are associated with life-threatening symptoms and sudden death (due to disease progression or acute complications), occurring mostly in hospitals. Solid tumors are more common among adolescents, may have a chronic evolution, have a relevant social burden due to the long course of the diseases, and often present with a progressive deterioration before death [30].

Children and adolescents in advanced stages of the disease have the undeniable right to receive palliative treatment as the best option to guarantee a quality of life until their death, which is nothing more than guaranteeing the right to a good death; For this, it is necessary to stop at the curative approach and move on to a more realistic and hopeful one based on the specific conditions of existence of each patient and their family, which undoubtedly guarantees personalized care [36].

Palliative care in Oncopediatrics implies assuming not only the vulnerability due to the disease but also that imposed by the very status of a minor. Minors are considered vulnerable groups that require social protection, where the state, the family and the treating team have unavoidable responsibilities without violating the development of the right to their autonomy. This assertion finds its genesis in the different contributions of disciplines such as Pedagogy, Psychology, Pediatrics, Psychiatry, Sociology, Legal Sciences, where the importance and concern for integral and harmonious development in childhood and adolescence [37].

2.2 Pediatric palliative care and their application in pediatric oncology

Several conditions fall into the domain of PPC applications and can be classified as life-threatening (high probability of premature death, but also a chance of long-term survival), life-limiting (where there is no reasonable hope of cure; both definitions also refer to serious illness), and terminal [9]. PPC is different from palliative care in the adult patient as it has to take into account the particular characteristics of the pediatric patient at a physical, developmental, psychosocial, ethical, and spiritual level [9, 38]. Furthermore, parents have a major role in all decisions and retain legal responsibilities regarding their children [38].

Therefore, patients in PPC and their families should be integrated into specific care programs according to the available resources [21, 29, 30]. These programs should be implemented at diagnosis or even before diagnosis when this is uncertain [9]. Three levels of PPC delivery can be identified, as follows: (I) palliative approach provided by all healthcare providers; (II) generalized PPC provided by the oncologist with training in PPC; or (III) specialized PPC, provided in a dedicated setting by a team of interdisciplinary PPC experts [31–33]. The level of PPC delivery can change along the entire disease trajectory [39].

Care can be provided in various settings, e.g., at home, in hospitals, in ambulatory care, or in a pediatric hospice, according to the clinical severity and complexity of needs. Current evidence emphasizes the importance of ensuring care in the setting of the preference of the child and family, but there is no univocal system applicable to all. A "floating" activity, as described by Brock et al., in which the specialized pediatric palliative care team performs a continuous activity divided between the hospice inpatient, hospitalized inpatient with consultation, and home assistance with 24/7 phone consultation plus domiciliary access could be the response to guarantee the continuum of care, which is unusual for PPC [40, 41]. Nevertheless, care at home is generally a common desire of both children and families. Home care ensures a family environment without the additional discomfort of moving to a less familiar and friendly environment, such as a hospital or hospice. Moreover, home care allows for social inclusion in the family's and friends' network, counteracting the loneliness that often affects families of seriously ill children [40–42].

A general palliative approach and supportive care are mandatory in all cancer children. Of note, specialized PPC should be provided well before the EoL period in a child with an incurable or potentially incurable oncological disease, considering the prognosis, the physiological changes related to growth, and the complexity of care [16, 39]. Indeed, the earlier introduction of PPC support in oncological patients has improved QoL and symptom burden [43]. The early integration of PPC also helps in the development of a trusting relationship between healthcare providers and families, thus improving the decision-making process [9].

To help understand when to seek a specialized level of PPC service, some "green lights" have been proposed:

At diagnosis:

- Life-threatening illness (e.g., extended brain glioma) or advanced-stage cancer (e.g., stage IV neuroblastoma; solid metastatic tumor)
- Diagnosis of a tumor with an event-free survival rate estimation <40% with current therapies.
- During illness:
- Progressive metastatic disease
- Recurrent or resistant diseases, also after organ failure
- Major toxicity during treatment
- In case of prolonged hospitalization (>3 weeks) or prolonged admission to intensive care unit (>1 week) without signs of improvement
- In case of three or more unplanned hospitalizations for serious medical issues within a 6-month period [39, 43].

In addition to the "green lights", pediatric oncologists may benefit from using dedicated tools to define the complexity of needs. The pediatric palliative screening scale (PaPas) helps identify children with cancer in need of PPC support by assessing five domains (trajectory of disease, expected outcome and burden from treatments, symptoms burden, preference of care of the child/family, and estimated life expectancy) [44, 45]. Its regular use has been associated with an earlier introduction of PPC and subsequent improvement in QoL [46]. Another example is the ACCAPED scale, which defines eligibility to the different levels of PPC delivery by measuring the grade of the complexity of medical needs and the risk of life-threatening events [47]. Nevertheless, using these instruments should not replace the specific evaluation of each case and the development of a trusting relationship. The investigation of the "needs of care" still represents the best approach to understanding the actual needs of the child and family.

Time of life and quality of life must form a binomial, which may not be perfect. When talking about cancer in the early stages of life, life to the full must become the objective of health care and this implies maintaining the personal principle of priority to life or inviolability of life, which cannot be interpreted as the use of disproportionate measures to maintain life, which is why a frame of reference from anthropological philosophy and bioethics is necessary to be able to offer care for life at the end of life. The moral ethical imperative to promote life with the support that this is the first and most sacred right and a necessary condition to be able to exercise any other type of right, determines that the relief of suffering constitutes a goal that gives real meaning to the action and thus be able to potentiate or preserve the quality of life of the little sufferer and his family. The recognition of the rights of pediatric patients and their comprehensive care under a bioethical approach becomes a great challenge for health professionals: due to the very characteristics imposed by the ontogenetic development of children and its main psychological determinants, (the pediatric patient is in a process of growth and development that definitely affects their understanding of the disease, life and death); due to the still prevailing paternalistic biomedical model, due to the great impact that care work can generate with these children and adolescents, as well as the deficit in their curricular training in such important aspects as the communication of bad news, attention to pain, suffering, mourning, death, hope, family surrender crises, the conspiracy of silence, and coping with the different bioethical dilemmas that they have to face in their professional practice. It is a reality that issues such as euthanasia, dysthanasia, orthothanasia, assisted suicide, therapeutic effort limit, palliative care, pain and suffering, are the order of the day when we talk about care for children and adolescents with cancer, which is why it is required of an axiological line that helps us in the process of humanization of Medicine and of life [48].

The considerations around childhood, adolescence and youth have varied through the different times and knowing and interpreting them allows professionals to locate themselves contextually when making decisions and resolving conflicts that entail ethical dilemmas in pediatric care. Diego Gracia [49] expressed that in the practice of Pediatrics there are two different ways of approaching ethical problems: one called paternalistic and the other autonomist. He says that autonomy should never be valued as a radical autonomy, but that its consideration will help to avoid excesses in which the traditional way of resolving ethical problems in childhood has incurred. In this regard, Claramonte Fuster [50] expresses "...the idea that minors are totally devoid of personal autonomy and, therefore, are incapable of making health decisions, enters into crisis from the sixties."

Several researchers assume that depending on its definition it will lead to immediate moral consequences. Knowledge of the evolutionary development, in general, of children and their moral development qualify a helping relationship that, according to Claramonte Fuster, can characterize a paternalistic doctor-patient relationship or a helping relationship based on autonomy [51].

It is necessary to frame the considerations on autonomy and moral competences in this age group. Autonomy at this stage cannot be governed by the law of all or nothing, that would be assuming a mechanistic attitude towards a problem as complex as the possibility of deciding on life, not even in the adult stage does it manifest itself in this way, since there are different degrees of autonomy and very well, they could be a function of the specific situation rather than the capacity of the subject. For example, should not a child be consulted when a foot has to be amputated? Shouldn't a child be explained when they must stay in a hospital for months, away from their siblings and other family members or when they request go home because you feel that the treatments are not taking away "this thing that I have"? We cannot continue with the belief that children do not realize their situation, nor its complexity. The same doctors and family members, with their actions, are the ones that very frequently generate negative emotional states, closely linked to inadequate communication. Like other researchers, I believe that age is an important aspect when evaluating the moral competencies of children, but not far from their expertise and experiences, especially when it is a child with cancer. Therefore, it would be opportune to ask ourselves autonomy for what, by whom and under what circumstances. Autonomy, freedom and responsibility are concepts that complement each other. The rights of the child have been universally proclaimed and accepted, which reinforces their recognition as a person, so they cannot be sullied or violated. The Convention on the Rights of the Child, adopted by the General Assembly of the United Nations on November 20, 1989, states that: a child is understood to be any human being under the age of 18, unless by virtue of the law that applicable to him, has previously reached the age of majority and said convention promulgates the constitutive rights of people at these ages [52].

The right to have their opinions valued and respect for them is also conditioned because many of these patients come into contact with illness and suffering from a very early age, which can lead to more mature behaviors than other children of similar ages [53]. From the experience of working with these patients, we can refer that many patients adopt behaviors that protect the suffering of their relatives. The attempt by family members to hide the reality from their children and protect them from information that could cause them suffering does not guarantee that it will be achieved because on many occasions children have more information than parents and professionals suppose.

In **Table 1** shows the frequency with which ethical dilemmas arise in clinical care practice and their consideration of whether they are prepared to face them. In it, it can be seen that 56.5% report that it is very common and in the category of common and uncommon, five doctors were located in each one for 21.7% respectively. In relation to the assessment of whether they are prepared to face them, 52.2% expressed that they were not prepared and 47.8% expressed that they were.

Of the 13 doctors (56.5%) who say they face ethical dilemmas very frequently, 30.4% say they are not prepared and of the 3 who were at the frequent level, 2 professionals said they were not prepared. If we combine the levels of Very frequent and Frequent responses, we find 18 doctors (78.2%) who are exposed to ethical dilemmas with some frequency and 9 (50%) are not prepared.

These results reflect the recognition of our professionals of their lack of preparation to face ethical dilemmas that become frequent in their practical actions. This information and the results reflected in other tables express the importance and need for training in Bioethics [37].

Frequency of ethical dilemmas	Preparation to face dilemmas				Total	
	Yes		No			
	n	%	n	%	n	%
Very common	6	26,1	7	30,4	13	56,5
Frequent	3	13,0	2	8,7	5	21,7
Infrequent	2	8,7	3	13,0	5	21,7
Never	0	0	0	0	0	0
Total	11	47,8	12	52,2	23	100

Table 1.
Doctors according to their opinions on the frequency of ethical dilemmas and preparation to face them.

Self-assessments in areas of performance in Pediatric Oncophysics, for which professional competencies are required in terms of knowledge, skills, and attitudes, are very important. The appropriation of an ethic of care sustained or based on an ethic of virtues is essential in performing in these areas. The virtues constitute a disposition to do well and should not be governed only by pure altruism, but rather organized in a health system and in the functional performance of any specialty. These "habits of the heart" are formed from undergraduate and are consolidated in postgraduate. If these issues are absent in the training of specialists, they will express knowledge and skills in care, but they will lack attitudes, which will lead to an "ethics of abandonment", instead of leading to an "ethics of non-abandonment". Ethical problem that has been reflected in the literature as "dispersion of responsibility" or "collusion in anonymity" [54]. Training in Bioethical issues in Oncopediatrics professionals is insufficient and does not allow the approach to quality of life through all sources, nor considering all the bioethical foundations and principles.

2.3 Reality, barriers and challenges

A study was carried out to find out when the PC started. 54.4% of oncopediatric patients had received palliative services before death [17]. The mean time from cancer diagnosis to palliative consultation was 509.6 days. Therefore, it did not occur at the time of diagnosis as recommended by the WHO. In part it is due to the fear of the professionals themselves; starting palliative care so early may provoke a feeling of hopelessness both in the child and the family. Related to this, a study of 1.2 million subjects revealed of between 33–38% of patients received treatment with curative intent, but with no beneficial effects, in the last 6 months of life [55]. It is better to alleviate and not be stubborn in these cases. Finding the best comfort conditions for the patient. In addition to the above, there are numerous barriers to the effective implementation of Palliative Care: policy (many countries do not include the need for this care in their legislation), education (professionals around the world are poorly trained in these subjects), availability of medicines (many countries have limited access to opioids. Developed countries consume 90% of painkillers [56]. If this is added that more than 97% of the children who need PC are in the latter countries), implementation, need for health personnel, psychological, social and cultural (people tend to avoid everything associated with the word death), financial...

Palliative care for pediatric cancer patients is widely recognized by different countries, organizations and international organizations, which does not imply that they have the same development in all the nations in which they are established. At the IV International Meeting of Pediatric Psychology, held in Mexico City, in 2019, a conference entitled "Reality of Pediatric Palliative Care in Latin America" was presented, conditioned by the review of updated works on the subject and by the The authors' experience, where reference is made to the fact that there is greater experience in cancer patients than with other diseases, the existence of uneven development in the region between countries, as well as the lack of consensus on CPP programs. 98% of children who need palliative care live in low- and middle-income countries, with little development of the hospice model for children and adolescents and of home care, as well as a lack of interrelation between the different levels of health care. The lack of public strategies that focus on the training of professionals and not only on policies and material resources is exposed, which, moreover, do not cover the needs of the demands of patients and family members, and are still focused on a biologist and paternalistic model. Lack of a palliative approach for curricular training versus technological development [57].

They were presented as challenges or challenges:

- Achieve more equitable and universal coverage for children with life-threatening/limiting conditions and their families.

- Strengthen social health policies and systems at all levels.

- Promote the development of different models of Pediatric Palliative Care.

- Adequately incorporate the religious and spiritual dimension.

- Recognize them as an essential right and not a resource for losers.

- Offer a service focused on quality and warmth of care.

- Evaluate the same CPP but at the same time differently than in adults.

- Define the role of children and adolescents in decision-making and the role of informed consent in Pediatrics.

- Develop intervention strategies to meet the needs of the child, the family and the care team.

- Recognize communication, support and teamwork as irreplaceable tools.

- Take advantage of the benefits of technology and social networks in their development.

- Generate training and professional training activities.

- Implement national and intercultural research

It concludes with the need for an unavoidable commitment from the governments for the development of the CPP, to stimulate international cooperation in assistance, teaching and research, and the development of scientific events that allow sharing experiences and socializing knowledge as well as promoting the development of multi-centre and international scientific productions [57].

2.4 Pediatric palliative care and death

2.4.1 Ethics and autonomy

There is a question we must ask ourselves: who should decide? The decision should be a joint one between the patient, the relatives and the healthcare personnel. The child, if he/she is somewhat older, has the right to know the situation and to be well informed [58]. The child, regardless of age, must be adequately informed and adapted to his or her age.

The knowledge of the doctors about the terms of mature minor, emancipated minor and majority is reflected in **Table 2**. The results show that only 5 doctors frame the age of the mature minor between 12 and 14 years and of them, one places them at 14 years old and the remaining four at 12 years old. These data tell us that, if we consider this range of ages as appropriate, then only 21.7% adequately locate the age at which the minor is considered mature; the others misplace them or say they do not know the term.

Ignorance of this theory or doctrine could cause many professionals not to maintain a more flexible position in relation to considerations of capabilities and self-determination in these patients, despite the fact that it is not institutionalized in our country. Although in our country this term is not supported by law, it is at least important to highlight that the Civil Code [59] in force in our country expresses in its Article 29 that the full capacity to exercise rights and carry out legal acts is acquired by: (a) when the age of majority is reached, which begins at 18 years of age and in section (b) when the minor gets married.

Article 3 of the Family Code states that exceptionally, and for justified reasons, minors under 18 years of age may be granted authorization to formalize the marriage, provided that the female is at least 14 years old and the male is 16 years old, also compliments.

This reflection is made to draw attention to the "age" variable to assume responsibilities towards some things and not towards others. I wonder, will not the condition of illness be an important factor for adolescents to also assume other responsibilities for very justified reasons in relation to their health?

Age	Mature minor		Emancipated minor		Majority of age	
	n	%	n	%	n	%
1–6	1	4,3	0	0	0	0
7–11	5	21,7	2	8,7	0	0
12–14	5	21,7	1	4,3	0	0
15–17	2	8,7	6	26,1	4	17,4
18 and over	2	8,7	2	8,7	18	78,3
Does not know	8	34,8	12	52,2	1	4,3
Total	23	100	23	100	23	100

Table 2.
Opinion of doctors in relation to age to define the categories of: Mature minor, emancipated minor and majority.

The term emancipated minor is unknown to 52.2% and 6 doctors (26.1%) placed it at ages between 15 and 17 years and of these only 4 at the age of 16 years; therefore, 82.7% do not place it appropriately due to the age variable.

The knowledge of when the age of majority is acquired is more adjusted to reality, with 78.3% of doctors stating that the age of majority is reached at 18 years of age and older; of them, only two cases refer to 19 years of age and one to 21. It is important to highlight the significance that this concept has for pediatric practice in adolescents with cancer where, as they themselves express, they very often face ethical dilemmas that arise due to conflicts. Decision between the professionals and the patient or between the patient and their parents or between the professionals and the minor's parents [37].

These data are very important for the topic discussed where it is ultimately assessed whether children with cancer can and should evaluate their quality of life [60].

2.4.2 Death awareness

Seriously ill children who know that death is irreversible are afraid of not leaving a legacy, of being forgotten. They also tend to think about death, even if they do not communicate it. From 18 months to 5 years of age, children do not understand the concept of the future, they live only in the present and associate death with sleep and immobility. From 5 to 10 years of age, they begin to be curious about death, and it implies separation not only from parents but also from friends and school. The irreversible nature of death is acquired around the age of 9 years, especially the fear of the death of parents appears [61].

Death is, therefore, a reality faced by the teams that care for children with cancer, so it is a situation that can be conceived as a failure at work or as the loss of someone significant [55]. It is this feeling of loss and the perception of less effective care or attention provision that can generate impotence, suffering, anger, sadness and insecurity, leading the professional to greater emotional exhaustion [57]. This is added to the appearance of physical health problems such as headaches, excessive nervousness, abdominal disorders and sleep disturbances, which translates into a decrease in the quality of care, job dissatisfaction and increased absenteeism. For some participants, this problem responds both to the lack of professional training in the areas of palliative care and grief support as well as to the inadequate support that exists from the health institutions themselves to the health teams, in the process of coping with the loss of patients [61].

In the case of pediatric cancer care, it must be taken into account that treatments are long and have many side effects for patients, requiring a growing demand for care, to which are added organizational factors such as fatigue due to lack of personnel, communication deficits, surrogate decision-making, role conflicts, and insufficient vacation time [61].

In contrast to the above, some nursing studies have revealed that the death of a patient can also generate positive attitudes, which are related to the satisfaction generated by the delivery of quality care to people at the end of life, which is considered rewarding and a learning situation, reducing the risk of emotional fatigue and with it, the burnout syndrome [62, 63]. Following what has been described, several studies have indicated that social support for health professionals can be an important mediator in coping with the death of patients, especially in the field of child health care [64, 65]. However, this support must not only be mediated by the recognition of the emotional bond with the patient, but also by the possibility of expressing the pain of the loss and feeling real support that responds to expectations and needs [22].

Llantá (2011), states that the diagnosis of Cancer in a child or adolescent, even when cancers in these age groups present a different behavior in terms of morbidity and mortality statistics in relation to Cancer in adults (70% of diagnosed patients may be survivors of childhood cancer) It is no less sad that 30% will die from the disease and/or complications throughout the treatment, so death must be considered within the natural course of the neoplastic disease [66].

In **Table 3** we have grouped different areas of performance that can in themselves be established as indispensable instruments of commitment in Oncology and especially in Oncopediatrics. As can be seen, the highest frequency percentages located in the Very category were: communication of treatments, with 11 professionals (47.8%) and communication of the diagnosis, with 9 (39.1%). In the Quite category, the best results were achieved by: communication of change from curative to palliative treatment and in attention to death, with 15 doctors (65.2%) respectively, followed in descending order by attention to suffering with 14 doctors. (60.9%), therapeutic care of hopes and knowledge in palliative care with 13 physicians (56.5%) respectively. More than half consider that they have little or no preparation in caring for grief with 12 professionals (52.1%), nor for caring for crises of family claudication with 14 (60.8%) and for the conspiracy of silence with 13 (56.5%).

Illustrative statements extracted from the interviews are expressed that denote the lack of preparation on these issues.

"I do not have the courage to tell a teenager or someone who is 8 or 10 years old who considers themselves a teenager: you have osteosarcoma or you are full of metastases and you are going to die soon, I do not have the courage to say that, Now, to the family yes, to the mother, to the father but not to the child, I do not have the courage for that"; "...ah look, you have a little cyst on your leg that we are going to take care of and since you are going to get a little short of breath at times, we are going to give a little bit of oxygen to help you but you are going to see that everything It's going to get better soon... you are going to see that soon, now it's not immediate, it takes a little while, it could be 15 days, it could be 20 days, you are going to get the oxygen when you need it... I do not have the courage."

"...I do many things because I have been learning from you...".

All the contents addressed are related to the topic of palliative care and its therapeutic management, where the majority of researchers and experts on the subject refer that there has been and still is a lack of curricular training, both from undergraduate and postgraduate levels [67]. In Cuba, the Special Working Group on Palliative Care, of which the author of this research is a member, has carried out training on these topics in different provinces of the country, but in the area of adults. Training on these topics of pediatric palliative care is a debt to our professionals and to our little mourners that must be resolved [37].

The author of this research [37] states that "The current medical model emphasizes the cure much more than the relief of suffering and this same paternalistic and even biological model makes us feel like losers when we cannot save a life and even guilty, so we perform heroic acts that have no other result than affecting the quality of life and a good death.

The doctor fails when he puts stubbornness into practice by maintaining obstinate behavior; what we consider inhuman, on many occasions demeaning and always a costly mistake that our little sufferers have to pay for as well as their families, but the professionals who care for children and adolescents with cancer do not fail when they appropriate the approach in their professional clinical practice. of palliative care, which presents among its basic strategies not to shorten but not to lengthen life, not

Performance areas	Preparation level							
	A lot		Quite		Bit		Nothing	
	n	**%**	**n**	**%**	**n**	**%**	**n**	**%**
Communication of the diagnosis	9	39,1	11	47,8	1	4,3	2	8,7
Communication of treatments	11	47,8	9	39,1	1	4,3	2	8,7
Communication of change from curative to palliative treatment	5	21,7	15	65,2	0	0	3	13,0
Attention to the dying process	2	8,7	15	65,2	4	17,4	2	8,7
Pay attention to fears and worries	3	13,0	11	47,8	6	26,1	3	13,0
Attention to suffering	4	17,4	14	60,9	3	13,0	2	8,7
Pay attention to hopes	4	17,4	13	56,5	4	17,4	2	8,7
Grief care	2	8,7	9	39,1	10	43,5	2	8,7
Prevention of family claudication crises	2	8,7	7	30,4	9	39,1	5	21,7
Prevention of the conspiracy of silence	1	4,3	9	39,1	8	34,8	5	21,7
Limit therapeutic effort	4	17,4	11	47,8	5	21,7	3	13,0
Palliative Care	2	8,7	13	56,5	6	26,1	2	8,7

Table 3.
Level of preparation for performance in difficult situations.

to advance death but not to delay it, not to favor death but not to make it difficult, not to kill but to let go, not to isolation, abandonment, emotional distancing, inadequate management of hopes and the conspiracy of silence, which implies proper management of information, promoting a quality death that is nothing more than giving quality of life until the last moment of existence. This aspect entails ethical dilemmas that are difficult to resolve and as Dr. Gómez Sancho would say "The doctor must learn that everything that can be done... should not be done" [68].

The CPPs and their establishment need to be in tune with the needs of patients, families and the team that provide health care in a specific sociocultural context, policies and institutional and state strategies cannot be unrelated to their implementation. Pediatric patients receiving palliative care are in a stage of development in all its aspects, where their psychological needs are related to the evolutionary stage within their ontogenetic development, but there are also needs conditioned by the disease, its treatments, frequent hospitalizations, changes in the family, social, school dynamics, the separation from their siblings, relatives and friends, which will undoubtedly influence their adaptation process. Their cognitive and emotional development condition the assessments they will have about their symptoms, worries, limitations and about the conception of the process of dying, which has meant that today it is the patients themselves who offer more accurate assessments about indicators of a subjective-emotional nature so their assessments should not be excluded. Symptom control, minimizing experiences of suffering and preserving and/or enhancing their quality of life and well-being cannot be outside of the own considerations and assessments of these patients [69].

The issue of communication and teamwork are irreplaceable tools for achieving objectives throughout the entire process and much more at the end of life.

Affectations in caregivers of children and adolescents with cancer are confirmed -more specifically in parents- while the reports on the QoL of their children are worse than the reports of the patients themselves, which places parents and family members as vulnerable groups in need of psychological support. Identifying the needs of these families, their preparation for the process of dying of their children, how to avoid the conspiracy of silence, crises of family claudication and preparation for mourning are tasks of the first order within the framework of a humanized medicine. If caregivers are affected, this will have an impact on care, so it is essential to work with them to alleviate their suffering, improve their coping styles and provide them with personological resources that allow them to fulfill the painful task of caring for a child with cancer [69].

The conspiracy of silence, under the pretext of protecting the minor, only achieves an atmosphere of mystery and loneliness and this is very common in pediatric and adult practice. If we take what happens with adults with cancer as a reference, it is impossible not to think that this phenomenon is much more exacerbated in children and adolescents. Doctors believe that children are unaware of the situation, ignoring the experiences that they are accumulating in their own hospital wards and the behaviors and attitudes of family members and that of the professionals themselves. Family surrender crises and grief are issues that require solid professional training and a deep ethical commitment that we cannot leave to spontaneity and common sense. When a person like this is asked and demanded to "do their part" or to "fight for life", to "be strong", when they are deceived by promising an improvement that does not come, when they are treated with pity that lacerates self-esteem, when we are asked questions for which we have no answers for fear of hurting them and making them suffer, when silence and silence as an answer is our behavior, we are generating unnecessary suffering and for this we are responsible. We must be very careful with the information, which cannot be translated into the absence of communication [70].

The illustrative statements that were expressed in the interviews.

"...in my opinion, you can say, well, someone who can come close to what I would classify as well prepared, in that someone I am talking about perhaps 5–10% of doctors, I cannot tell you more honestly. Because I think there is nothing more to it than that."

"To give you examples that I have had, I have had to assume this support role and remove the professional because that professional is participating in that moment in the duel as if he were a family member and therefore, loses the role."

"...generally the palliative part belongs to what is primary care, we are here to cure."

"You see the children, you know that they are going to die, that they no longer have a solution and you continue with the palliative treatment and things like that..., personally I reject him a little, I no longer want to go in to see him, now I do not want to... since I know that this is the reality in me, in my person, when I know that they are in this phase and I have to go see it, it's my turn, but I would not want to go see it, I would not want to enter. To that cubicle, I would not want to anymore, do you understand me?... I already see the parents with pity... sometimes I would not want to look at them in front of them."

"There are people who continue to make the same mistakes when it comes to managing grief. Do you want something more difficult than seeing the professional give elements to perpetuate the grief?..."; "You as a professional have to know that grief does not exist until the patient dies."

The author's criteria, supported by reviews on the subject and by her work experience with children with cancer for 17 years, is in favor of children who die of cancer receiving aggressive treatments at the end of their lives, experiencing suffering without adequate control of symptoms, they die in health institutions, in intensive care rooms full of technology and do not receive the benefits of home care at all.

In professionals, it is important to stimulate the development of competencies for this type of care, from the development of knowledge, skills and attitudes, since they frequently complain about the lack of curricular training. It is also necessary to prevent and control burnout or burnout syndrome, compassion fatigue, the development of strategies for teamwork, the work-family relationship, and emotional self-regulation in the face of the suffering of others. The evaluation of professional burnout emerges as an important task to develop since in reality it is not a myth, but a reality in our environment. It is not ethical, nor human, to be treated by a professional who is affected by the so-called Burnout Syndrome (depersonalization, emotional exhaustion and lack of personal fulfillment); neither is working in those conditions were not only the health of the worker is affected, but also the health of the family. This was studied in these caregivers, also as part of the "Quality of life in Oncopediatrics" Project [71]. Different investigations support the need to pay attention to this syndrome [72]. The therapeutic relentlessness or the use of disproportionate means are conceived as a transgression to the quality of life, although it is recognized that it occurs in clinical practice. For this group of professionals, the concept of quality of life in patients with advanced or terminal disease is not renounced, a very important aspect in light of the current controversies within Bioethics between utilitarian and personality perspectives around this concept and its misuse as a justification for ending a life when it is considered without quality [72].

"There are people who continue to make the same mistakes when it comes to handling the duel, do you want something more difficult than seeing that the professional gives elements to perpetuate the duel?..."; "You, as a professional, have to know that the duel does not exist yet until the patient dies." This constitutes an erroneous conceptualization of mourning. There is anticipatory mourning that, when well-managed, helps family members in coping with the death of a loved one [73].

The training of these pediatric palliative care issues is a debt with our professionals and with our little mourners that must be resolved.

2.5 Professionals

The non-inclusion of value ethics in their conceptions leads to a reductionist use of the term. The professionals recognize that if they offered information provided to patients in relation to their diagnosis, treatment, and side effects, if they listened to their worries or concerns, and if they provided psychological support, they would contribute to preserving or enhancing the quality of life of their patients.

These same researchers, like Cassem [74], report that telling the truth, adapted to the strength of each patient and maintaining hope, is a firm basis for a relationship of trust and will facilitate the resolution of problems that arise in the cancer patient journey.

The communication of the diagnosis is a dynamic process, where the correct use of the information is therapeutic and where the main principles to inform are those of the bearable truth and the truth desirable.

Teamwork and psychological support were recognized as favorable factors that influence the quality of life of these children and adolescents.

Teamwork, the work of the psychologist and emotional support are resources that promote quality of life as buffers against emotional distress in children, family members and the work team itself.

3. Conclusions and future directions

A child with cancer needs care beyond cancer treatment, such as treating complex symptoms, psychosocial support, and sharing existential and spiritual issues. The goal of PPC is to share strategies, tools, and skills with pediatric oncologists to guarantee a continuous and multidimensional assessment and management of those needs, and taking care of the patient–family unit. Early involvement of a PPC team and the application of the PPC principles has been shown to positively impact the QoL of pediatric cancer patients at all stages of the disease.

Unfortunately, there is still a gap between what could be done and what is being done in clinical practice. Indeed, there are several areas to be addressed to allow all children with cancer an integrated and effective approach to palliative care: first, training that allows and stimulates integration between pediatric oncologists and PPC experts, through the acquisition and sharing of skills on the fundamental principles of palliative care and teamwork. Another important need is research: collecting and sharing data, strategies, and tools can lead to new strategies and more effective models of care. To reach all children eligible for PPC and their families, new technologies and tools, such as telemedicine, should be implemented.

With the hope that the availability of PPC services will increase worldwide, we believe that it is now essential that the application of palliative care principles becomes familiar to all healthcare professionals. Today in pediatric oncology, holistic care of the child with cancer and their family represents a standard of care that must be guaranteed to every child in every setting.

Moreover, a constantly evolving field, the challenge for the future will be to harmonize the interaction between PPC specialists and oncologists in order to provide truly holistic patient care.

Despite medical advances, pediatric palliative patients still continue to suffer significantly.

One of the most important goals of PCs focuses on the need to initiate this aspect of care as soon as possible, as well as to work in a multidisciplinary manner, delving into the latest quality information in order to improve the health care of our patients. A fundamental point is the doctor-patient relationship and the doctor-family relationship, in order to achieve a global approach to the patient's problems. To this end, it is essential to work on the psychosocial, emotional and spiritual aspects, as well as to provide the necessary and fair information to both the patient and the family members in order to facilitate the assimilation of the process. Another very influential aspect is the international inequality in terms of recognition of this right and the material and drug availability of the countries. Governments must cooperate and help less wealthy countries to achieve the objectives proposed by the WHO.

Author contributions

Data collection, F.M., and LL. MC.; manuscript writing: F.M., and LL.MC.; manuscript revision, F.M., and LL.MC.; approval to submit: F.M., and LL.MC. All authors have read and agreed to the published version of the manuscript.

Funding

This research received no external funding.

Conflicts of interest

The authors declare no conflict of interest.

Author details

Mariuska Forteza Sáez* and Marìa del Carmen Llantà
Institute of Oncology and Radiobiology of Havana, Cuba

*Address all correspondence to: mforteza8324@gmail.com

References

[1] Siegel RL, Miller KD, Fuchs HE, Jemal A. Cancer statistics, 2021. CA: A Cancer Journal for Clinicians. 2021;**71**(1):7-33

[2] Connor SR, Downing J, Marston J. Estimating the global need for palliative care for children: A cross-sectional analysis. Journal of Pain and Symptom Management. 2017;**53**:171-177. DOI: 10.1016/j.jpainsymman.2016.08.020

[3] Make Every Child Count. Available from: https://www.togetherforshortlives.org.uk/resource/make-every-child-count/ [Accessed: February 22, 2022]

[4] Feudtner C, Kang TI, Hexem KR, Friedrichsdorf SJ, Osenga K, Siden H, et al. Pediatric palliative care patients: A prospective multicenter cohort study. Pediatrics. 2011;**127**:094-101. DOI: 10.1542/peds.2010-3225

[5] World Health Organization. WHO definition of palliative care. 2002. Disponible en: http://www.whoint/cancer/palliative/definition/en [Acceso marzo 2007]

[6] Organización Mundial de la Salud. WHO Definition of Palliative Care. Organización Mundial de la Salud; 2004

[7] Committee on Bioethics and Committee on Hospital Car. Palliative care for children. Pediatrics. 2000;**106**(2):351-357. DOI: 10.1542/peds.106.2.351

[8] World Health Organization Integrating Palliative Care and Symptom Relief in Paediatrics. 2018. Available from: https://apps.who.int/iris/handle/10665/274561 [Accessed: February 23, 2022]

[9] Benini F, Pappadatou D, Bernadá M, Craig F, De Zen L, Downing J, et al. International standards for pediatric palliative care: From IMPaCCT to GO-PPaCS. Journal of Pain and Symptom Management. 2022;**63**:e529-e543. DOI: 10.1016/j.jpainsymman.2021.12.031

[10] Snaman J, McCarthy S, Wiener L, Wolfe J. Pediatric palliative care in oncology. Journal of Clinical Oncology. 2020;**38**:954-962. DOI: 10.1200/JCO.18.02331

[11] Salins N, Hughes S, Preston N. Palliative care in paediatric oncology: An update. Current Oncology Reports. 2022;**24**:175-186. DOI: 10.1007/s11912-021-01170-3

[12] Kaye EC, Weaver MS, DeWitt LH, Byers E, Stevens SE, Lukowski J, et al. The impact of specialty palliative care in pediatric oncology: A systematic review. Journal of Pain and Symptom Management. 2021;**61**:1060-1079.e2. DOI: 10.1016/j.jpainsymman.2020.12.003

[13] Friedrichsdorf SJ, Postier A, Dreyfus J, Osenga K, Sencer S, Wolfe J. Improved quality of life at end of life related to home-based palliative care in children with cancer. Journal of Palliative Medicine. 2015;**18**:143-150. DOI: 10.1089/jpm.2014.0285

[14] Snaman JM, Kaye EC, Lu JJ, Sykes A, Baker JN. Palliative care involvement is associated with less intensive end-of-life care in adolescent and young adult oncology patients. Journal of Palliative Medicine. 2017;**20**:509-516. DOI: 10.1089/jpm.2016.0451

[15] Keim-Malpass J, Erickson JM, Malpass HC. End-of-life care characteristics for young adults with

cancer who die in the hospital. Journal of Palliative Medicine. 2014;**17**:1359-1364. DOI: 10.1089/jpm.2013.0661

[16] Cuviello A, Raisanen JC, Donohue PK, Wiener L, Boss RD. Defining the boundaries of palliative care in pediatric oncology. Journal of Pain and Symptom Management. 2020;**59**:1033-1042.e1. DOI: 10.1016/j.jpainsymman.2019.11.022

[17] Cheng BT, Rost M, De Clercq E, Arnold L, Elger BS, Wangmo T. Palliative care initiation in pediatric oncology patients: A systematic review. Cancer Medicine. 2019;**8**:3-12. DOI: 10.1002/cam4.1907

[18] Thompson LA, Knapp C, Madden V, Shenkman E. Pediatricians' perceptions of and preferred timing for pediatric palliative care. Pediatrics. 2009;**123**:e777-e782. DOI: 10.1542/peds.2008-2721

[19] Kaye EC, Woods C, Kennedy K, Velrajan S, Gattas M, Bilbeisi T, et al. Communication around palliative care principles and advance care planning between oncologists, children with advancing cancer and families. British Journal of Cancer. 2021;**125**:1089-1099. DOI: 10.1038/s41416-021-01512-9

[20] Benini F, Orzalesi M, de Santi A, Congedi S, Lazzarin P, Pellegatta F, et al. Barriers to the development of pediatric palliative care in Italy. Annali dell'Istituto Superiore di Sanità. 2016;**52**:558-564. DOI: 10.4415/ANN_16_04_16

[21] Ehrlich BS, Movsisyan N, Batmunkh T, Kumirova E, Borisevich MV, Kirgizov K, et al. Barriers to the early integration of palliative care in pediatric oncology in 11 Eurasian countries. Cancer. 2020;**126**:4984-4993. DOI: 10.1002/cncr.33151

[22] Parisio KN, Levy CD, Lewis AM, Schultz CL. Attitudes and practices of pediatric oncologists regarding palliative care consultation for pediatric oncology patients. Journal of Pediatric Hematology/Oncology. 2021;**44**(5):230-236. DOI: 10.1097/MPH.0000000000002276. Epub ahead of print

[23] Bogetz JF, Root MC, Purser L, Torkildson C. Comparing health care provider-perceived barriers to pediatric palliative care fifteen years ago and today. Journal of Palliative Medicine. 2019;**22**:145-151. DOI: 10.1089/jpm.2018.0367

[24] Drach LL, Cook M, Shields S, Burger KJ. Changing the culture of pediatric palliative care at the bedside. Journal of Hospice and Palliative Nursing. 2021;**23**:20-27. DOI: 10.1097/NJH.0000000000000707

[25] Marcus KL, Santos G, Ciapponi A, Comandé D, Bilodeau M, Wolfe J, et al. Impact of specialized pediatric palliative care: A systematic review. Journal of Pain and Symptom Management. 2020;**59**:339-364.e10. DOI: 10.1016/j.jpainsymman.2019.08.005

[26] Benini F, Cauzzo C, Congedi S, Da Dalt L, Cogo P, Biscaglia L, et al. Training in pediatric palliative care in Italy: Still much to do. Annali dell'Istituto Superiore di Sanità. 2019;**55**:240-245. DOI: 10.4415/ANN_19_03_07

[27] Bayés R. The Psychology of Suffering and Death. Vol. 14, 2. Barcelona: Martínez Roca Editions; 2001. pp. 93-99

[28] Organización Mundial de la Salud. WHO Definition of Palliative Care. Organización Mundial de la Salud; 1998

[29] Chambers Association for Children's Palliative Care. A Guide to the

Development of children's Palliative Care Services. ACT; 2009

[30] Bhakta N, Force LM, Allemani C, Atun R, Bray F, Coleman MP, et al. Childhood cancer burden: A review of global estimates. The Lancet Oncology. 2019;**20**:e42-e53. DOI: 10.1016/S1470-2045(18)30761-7

[31] Hudson MM, Link MP, Simone JV. Milestones in the curability of pediatric cancers. Journal of Clinical Oncology. 2014;**32**:2391-2397. DOI: 10.1200/JCO.2014.55.6571

[32] Donnelly DW, Gavin AT. Mortality among children and young people who survive cancer in Northern Ireland. The Ulster Medical Journal. 2016;**85**:158-163

[33] Ward E, DeSantis C, Robbins A, Kohler B, Jemal A. Childhood and adolescent cancer statistics, 2014. CA: A Cancer Journal for Clinicians. 2014;**64**:83-103. DOI: 10.3322/caac.21219

[34] Snaman JM, Kaye EC, Baker JN, Wolfe J. Pediatric palliative oncology: The state of the science and art of caring for children with cancer. Current Opinion in Pediatrics. 2018;**30**:40-48. DOI: 10.1097/MOP.0000000000000573

[35] Rosenberg AR, Wolfe J. Approaching the third decade of paediatric palliative oncology investigation: Historical progress and future directions. The Lancet Child & Adolescent Health. 2017;**1**:56-67. DOI: 10.1016/S2352-4642(17)30014-7

[36] AMC L. Enfoque interdisciplinar a la calidad de vida y de muerte en oncopediatría. Rev Cuba Enf. 2011;**27**(1):98-105. Disponible en: http://bvs.sld.cu/revistas/enf

[37] Llantá MC. Calidad de vida en Oncopediatrìa: una reflexión desde la Bioética [thesis]. Tesis para optar por el grado científico de Master en Bioética. La Habana, Cuba: Universidad Católica de Valencia y Centro Juan Pablo II; 2013. Available from: http://scielo.sld.cu/scielo

[38] Kattner P, Strobel H, Khoshnevis N, Grunert M, Bartholomae S, Pruss M, et al. Compare and contrast: Pediatric cancer versus adult malignancies. Cancer Metastasis Reviews. 2019;**38**:673-682. DOI: 10.1007/s10555-019-09836-y

[39] Jankovic M, De Zen L, Pellegatta F, Lazzarin P, Bertolotti M, Manfredini L, et al. A consensus conference report on defining the eligibility criteria for pediatric palliative care in Italy. Italian Journal of Pediatrics. 2019;**45**:89. DOI: 10.1186/s13052-019-0681-3

[40] Brock KE, Snaman JM, Kaye EC, Bower KA, Weaver MS, Baker JN, et al. Models of pediatric palliative oncology outpatient care-benefits, challenges, and opportunities. Journal of Oncology Practice/ American Society of Clinical Oncology. 2019;**15**:476-487. DOI: 10.1200/JOP.19.00100

[41] American Academy of Pediatrics Committee on Bioethics and Committee on Hospital Care. Palliative care for children. Pediatrics. 2000;**106**:351-357

[42] Chong PH, De Castro Molina JA, Teo K, Tan WS. Paediatric palliative care improves patient outcomes and reduces healthcare costs: Evaluation of a home-based program. BMC Palliative Care. 2018;**17**:11. DOI: 10.1186/s12904-017-0267-z

[43] Kaye EC, Friebert S, Baker JN. Early integration of palliative care for children with high-risk cancer and their families. Pediatric Blood & Cancer. 2016;**63**:593-597. DOI: 10.1002/pbc.25848

[44] Bergstraesser E, Hain RD, Pereira JL. The development of an instrument

that can identify children with palliative care needs: The Paediatric palliative screening scale (PaPaS scale): A qualitative study approach. BMC Palliative Care. 2013;**12**:20. DOI: 10.1186/1472-684X-12-20

[45] Song IG, Kwon SY, Chang YJ, Kim MS, Jeong SH, Hahn SM, et al. Paediatric palliative screening scale as a useful tool for clinicians' assessment of palliative care needs of pediatric patients: A retrospective cohort study. BMC Palliative Care. 2021;**20**:73. DOI: 10.1186/s12904-021-00765-8

[46] Andriastuti M, Halim PG, Kusrini E, Bangun M. Correlation of pediatric palliative screening scale and quality of life in pediatric cancer patients. Indian Journal of Palliative Care. 2020;**26**:338-341. DOI: 10.4103/IJPC.IJPC_197_19

[47] Lazzarin P, Giacomelli L, Terrenato I, Benini F. On behalf of the ACCAPED study group a tool for the evaluation of clinical needs and eligibility to pediatric palliative care: The validation of the ACCAPED scale. Journal of Palliative Medicine. 2021;**24**:205-210. DOI: 10.1089/jpm.2020.0148

[48] Abreu L. Calidad de vida relacionada con la salud en pacientes oncopediátricos: La Habana, 2011-2013. Editorial Universitaria; 2016. Available from: https://indaga.ual.es/permalink/34CBUA_UAL/12cive/alma991001886671204991

[49] Gracia D. Ética de los confines de la Vida. Colección Ética y vida. Cap. 9. In: Estudios de Bioética. 1a. ed. Vol. Tomo 3. El Buho; 1998. pp. 193-205

[50] Claramonte Fuster MA. El principio de la autonomía en el niño y el adolescente En: Ensayos de Bioética-3. España: Ed. Mapfre, S. A. Institut. Borja de Bioética; 2003:253

[51] Llantá AMC, Grau AJ, Bayarre VH. Calidad de Vida relacionada con la Salud en Oncopediatría: Hacia una reflexión del tema. Revista Habanera de Ciencias Médicas. 2014;**13**(3):528-536. Available from: http://scielo.sld.cu

[52] General Assembly of the United Nations. Ratification and Accession by General Assembly Resolution 44/25 of 20 November 1989. Vol. 1577. United Nations, Treaty Series; 1987. p. 3. Available from: https://www.refworld.org/docid/3ae6b38f0.html [Accessed: July 19, 2023]

[53] Hendricks-Ferguson V. Relationships of age and gender to hope and spiritual well-being among adolescents with cancer. Journal of Pediatric Oncology Nursing. 2006;**23**:189-199. DOI: 10.1177/1043454206289757

[54] Grau JA, Chacón M, Llanta MC. Psicología de la salud: diversas perspectivas para mejorar la calidad de vida. In: La Evaluación Psicológica del Sufrimiento y de la calidad de vida al final de la vida: una revisión. Puebla, México: Editora de la Universidad Autónoma de Puebla; 2015. pp. 172-218, ISBN 978-607-96675-5-9. Available from: https://dialnet.unirioja.es/servlet/articulo?codigo=5634119

[55] Cardona-Morrell M, Kim J, Turner RM, Anstey M, Mitchell IA, Hillman K. Non-beneficial treatments in hospital at the end of life: A systematic review on extent of the problem. International Journal for Quality in Health Care. 2016;**28**(4):456-469. DOI: 10.1093/intqhc/mzw060. Epub 2016 Jun 27

[56] WHO. Global Atlas of Palliative Care. 2nd ed. Geneva, Switzerland: World Health Organization; 2020. COPYRIGHT © 2020 by Worldwide Palliative Care ISBN: 978-0-9928277-2-4

[57] Gómez García WC, Rivas S, Paz G, Bustamante M, Castro G, Gutiérrez H. Pediatric oncology palliative care programs in Central America: Pathways to success. Children (Basel). 2021;**8**(11):1031. DOI: 10.3390/children8111031

[58] Weaver MS, Mooney-Doyle K, Kelly KP, Montgomery K, Newman AR, Fortney CA, et al. The benefits and burdens of pediatric palliative care and end-of-life research: A systematic review. Journal of Palliative Medicine. 2019;**22**(8):915-926. DOI: 10.1089/jpm.2018.0483. Epub 2019 Mar 5

[59] Código civil cubano. Gaceta Oficial de la República de Cuba. L No. 59. Código civil cubano; 1987. Disponible en: http://www.gacetaoficial.cu/html/codigo%20civil%20lib1.html [Consultado 3 ene 2013]

[60] Gijsberts MHE, Liefbroer AI, Otten R, Olsman E. Spiritual care in palliative care: A systematic review of the recent European literature. Medical Sciences (Basel). 2019;7(2):25. DOI: 10.3390/medsci7020025

[61] Chew Y, Ang S, Shorey S. Experiences of new nurses dealing with death in a paediatric setting: A descriptive qualitative study. The Journal of Advanced Nursing (Internet). 2021;**77**:343-354. DOI: 10.1111/jan.14602

[62] Papadatou D, Kalliani V, Karakosta E, Liakopoulou P, Bluebond-Langner M. Home or hospital as the place of end-of-life care and death: A grounded theory study of parents' decision-making. Palliative Medicine. 2021;**35**:219-230

[63] Fernández M, García M, Pérez M, Cruz F. Experiences, and obstacles of psychologists in the accompaniment of processes at the end of life. Annals of Psychology. (Internet). 2013;**16**(1):1-8. DOI: 10.6018/analesps.29.1.139121

[64] Betriana F, Kongsuwan W. Nurses' grief in caring for patients with advanced cancer: A literature review. Songklanagarind Journal of Nursing (Internet). 2019;**39**(1):138-134. Disponible en: https://he02.tci-thaijo.org/index.php/nur-psu/article/view/181323

[65] Anderson K, Ewen H, Miles E. The grief support in healthcare scale. Nursing Research. (Internet). 2010;**59**(6):372-379. DOI: 10.1097/NNR.0b013e3181fca9de

[66] Llantá MC. Calidad de vida y calidad de muerte en oncopediatría. Revista Cubana de Enfermería. 2011;**27**(1):98-105. Disponible en: http://scielo.sld.cu http://bvs.sld.cu/revistas/enf

[67] Llantá Abreu MC, Grau Abalo JA, Massip Pérez C. Psicología de la Salud y la lucha contra el cáncer. En: Grau J, Hernández E (Eds.). Psicología de la Salud: Fundamentos y aplicaciones. Guadalajara: Centro Universitario de Ciencias de la Salud, 2005, II Parte, Cap. 7, p. 467-506. ISBN: 9702708079, 9789702708070

[68] Gómez S. Cuidados Paliativos: atención integral a enfermos terminales. Published by ICEPSS (1998). vol I. p. 221-237. ISBN-10: 8489151091 ISBN-13: 978-8489151093

[69] Montgomery KE, Raybin JL, Ward J, Balian C, Gilger E, Murray P, et al. Using patient-reported outcomes to measure symptoms in children with advanced cancer. Cancer Nursing. 2020;**43**:281-289. DOI: 10.1097/NCC.0000000000000721

[70] Montgomery K, Sawin KJ, Hendricks-Ferguson VL. Experiences of pediatric oncology patients and their parents at end of life:

A systematic review. Journal of Pediatric Oncology Nursing. 2016;**33**:85-104. DOI: 10.1177/1043454215589715

[71] Llantá Abreu MC. Factores asociados con la calidad de vida relacionada con la salud en niños y adolescentes con cáncer. La Habana, Cuba. 2011-2013. Salud & Sociedad. 2018;**9**(2):192-205. DOI: 10.22199/S07187475.2018.0002.00006

[72] Balch CM, Shanafelt TD, Sloan J, et al. Burnout and career satisfaction among surgical oncologist compared with other surgical specialties. Annals of Surgical Oncology. 2011;**18**:16-25

[73] Ferrell BR, Temel JS, Temin S, et al. Integration of palliative care into standard oncology care: American Society of Clinical Oncology clinical practice guideline update. Journal of Clinical Oncology. 2017;**35**(1):96-112

[74] Cassem NH, editors. Psiquiatría de Enlace en el Hospital General. 3rd ed. Madrid: Published by Ed. Díez de Santos, S.A.; 1994; 834 p. ISBN-10: 847978119X, ISBN-13: 978-8479781194

Chapter 14

Endoscopic Palliation of Gastrointestinal Disease

Karthik Chandrasekaran, Navim Mobin and Nicholas Gregory Brown

Abstract

Gastrointestinal malignancies account for over 35% of cancer-related deaths with a projected 73% increase by 2040. Recent advances in endoscopic technique and devices have created exponential growth in the field of therapeutic gastroenterology and have enhanced diagnostic and treatment potential. As a result, palliative endoscopic therapies have experienced an equally tremendous amount of gain. Palliative endoscopy refers to maneuvers performed during gastrointestinal procedures with the intent to minimize patient suffering and discomfort. These procedures can be highly effective in providing rapid, non-operative relief and, as such, occupy an important role in the ability to alleviate symptoms of advanced malignancies throughout the gastrointestinal tract. Complications of end-stage malignances can result in tremendous discomfort, emotional trauma, and social embarrassment for the patient. Throughout the length of the gastrointestinal tract, there are a wide variety of endoscopic procedures that can provide relief in a minimally invasive fashion. The aim of this chapter is to provide insight into the current landscape of endoscopic procedures with the intent to minimize suffering, and provide a review of the indications, practice, and outcomes of endoscopic palliative therapies available.

Keywords: endoscopic ultrasound, endoscopic retrograde cholangiopancreatography, enteric stenting, endoscopic palliation, gastric outlet obstruction, percutaneous endoscopic gastrostomy, biliary drainage, radiofrequency ablation, photodynamic therapy, celiac plexus neurolysis, large bowel obstruction

1. Introduction

Gastrointestinal malignancies account for over 35% of cancer-related deaths with a projected 73% increase by 2040 [1]. Recent advances in endoscopic technique and devices have created exponential growth in the field of therapeutic gastroenterology and have enhanced diagnostic and treatment potential. As a result, palliative endoscopic therapies have experienced an equally tremendous amount of gain. Palliative endoscopy refers to maneuvers performed during gastrointestinal procedures with the intent to minimize patient suffering and discomfort. These procedures can be highly effective in providing rapid, non-operative relief and, as such, occupy an important role in the ability to alleviate symptoms of advanced malignancies throughout the gastrointestinal tract. Complications of end-stage malignances can result in tremendous discomfort, emotional trauma, and social embarrassment for the patient. Throughout the length of the gastrointestinal tract, there are a wide variety of endoscopic procedures that can provide relief in a minimally invasive fashion. The aim of this chapter is to provide insight into the current landscape of endoscopic procedures with the intent to minimize suffering, and provide a review of the indications, practice, and outcomes of endoscopic palliative therapies available.

2. Esophagus

Esophageal cancer is the 7th leading cancer worldwide, with over 600,000 cases in 2020 [2]. Squamous cell carcinoma accounts for 85% of disease burden with the remaining 15% attributed to adenocarcinoma. The highest incidence of esophageal cancer has been reported in Eastern Asia and Africa, with the lowest incidence being reported in Central America and Western Africa [3].

Dysphagia, due to either intrinsic esophageal tumor or extrinsic compression, occurs in up to three-fourth of all patients and is increasingly pronounced as the disease progresses [4]. Solid food dysphagia can be severe though compensatory patient mechanisms can also make this a challenging symptom to uncover. Dysphagia to liquids typically occurs during the end-stage of the disease, hence, malnutrition is a common concern in these patients [5]. In fact, dysphagia and loss of appetite are independent predictors of poor quality of life and potential targets for endoscopic therapy [6]. Endoscopic techniques such as placement of a self-expanding metal stent (SEMS) allows patients with esophageal cancer to maintain oral food intake and improve their quality of life [7].

2.1 Self-expanding metal stents

Esophageal stent placement is preferred in patients with a short-term survival as it has been shown to induce rapid relief of dysphagia symptoms [8]. A variety of esophageal stents are available and ordinarily consist of self-expanding metal stents (SEMS), which come with an array of diameters, anti-migration features and can be covered or uncovered. Fully covered self-expandable stents (FCSEMS) and partially covered self-expandable stents (PCSEMS) are the most commonly available and are the only stents recommended for clinical practice in patients suffering from malignant dysphagia [9]. Placement of either a partially or fully covered SEMS is the core palliative therapy for these patients, however, adjunct therapies exist, including photodynamic therapy [2].

When considering placement of an esophageal stent, SEMS are generally preferred over self-expanding plastic stents (SEPSs) as they carry lower rates of symptom recurrence and adverse events [10]. There has been no difference in outcome when comparing FCSEMS and PCSEMS placement, and choice of either stent should be performed based on endoscopist preference and availability [11]. In addition, the endoscopist must also consider proximity of the malignant lesion to the airways as well as the upper esophageal sphincter. Lesions near the upper esophageal sphincter may not accommodate the proximal flange of the stent and can elevate the risk for aspiration, contributing to morbidity. Lesions with compression of, or risk of post-stent compression of the mainstem bronchus, should have collaboration with interventional pulmonary for prophylactic endobronchial stent placement in the affected airways.

Established recommendations also include SEMS placement alone with or without brachytherapy as first line therapy. Alternatively, brachytherapy alone could be considered for patients who present with dysphagia who are not candidates for resection [2, 12]. To add, a 2018 meta-analysis and systematic review of 8 RCTs found that placement of a SEMS in combination with either radiation or chemotherapy resulted in more rapid relief of dysphagia [12, 13]. Despite success in the literature, access to brachytherapy may be limited and the availability of regional services will influence the clinical treatment algorithms.

The role of esophageal stent placement in operative candidates currently is limited. A landmark 2015 study by Mariette and colleagues compared 38 candidates with resectable disease, who underwent SEMS placement compared to 152 placebo-controlled candidates found SEMS negatively impacted surgical and oncologic outcomes [14]. Palliative stent placement prior to considering resection also has temperate data and is not generally recommended [2].

In addition to obstruction, a tracheoesophageal fistula (TEF) is a common occurrence in up to 5–15% of patients with esophageal cancer and is a result of direct penetration of tumor into the airway or as a complication of radiation therapy [15]. Placement of a covered SEMS can be used to provide palliation of malignant tracheoesophageal fistulas as SEMS placement occludes the fistula and prevents extravasation of esophageal contents to the airways [16]. Clinical success rates of SEMS placement for TEF range widely, between 56 and 100%. Factors associated with potential stent failure include large fistula (>1 cm), and a proximal fistula location [17]. TEF recurrence has been reported to occur in up to 39% of cases after initial SEMS placement, though this is typically successfully managed endoscopically with repositioning or replacement of the stent [18].

Finally, placement of SEMS for relief of malignant extrinsic compression of the gut lumen is often considered less than for intrinsic disease. Although, retrospective data of 105 patients (85 intrinsic, 20 extrinsic) demonstrated the 4, 8, and 12-week patency rates of SEMSs were 90.5%, 78.8%, and 63.9%, in patients with intrinsic malignant obstruction, while the stents in the extrinsic compression group were patent until the patient expired. Thus, SEMSs in the esophagus should be considered effective management for both malignant intrinsic and extrinsic compression [19].

2.2 Adverse events

Though generally safe, adverse events must be considered when counseling patients about esophageal SEMS, including chest pain, heartburn, stent migration, tumor ingrowth, bleeding, fistula formation, food impaction and perforation [18, 20, 21]. Though tumor ingrowth and overgrowth are common in up to 14% of cases, successful management can be achieved with the stent-in-stent technique which involves placement of a covered SEMS within the existing stent to restore patency [22].

As mentioned, SEPS are not recommended due to increased incidence of stent migration when compared to their metal counterparts. To mitigate risks of reintervention due to SEMS migration, which has been estimated as high as 50% for cSEMS, partially covered SEMS and/or stent fixation should be considered. Technical and clinical success rates of fixation are high with significant reduction in migration, which can reach a nadir of 9% [23, 24].

Lastly, gastroesophageal reflux has been reported in 70–100% of patients after SEMS placement. Heartburn is a result of gastric contents refluxing into the esophagus and can especially be a concern if the SEMS spans the GE junction and disrupts the barrier of the diaphragmatic pinch and lower-esophageal sphincter. Management is with acid-suppression is effective, though SEMS with anti-reflux valves are under investigation [25].

2.3 Palliative dilatation

Palliative stent placement for benign strictures in patients who fail to reach a target diameter of 14 mm after dilation every other week over 5 sessions or fail to maintain the target diameter up to 4 weeks after the last dilation could be considered [26]. No such recommendation exists for malignant disease and dilation for malignant strictures is recommended against due to high complication rates [27].

3. Gastroduodenal obstruction

Gastric outlet obstruction is a reduction in the caliber of the gut lumen at the level of the pylorus or duodenum. Malignant tumor invasion is one of the most common causes of GOO in the United States and it unfortunately occurs with distressing frequency in up to in up to 70% of pancreatic cancer cases and as many as 15% of patients with gastric cancer [28–30]. Symptoms include nausea/vomiting, early satiety, weight loss and heartburn are often nonspecific and require a sensitive clinician. Re-establishing continuity of the gut lumen for these patients can improve quality of life, nutritional status, discomfort, and may allow for resumption of systemic therapy [31].

3.1 Gastroduodenal stenting

As described above for symptomatic esophageal malignancy, self-expanding metal stent placement is also the mainstay therapy used to alleviate a solitary malignant gastroduodenal obstruction. Endoscopic stent placement is highly technically successful in up to 97% of cases with a near 90% clinical success, defined as symptom resolution and ability to tolerate soft solid or full liquid diet [32]. When compared to surgical gastrojejunostomy, which was the preferred therapy for malignant GOO in years past, gastroduodenal SEMS placement provides more rapid symptom relief with an average of 1.5 days to oral intake compared to 8.1 days in patients who underwent operative management. Endoscopic stent placement also results in shorter duration of hospital stay at 5.1 days vs. 12.1 days in the surgically managed cohort [33–35].

Gastroduodenal stents are manufactured as covered (cSEMS) and uncovered SEMS (uSEMS) varieties. The advantages of cSEMS and uSEMS are predictable, with higher rates of stent migration utilizing cSEMS, up to 28%, compared to 3% in uSEMS. The advantage of a cSEMS is reduced obstruction due to tumor ingrowth through the stent struts at 6.9% and 7.2% with cSEMS and uSEMS, respectively [36]. Though uSEMS are the cornerstone of therapy, stent selection varies regionally. During pre-procedure preparation, concomitant biliary stenting should be considered at the time of enteric stent placement due to difficulty of reaching the ampulla following SEMS insertion and the potential for biliary occlusion after SEMS placement. Mean hospital stays after insertion of luminal stents are typically 7 days with a mean overall survival of 100 days after stent placement [37].

Adverse events of gastroduodenal stenting are rare but including bleeding (4%), perforation, (2%), stent migration (5%), pancreatitis (<1%), and stent obstruction due to tumor ingrowth, overgrowth, or food impaction (18%) [32, 38]. When compared to surgical gastrojejunostomy, delayed complications occurred at a rate of 6.7% in the SEMS group and 13.8% in surgical group, which included post-surgical bowel obstruction, and wound infections [39].

Comparisons to surgical bypass have long been made. SEMS afford patients shorter procedure duration, more rapid symptom relief and shorter duration of hospitalization but with caveat of more frequent intervention due to stent dysfunction [39–42]. Retrospective data is mixed and unsettled on which method offers increased survival, with vacillating data touting survival of one method over the other, a definitive conclusion cannot be reached. Yet, in the retrospective literature that implies a survival benefit of surgical gastrojejunostomy over SEMS, the surgical cohorts are comprised of significantly higher functional status and lower Eastern Cooperative Oncology Group (ECOG) scores with a mean ECOG of only 1 [43]. Therefore, SEMS placement remains the pillar of therapy but, in patients with excellent functional status or those with multi-focal obstruction, surgical bypass could be considered as an alternative to endoscopic SEMS placement.

3.2 Additional management strategies

Most patients with malignant gastroduodenal obstruction are appropriately managed with either SEMS placement or surgical gastroenterostomy. In clinical practice, though, situations arise where both SEMS and surgical management are either not effective or advisable. In these challenging cases, alternative therapies such as decompressive gastrostomy tube insertion or EUS-directed gastroenterostomy may be offered.

Placement of a percutaneous endoscopic gastrostomy (PEG) tube for bowel decompression is an established therapeutic option for gastric outlet obstruction. This is accomplished during an upper endoscopy following a small skin incision on the abdominal wall. A trocar and guidewire are introduced, the wire is grasped endoscopically and fastened to the PEG tube which is then withdrawn through the abdominal wall. PEG placement obviates the need for nasogastric tube decompression which is a source of significant physical and social discomfort for the patient. Gastric decompression tubes provide relief of obstructive symptoms in 95% of cases with median survival of 63 days following PEG insertion [44].

An EUS-directed gastroenterostomy is the creation of a fistulous tract under the guidance of endoscopic ultrasound between portions of the gut lumen, typically stomach and jejunum. This fistulous tract bypasses the malignant obstruction via placement of a fully covered lumen-apposing metal stent (LAMS) which connects the stomach and the loop of bowel distal to the diseased portion of the gut lumen [45]. Mounting evidence has demonstrated the safety and efficacy of EUS-guided gastroenterostomy in these clinical scenarios and it has been shown can be a technical success in over 90% of GOO cases with comparable morbidity, mortality, and hospital length of stay to a surgical gastrojejunostomy [46, 47]. It should be noted that use of LAMS in these cases, though supported by a growing body of evidence, remains an off-label indication. After multidisciplinary discussion, in cases where conventional methods of relieving GOO are not in the patient's best interest, the treatment team should consider either decompressive gastrostomy tube or referral to a high-volume center for EUS-guided gastroenterostomy for this unique patient population near the end-of-life.

3.3 Enteral access

The decision to pursue artificial enteric nutrition in patients with advanced malignancy with late-stage malignancy can include ethical dilemmas, especially when the prospect of recovering from illness does not exist. Nutritional supplementation is provided with the intent to ameliorate suffering involved with starvation; however, it is not clear feeding via PEG tubes achieve this goal in patients with terminal malignancy [44, 48, 49]. Supporting literature in this setting also suggests that artificial enteric nutrition via PEG or NG tube also do not prolong survival, though again, data is a bit varied. Thus, with respect to achieving the goal of providing comfort and ameliorating suffering and providing comfort to family members, PEG placement for nutritional supplementation may fall short and unduly prolong suffering.

However, if enteric nutrition is desired, it can be accomplished via a nasogastric tube or a percutaneous tube such as a PEG with or without jejunal extension (PEG-J) or direct percutaneous endoscopic jejunostomy (PEJ). The method for PEG placement is briefly described earlier. PEJ tube placement mirrors that of a PEG tube placement with the exception that the percutaneous tube is placed in the jejunum rather than the anterior wall of the gastric body, a higher risk procedure with more technical challenges. A PEG-J is a PEG tube that has an external Y-port with access for venting and the other leads to a small caliber (often 9Fr or 12Fr) tube that is guided into the small bowel for feeding.

The use of a PEG-J or PEJ is reserved for patients with delayed gastric emptying and/or to theoretically decrease the risk of aspiration. Robust data is lacking and mixed, though, very small retrospective studies suggest distal feeds via a PEG-J or PEJ may potentially decrease the risk for aspiration, though more sturdy data is certainly needed to inform decision-making [48].

Minor complications after a PEG placement include PEG site pain, and cellulitis. Major complications can include bleeding, peritonitis, aspiration pneumonia, and perforation. Adverse events after PEG placement in this scenario is accompanied by major and minor complication incidence of 8.7% and 37%, respectively, with high ASA score (>/=4) as a significant predictor of adverse events [49]. Lastly, tumor seeding must be considered as well in patients with pharyngoesophageal malignancy with varying reports of tumor seeding rates to the PEG site (<0.5 to 3%) [50]. Direct access PEG or gastrostomy tube placement should be considered in these patients.

Like all medical interventions, the potential burdens and benefits, the care goals, religious practices, and medical situation must be weighed when considering PEG placement for artificial nutrition in this vulnerable patient population. Like all medical interventions, percutaneous enteral access can be ethically withheld in the proper clinical environment.

4. Pancreatic and hepatobiliary

Unresectable pancreatic and hepatobiliary malignancies create unabating difficulties including debilitating pain, obstructive pruritis and jaundice, which often require intervention. Historically, surgical and percutaneous modalities were the mainstay of palliation. However, since the first endoscopic retrograde cholangiopancreatography (ERCP) in 1988 for biliary stenting of malignant bile duct obstruction, the applications of endoscopic therapies have continued to expand as have their role in palliation.

With 78% of pancreatic malignancy located in the pancreatic and a rising incidence of pancreatic head malignancy, especially in you women, early identification and management of local complications is critical [51–53]. Alleviating biliary obstruction and the associated symptoms of jaundice and pruritis can have a profound improvement on quality of life and the accompanying social discomfort. ERCP-directed therapy is the foundation of managing malignant biliary disease. In this section, we will review endoscopic management strategies in pancreatic and hepatobiliary malignancies.

4.1 Palliation with plastic stents

Since the 1970's, plastic stents (PS) have been used for relief of malignant biliary obstruction and, over the years, have evolved into various materials including polyurethane, polyethylene, and Teflon [54]. Sizes and shapes of plastic stents range from 5 Fr to 12 Fr in diameter to up to 22 cm in length with varying shapes from straight, single, and double pigtail [55]. Plastic stents are low-cost and effective for short-term drainage with an average time to stent dysfunction being 73 days (median 62–165 days) [56–58]. Thus, they are typically used for patients with for patients with overall expected survival of less than 3–4 months, or those patients who prefer to avoid repeat ERCP and stent exchange within this time frame [57]. Plastic stent exchange is usually recommended within 3 months, though alternatively, patients may elect for "on-demand" stent changes, which can diminish the burden to the patient and the cost associated with elective ERCP.

Stent dysfunction can occur for a variety of reasons, most commonly due to lumen occlusion by biliary sludge and bacterial biofilm, with stent migration being the second most likely cause of stent-related dysfunction. PS have a significantly higher stent dysfunction rate (41%) compared to alternative options (SEMS) [59]. Most commonly, PS accumulate biliary debris and sludge, resulting clogging of the small-caliber stent lumen (33%) [59].

4.2 Palliation with self-expanding metal biliary stents

In addition to PS above, the endoscopist may also select from a variety of metal options. Self-expanding metal stents (SEMS), which have demonstrated superior patency compared to plastic stents, are available in a variety of different forms including covered (cSEMS), partially covered (pcSEMS) and uncovered (uSEMS) [60–64]. The primary difference between the types of self-expanding metal stents is the ability and time to removal or exchange. Placement of uSEMS is typically reserved for patients with unresectable disease as uSEMS are permanent; pcSEMS are also not indicated for removal. The chronic inflammatory response to the stent mesh along with tumor ingrowth through the wire struts, prohibits stent removal, but with the added benefit of reduced stent migration. Conversely, cSEMS have an interior coating that prevents tumor infiltration, though they are more prone to stent migration.

Stent patency of uSEMS is typically 111–273 days. uSEMS dysfunction includes a low migration rate at 0–2%, though higher occlusion rates (due to tumor ingrowth) in approximately 17% [58, 59, 62, 65–70]. Overall uSEMS dysfunction rate is 27% [59].

A variety of remedies exist to address stent occlusion, including a stent-in-stent technique and intraductal radiofrequency ablation [61]. Other complications include acute cholangitis, persistent abdominal pain, liver abscess at 0.6–1% [61].

In contrast, cSEMS and pcSEMS have a coating to prevent infiltration of tumor and thereby prolonging lumen patency and avoiding repetitive endoscopic manipulation [8]. Covered SEMS are indicated in benign and malignant disease, and most are approved for removal. Stent patency of cSEMS is comparable to uSEMS with different mechanisms of dysfunction. Tumor ingrowth rate is nearly 0% with very few reported cases, tumor overgrowth can occur [59, 62–71]. However, cSEMS dysfunction includes a higher migration rate at 17% of patients [59, 67]. Overall cSEMS stent dysfunction rate is 20% [59].

Historically, cSEMS were selected for benign or resectable malignancies and uSEMS had been reserved for patients with unresectable disease. This notion has been overturned more recently and has liberated the endoscopist to select either covered or uncovered SEMS for palliation as adverse events are similar (**Figure 1** and **Table 1**) [58, 59, 65–70, 72, 73]. Appropriate stent selection requires consideration of patient factors (stricture size and location, presence of metastatic disease, performance status) that predict patient survival, anatomic factors and endoscopist preference. SEMS placement is not always feasible or advisable in each patient and each situation is individualized. As such, there are no universally accepted recommendations for stent selection based on survival benefit. Traditionally, endoscopists favored SEMS in patients expected to survive more than 3–6 months (**Figure 1**). However, that has also been challenged more recently [58, 73]. Many endoscopists suggest that SEMS should be utilized regardless of life expectancy for malignant biliary obstruction as they possess superior patency even at 30 days, improve quality of life by curtailing reintervention, reduce hospitalization, and are the more cost-effective option (**Table 2** and **Figure 1**) [58, 61, 65–68, 71, 73–76].

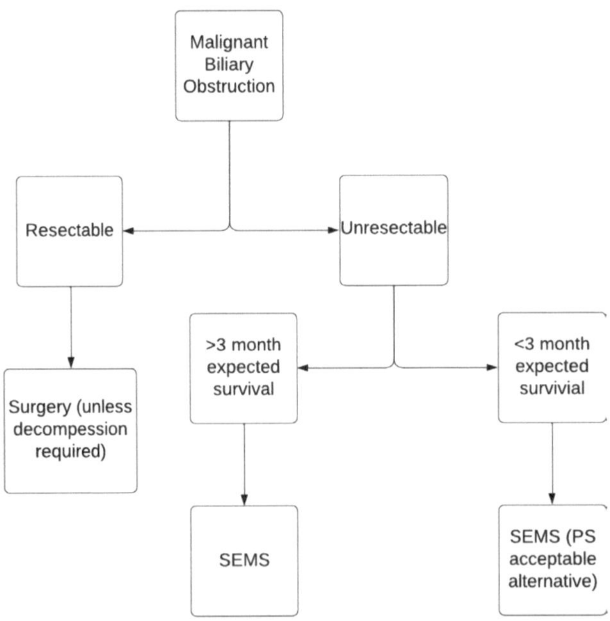

Figure 1.
Biliary stent algorithm for malignant obstruction.

	uSEMS	cSEMS
Successful biliary drainage*	No difference	
Mean stent patency	111–273 days, no difference**	
Incidence of stent dysfunction	27%	20%
Stent occlusion (due to tissue ingrowth)	17%	0–1%
Stent migration	0–2%	17%
Survival at 1 year	No difference	

**As defined by decrease in serum bilirubin [67].*
***Variable in multiple different RCTs, overall comparable mean stent patency duration (~111–273 days).*

Table 1.
Malignant biliary obstruction: Uncovered vs. covered SEMS.

	Plastic stent	SEMS
Average time to stent dysfunction (days)	62–165 days	111–273 days
Incidence of stent dysfunction	41%	24%
Stent clogging (due to debris, sludge)	33%	6%
Stent migration	6%	0–1% (uSEMS)
Tissue ingrowth	Not applicable	17% (uSEMS)
Recommended interval for reintervention*	Shorter time interval (within 3 months)*	Longer timer interval (6–12 months)*
30-day mortality rate	No difference	

**If proactive stent management is desired; PS = plastic stent; SEMS = self-expanding metal stent.*

Table 2.
Biliary PS vs. SEMS characteristics.

4.3 ERCP failures and alternative biliary drainage maneuvers

Due to its high success rate, ERCP remains the standard technique to restore biliary patency in malignant obstruction. However, failed ERCP can still occur in up to 40% of cases, particularly with surgically altered anatomy, tumor obstruction, duodenal diverticula, or gastroduodenal obstruction [77]. In such cases, percutaneous biliary drainage has been proven to be technically and clinically successful and is the most widely utilized next step in therapy. However, drain site discomfort and drain dysfunction, risk for recurrent infection and cholangitis, and the cosmetically unpleasant experience of having an external drainage bag have driven alternative methods [60, 78, 79]. Endoscopic ultrasound guided biliary drainage (EUS-BD) is a rapidly evolving therapeutic option in select cases not amenable to traditional biliary stenting [80, 81].

4.4 EUS-guided biliary drainage

EUS-BD has begun to emerge at the forefront of therapeutic options in patients who have had unsuccessful biliary drainage during ERCP [82, 83]. The method of achieve EUS-BD is highly dependent on patient anatomy with the intent of creating a fistulous tract from bowel to the biliary tree that cannot be decompressed with conventional methods. This often takes the form of choledochoduodenostomy or hepaticogastrostomy.

EUS-guided choledochoenterostomy is performed by puncturing the bile duct via either the gastric antrum (choledochogastrostomy) or the duodenal bulb (choledochoduodenostomy) under EUS and fluoroscopic guidance. A guidewire is passed into the bile duct, and a lumen-apposing metal stent (LAMS) or cSEMS is then placed to create a permanent fistulous connection, thus, permitting biliary drainage via the gut lumen, bypassing the obstructed or inaccessible portion of the biliary tree [84, 85].

For patients with hilar or intrahepatic obstruction, an EUS-guided hepaticogastrostomy may be applied as this utilizes a transgastric approach to puncture the left intrahepatic biliary system. The new connection between the stomach and the left intrahepatic system can then be stented in a similar manner as described above, with a covered biliary SEMS. EUS guidance can also be employed to drain the gallbladder in patients who are not candidates for cholecystectomy and place emphasis on avoiding percutaneous drainage [86].

Though informed by relatively few RCTs, current literature demonstrates high technical (94.1–100%) and clinical success (87.5%–94.0%) of EUS-BD when compared to a percutaneous approach [85, 87]. Additionally, EUS-BD procedures required fewer reinterventions (1.67 vs. 3.44) while resulting in lower adverse event rate. EUS-BD was associated has demonstrated safety with low rates of bleeding (2.7%), bile leaks (3%) and pain (1.5%) [88, 89]. Efficacy and safety of the EUS-BD approaches are not significantly different therefore, the most suitable method is dictated by patient anatomy (**Figure 2**) [90, 91].

EUS directed rendezvous is an additional therapeutic in the can be used to help achieve access to the biliary after conventional methods have failed. In an EUS guided rendezvous, the bile duct is accessed from either in the stomach or the duodenum under EUS guidance. Once confirmation of the puncture is made, a guidewire is passed into the bile duct and across the papilla into the duodenum. At this time, a standard ERCP can then be performed using the existing wire for transpapillary stent placement [60].

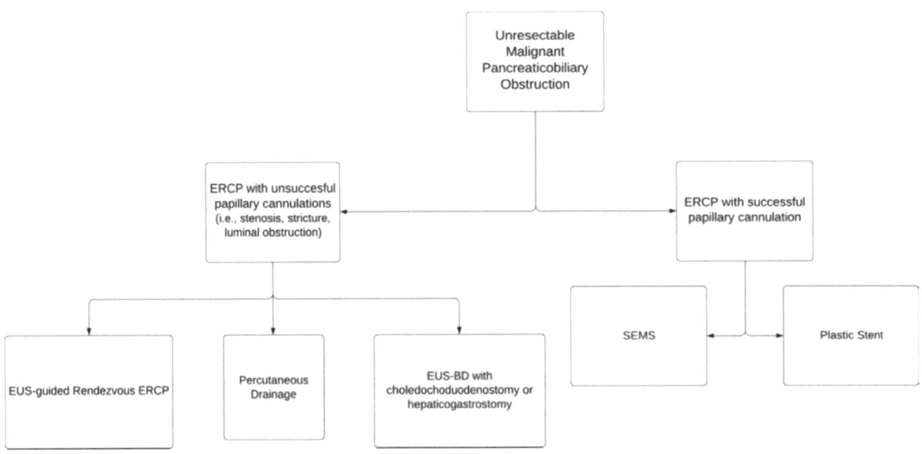

Figure 2.
Suggested algorithm to restore biliary patency.

Further studies are necessary to determine the optimal technique and tools maximize the potential of EUS-BD. Nevertheless, in established guidelines EUS-BD was substantiated as the recommended procedure of choice for biliary drainage in patients with failed ERCP—in the right clinical center, with appropriate endoscopist expertise [82, 83]. Percutaneous drainage remains an alternative if EUS-BD is unsuccessful, not feasible or not available [82]. A proposed treatment algorithm is below (**Figure 2**).

4.5 Radiofrequency ablation

Due to the relentless nature of pancreaticobiliary malignancies, the efforts above may be insufficient and adjunct therapies are often necessary. Radiofrequency ablation (RFA) may be used as a primary or adjunctive therapy to reduce tumor burden and improve quality of life. Endoscopic RFA utilizes radiofrequency waves at 450–500 kHz applied directly to malignant tissue to induce irreversible hyperthermic tissue injury and necrosis. Endobiliary RFA for the palliation of malignant biliary obstructions has been reported with successful restoration of biliary patency, reduced stent occlusion, and an increase in overall mean survival time [92–95]. There remains a need to collect further data comparing RFA to alternative therapies (plastic stent, SEMS) for malignant biliary obstruction.

Endoscopic RFA also appears to be an effective method for restoration of malignant biliary stent obstruction. RFA therapy alone compared to PS placement for the treatment of occluded metal stents showed a significant increase in biliary patency following RFA as well as low risk of short-term adverse events stents [96–98].

While the emerging data surround RFA has been largely positive, more recent data has moderated enthusiasm for endobiliary RFA for stent occlusion. Recent studies have not demonstrated any significant difference in biliary stent patency nor overall survival versus SEMS placement alone [99]. More importantly, life-threatening complications including cholangitis, hemobilia, hepatic infarction and fistula formation have been reported following use of RFA [93, 100–102]. The use of RFA is still a relatively novel concept and consideration for use should remain dependent on institution resources and endoscopist expertise. Although early data invited some hope, there remains a significant need for additional investigation before RFA can be regularly included in the standard of palliative endoscopic care.

4.6 Photodynamic therapy

Photodynamic therapy (PDT) is another adjunctive palliative option for patients with pancreatobiliary and hepatic malignancies. PDT is the creation of selective tissue injury by systemic injection of a photosensitizing agent. This agent is preferentially taken up by the target tumor, activated by light exposure, which induces tissue necrosis of the malignant lesion. Injection of the photosensitizing agent can be achieved by ERCP or EUS. PDT has been shown to be a safe and effective method for selective tumor tissue destruction in advanced biliary malignancies [103–105]. Randomized trials comparing PDT with stenting alone have demonstrated a significantly prolonged median survival time, improved biliary drainage and improved quality of life compared to those with stenting alone [103, 106, 107]. Additionally, the benefit of PDT can be maximized with SEMS placement immediately following PDT. The median survival time in patients who underwent PDT and stent placement was 493 days compared to 98 days in patients with stent placement alone [103, 106]. Notwithstanding the reported advantages of PDT, this therapy must be discussed with the care team and patient. It is not yet commonplace in most centers due to cost burdens and side effects and, in addition, data demonstrated comparable efficacy of RFA, which is more widely available [105, 106, 108].

5. Endoscopic pain management

Despite advances in medical and surgical oncology for pancreatic ductal adenocarcinoma, only 15% of patients have resectable disease at the time of presentation [109]. Over 90% of patients with stage IV pancreatic cancer experience intense, debilitating pain. The origin of pain is poorly understood but believed to be multifactorial and principally attributed to perineural infiltration, pancreatic duct obstruction, and nodal tumor metastases. The primary goal for both patient and caregivers is effective support with proper pain control. Following the WHO recommendations, the cornerstone of symptom management is pharmacologic and is often approached using a stepwise analgesic approach beginning with NSAIDs and acetaminophen, followed by escalating doses of opiates [110, 111]. Despite this, symptoms can remain difficult to control and treatment can be accompanied by side effects including kidney injury, altered sensorium, dry mouth, pruritus, and constipation, which can be distressing and have a profound impact on patient satisfaction. In such situations, EUS-guided celiac plexus neurolysis can be an effective adjunctive therapy [112].

5.1 Celiac plexus neurolysis

EUS-guided celiac plexus neurolysis (CPN) and celiac plexus block (CPB) are often used interchangeably though they carry different indications. CPB implies the injection of a local anesthetic and steroid (i.e., bupivacaine and triamcinolone) and is typically reserved for pain from benign disease, such as chronic pancreatitis. CPN involves the injection of a local anesthetic and a neurolytic agent (i.e., bupivacaine and ethanol) to defunctionalize pain signaling from the afferent nerves of the celiac plexus to the central nervous system and offer a more prolonged and effective interruption of pain transmission.

EUS-CPN has been shown to significantly reduce pain up to 3 months following the procedure and lower narcotic consumption. Though much of the data forming the foundation of this procedure is retrospective. RCT's have demonstrated small but significant reduction in pain 4 and 8 weeks as well as a significant reduction in narcotic use and its associated constipation without any serious adverse events [113, 114]. Successful pain reduction has also been demonstrated up to 12 weeks utilizing EUS-CPN but without any observed impact on survival or quality of life [114].

Despite decades of mostly positive data on efficacy, studies with rigorous methodology were somewhat lacking and the efficacy of CPN has now been called into question [115, 116]. A more recent RCT and retrospective study of EUS-CPN versus aggressive oral opiate dosing found a significant reduction in pain in both groups but no statistical difference appreciated between the two arms. Patients did not experience any benefit in quality or life nor reduction in narcotic consumption.

Though considered a low-risk procedure, it is important to be cognizant of the potential complications of CPN. Common procedure-related adverse events include back pain, experienced by up to 96% of patients post-procedure, transient hypotension, and diarrhea (40–60%) which are easily managed pharmacologically [114, 117, 118]. Due to the unopposed parasympathetic activity following CPN, bowel hypermobility is frequently reported and thus highlights bowel obstruction as a key contraindication to CPN [118]. Lastly, rare, but serious reported complications have been reported and include retroperitoneal bleeding, ischemia and nerve injury.

Despite recent, more humbling data for EUS-CPN, it remains a safe endoscopic modality with potential benefits. Patient factors are important to consider to maximize the benefit of CPN. Metastatic disease, pain originating from beyond the celiac plexus, and direct tumor invasion into the celiac plexus may be difficult to control, even with CPN [110, 118, 119]. During discussions with the patient and care team, EUS-CPN should be given consideration with the intent of augmenting pharmacologic therapy, reducing narcotic-induced side effects, and slowing the rate of narcotic escalation rather than with the ambition of obviating the need for pharmacologic therapy altogether.

6. Colorectal

Colorectal cancer presents as metastatic disease in up to 30% of patients, with up to 13% of all colorectal cancer patients experiencing obstructive symptoms [120–122]. Since 1991, when colonic stent placement was first introduced, reestablishing colonic patency with self-expanding metal stent has become the standard of care for malignant colonic obstruction owing to the high technical success, low complication rates, short hospitalization, improved quality of life and obviating the need for surgical management, including ostomy creation [120, 123].

The procedure mimics that of enteric stents previously described in this chapter. The endoscope is inserted to the level of the obstruction, a guidewire is used to traverse the culprit lesion and, over the wire a catheter containing a sheathed SEMS is deployed under fluoroscopic guidance. There are two main colonic stent considerations—covered and uncovered. In keeping with established guidelines, uSEMS are recommended due to lower rates of stent migration, more durable stent patency and reduced need for reintervention [122, 124].

Colonic stent placement is successful both technically and clinically, though randomized data for stent placement proximal to the splenic flexure is lacking [121, 125]. Stent patency in the palliative setting is also favorable, with median patency of 3–6 months and a robust 82% patency rate at 6 months and 50–65% at 12 months [122, 126–128].

Enteral stenting may also be feasible in patients with obstruction due to extracolonic malignancy (ECM). Though technical success rates may be high, clinical success rates, defined as resolution of obstructive symptoms, of 25–87.5%, are less impressive [129]. SEMS for ECMs are known to pose a higher risk for non-functioning immediately after placement and re-obstruction at shorter intervals compared to stenting for primary colonic malignancies [125]. In fact, given the lower clinical success rates, a larger portion of such patients will require surgical diversion [130]. Nonetheless, colonic stenting remains the cornerstone and first-line therapy which is consistent with practice guidelines [122].

Though colonic SEMS placement is a low-risk procedure adverse events can occur, including decompression failure, tumor ingrowth (3–29%), stent migration (1–10%), perforation (5–7%), bleeding (0–6%), pain [131–134]. When addressing stent migration or obstruction, endoscopic reassessment with stent-in-stent placement for stent obstruction is the first line choice though many endoscopists also recommend low-residue diet and indefinite laxative use to reduce the likelihood of stent obstruction [122]. Concurrent chemotherapy administration of anti-angiogenic chemotherapy (i.e., bevacizumab) may play a role in increased risk for stent migration due to ongoing shrinkage of the tumor. Additionally, bevacizumab has been reported to increase risk of stent perforation and its use during stent placement is generally regarded as a contraindication, though SEMS are safe following cessation of the medication [122, 135].

In the troublesome cases where luminal SEMS placement is not feasible, EUS-guided therapies, such as the previously mentioned EUS-guided enteroenterostomy, can be considered in the appropriate patient. In small series, tertiary care centers have demonstrated the efficacy of EUS-guided colo-colonic LAMS therapy to bypass the occluded large bowel [136, 137]. EUS-directed colo-colonic LAMS is part of a growing armamentarium of therapeutic options, and may be considered based on local expertise, multidisciplinary discussion, and patient wishes.

Colorectal cancer is one of the most common malignancies and complications related to this unfortunate disease are certain to be encountered. Fortunately, endoscopic management for symptomatic malignant large bowel obstruction is technically and clinically successful with few adverse events. The decision to proceed with stent placement should be made after multidisciplinary discussion and including the surgical and oncological teams. With exception of a pre-existing colonic perforation, SEMS placement is the preferred treatment for the palliation of malignant colonic obstruction with clear quality of life benefits and should be offered as first-line therapy [122].

7. Conclusion

Advanced gastrointestinal malignancies are a sobering set of diseases with intensely troublesome side effects. All such patients should be treated in multidisciplinary setting with early involvement of palliative care discussions. Owing to developments in technology and evolution of endoscopic interventions, we now have greater support than ever before for patients with gastrointestinal malignancies near the end of life. The above chapter should serve as a guide to understand the data and endoscopic treatment options available for compassionate and individualized care.

Author details

Karthik Chandrasekaran[1], Navim Mobin[1] and Nicholas Gregory Brown[1,2]*

1 NewYork-Presbyterian/Brooklyn Methodist Hospital, Brooklyn, NY, USA

2 Weill Cornell Medical College, New York, NY, USA

*Address all correspondence to: nb2931@cumc.columbia.edu

References

[1] Ferlay J, Ervik M, Lam F, Colombet M, Mery L, Piñeros M, et al. Global cancer observatory: Cancer today. Lyon, France: International Agency for Research on Cancer. 2018;**3**(20):2019

[2] Spaander MC et al. Esophageal stenting for benign and malignant disease: European Society of Gastrointestinal Endoscopy (ESGE) clinical guideline. Endoscopy. 2016;**48**(10):939-948

[3] Morgan E et al. The global landscape of esophageal squamous cell carcinoma and esophageal adenocarcinoma incidence and mortality in 2020 and projections to 2040: New estimates from GLOBOCAN 2020. Gastroenterology. 2022;**163**(3):649-658

[4] Daly JM et al. Esophageal cancer: Results of an American College of Surgeons patient care evaluation study. Journal of the American College of Surgeons. 2000;**190**(5):562-572

[5] Bower MR et al. Nutritional management during neoadjuvant therapy for esophageal cancer. Journal of Surgical Oncology. 2009;**100**(1):82-87

[6] Darling GE. Quality of life in patients with esophageal cancer. Thoracic Surgery Clinics. 2013;**23**(4):569-575

[7] Homs MY et al. Palliative therapy. Journal of Surgical Oncology. 2005;**92**(3):246-256

[8] Yang C et al. Interventions for dysphagia in oesophageal cancer. Cochrane Database of Systematic Reviews. 2014;**10**:1-127

[9] Vermeulen BD et al. Esophageal stenting in clinical practice: An overview. Current Treatment Options in Gastroenterology. 2018;**16**:260-273

[10] Aiolfi A et al. Stent-in-stent, a safe and effective technique to remove fully embedded esophageal metal stents: Case series and literature review. Endoscopy International Open. 2015;**3**(04):E296-E299

[11] Wang C et al. Comparison of fully-covered vs partially covered self-expanding metallic stents for palliative treatment of inoperable esophageal malignancy: A systematic review and meta-analysis. BMC Cancer. 2020;**20**(1):1-2

[12] Ahmed O et al. AGA clinical practice update on the optimal management of the malignant alimentary tract obstruction: Expert review. Clinical Gastroenterology and Hepatology. 2021;**19**(9):1780-1788

[13] Lai A et al. Role of esophageal metal stents placement and combination therapy in inoperable esophageal carcinoma: A systematic review and meta-analysis. Digestive Diseases and Sciences. 2018;**63**:1025-1034

[14] Mariette C et al. Self-expanding covered metallic stent as a bridge to surgery in esophageal cancer: Impact on oncologic outcomes. Journal of the American College of Surgeons. 2015;**220**(3):287-296

[15] Shamji FM et al. Management of malignant tracheoesophageal fistula. Thoracic Surgery Clinics. 2018;**28**(3):393-402

[16] Kim KR et al. Palliative treatment of malignant esophagopulmonary fistulas with covered expandable metallic stents.

American Journal of Roentgenology. 2009;**193**(4):W278-W282

[17] Kim PH et al. Self-expandable metal stent use to palliate malignant esophagorespiratory fistulas in 88 patients. Journal of Vascular and Interventional Radiology. 2018;**29**(3):320-327

[18] Shin JH et al. Esophagorespiratory fistula: Long-term results of palliative treatment with covered expandable metallic stents in 61 patients. Radiology. 2004;**232**(1):252-259

[19] Rhee K et al. Self-expandable metal stents for malignant esophageal obstruction: A comparative study between extrinsic and intrinsic compression. Diseases of the Esophagus. 2016;**29**(3):224-228

[20] Shenfine J et al. A randomized controlled clinical trial of palliative therapies for patients with inoperable esophageal cancer. Official Journal of the American College of Gastroenterology|ACG. 2009;**104**(7):1674-1685

[21] Conio M et al. A randomized prospective comparison of self-expandable plastic stents and partially covered self-expandable metal stents in the palliation of malignant esophageal dysphagia. Official Journal of the American College of Gastroenterology|ACG. 2007;**102**(12):2667-2677

[22] Sharma P et al. Practice Parameters Committee of the American College of Gastroenterology. Role of esophageal stents in benign and malignant diseases. Official Journal of the American College of Gastroenterology|ACG. 2010;**105**(2):258-273

[23] Law R et al. Stent migration following endoscopic suture fixation of esophageal self-expandable metal stents: A systematic review and meta-analysis. Surgical Endoscopy. 2018;**32**:675-681

[24] Bick BL et al. Endoscopic suturing of esophageal fully covered self-expanding metal stents reduces rates of stent migration. Gastrointestinal Endoscopy. 2017;**86**(6):1015-1021

[25] Dua KS et al. A phase III, multicenter, prospective, single-blinded, noninferiority, randomized controlled trial on the performance of a novel esophageal stent with an antireflux valve (with video). Gastrointestinal Endoscopy. 2019;**90**(1):64-74

[26] Kochman ML et al. The refractory and the recurrent esophageal stricture: A definition. Gastrointestinal Endoscopy. 2005;**62**(3):474-475

[27] Fan Y et al. Evaluation of the incidence of esophageal complications associated with balloon dilation and their management in patients with malignant esophageal strictures. American Journal of Roentgenology. 2012;**198**(1):213-218

[28] Brimhall B et al. Enteral stents for malignant gastric outlet obstruction. Gastrointestinal Endoscopy Clinics of North America. 2011;**21**(3):389-403

[29] Tsukada K. Metallic stent placement or gastroenterostomy for gastric outlet obstruction caused by gastric cancer? Journal of Gastroenterology. 2005;**40**:1007-1008

[30] Kim M et al. Interventional endoscopy for palliation of luminal gastrointestinal obstructions in management of cancer: Practical guide for oncologists. Journal of Clinical Medicine. 2022;**11**(6):1712

[31] Fujitani K et al. Multicentre observational study of quality of life

after surgical palliation of malignant gastric outlet obstruction for gastric cancer. BJS Open. 2017;**1**(6):165-174

[32] Dormann A et al. Self-expanding metal stents for gastroduodenal malignancies: Systematic review of their clinical effectiveness. Endoscopy. 2004;**36**(06):543-550

[33] Nagaraja V, Eslick GD, Cox MR. Endoscopic stenting versus operative gastrojejunostomy for malignant gastric outlet obstruction - A systematic review and meta-analysis of randomized and non-randomized trials. Journal of Gastrointestinal Oncology. 2014;**5**(2):92-98

[34] Jeurnink SM et al. Surgical gastrojejunostomy or endoscopic stent placement for the palliation of malignant gastric outlet obstruction (SUSTENT study): A multicenter randomized trial. Gastrointestinal Endoscopy. 2010;**71**(3):490-499

[35] Fiori E et al. Palliative management of malignant antro-pyloric strictures. Gastroenterostomy vs. endoscopic stenting. A randomized prospective trial. Anticancer Research. 2004;**24**(1):269-271

[36] Jeong SJ, Lee J. Management of gastric outlet obstruction: Focusing on endoscopic approach. World Journal of Gastrointestinal Pharmacology and Therapeutics. 2020;**11**(2):8-16. DOI: 10.4292/wjgpt.v11.i2.8

[37] Jeurnink SM et al. Stent versus gastrojejunostomy for the palliation of gastric outlet obstruction: A systematic review. BMC Gastroenterology. 2007;**7**(1):1

[38] Yamao K et al. Factors predicting through-the-scope gastroduodenal stenting outcomes in patients with gastric outlet obstruction: A large multicenter retrospective study in West Japan. Gastrointestinal Endoscopy. 2016;**84**(5):757-763 e6

[39] Roy A et al. Stenting versus gastrojejunostomy for management of malignant gastric outlet obstruction: Comparison of clinical outcomes and costs. Surgical Endoscopy. 2012;**26**:3114-3119

[40] Khashab M et al. Enteral stenting versus gastrojejunostomy for palliation of malignant gastric outlet obstruction. Surgical Endoscopy. 2013;**27**(6):2068-2075. DOI: 10.1007/s00464-012-2712-7. Epub 2013 Jan 9

[41] Del Piano M et al. Endoscopy or surgery for malignant GI outlet obstruction? Gastrointestinal Endoscopy. 2005;**61**(3):421-426. DOI: 10.1016/s0016-5107(04)02757-9

[42] Ly J et al. A systematic review of methods to palliate malignant gastric outlet obstruction. Surgical Endoscopy. 2010;**24**(2):290-297. DOI: 10.1007/s00464-009-0577-1. Epub 2009 Jun 24

[43] Chamberlain RS et al. Hepatic neuroendocrine metastases: Does intervention alter outcomes? Journal of the American College of Surgeons. 2000;**190**(4):432-445

[44] Kawata N et al. Percutaneous endoscopic gastrostomy for decompression of malignant bowel obstruction. Digestive Endoscopy. 2014;**26**(2):208-213

[45] Tyberg A et al. Endoscopic ultrasound-guided gastrojejunostomy with a lumen-apposing metal stent: A multicenter, international experience. Endoscopy International Open. 2016;**4**(03):E276-E281

[46] Iqbal U et al. EUS-guided gastroenterostomy for the management

of gastric outlet obstruction: A systematic review and meta-analysis. Endoscopic Ultrasound. 2020;**9**(1):16

[47] Khashab MA et al. International multicenter comparativetrial of endoscopic ultrasonography-guidedgastroenterostomy versus surgical gastrojejunostomyfor the treatment of malignantgastric outlet obstruction. Endoscopy International Open. 2017;5(4):E275-E281

[48] Panagiotakis PH et al. DPEJ tube placement prevents aspiration pneumonia in high-risk patients. Nutrition in Clinical Practice. 2008;**23**(2):172-175. DOI: 10.1177/0884533608314537

[49] Richards DM et al. Percutaneous endoscopic gastrostomy in cancer patients: Predictors of 30-day complications, 30-day mortality, and overall mortality. Digestive Diseases and Sciences. 2013;**58**:768-776

[50] Greaves JR. Head and neck cancer tumor seeding at the percutaneous endoscopic gastrostomy site. Nutrition in Clinical Practice. 2018;**33**(1):73-80

[51] Lau MK, Davila JA, Shaib YH. Incidence and survival of pancreatic head and body and tail cancers: A population-based study in the United States. Pancreas. 2010;**39**(4):458-462

[52] Saad AM, Turk T, Al-Husseini MJ, Abdel-Rahman O. Trends in pancreatic adenocarcinoma incidence and mortality in the United States in the last four decades; A SEER-based study. BMC Cancer. 2018;**18**(1):1-1

[53] Abboud Y, Samaan JS, Oh J, Jiang Y, Randhawa N, Lew D, et al. Increasing pancreatic cancer incidence in young women in the United States: A population-based time-trend analysis, 2001-2018. Gastroenterology. 2023;**164**(6):978-989

[54] Pereiras RV Jr, Rheingold OJ, et al. Relief of malignant obstructive jaundice by percutaneous insertion of a permanent prosthesis in the biliary tree. Annals of Internal Medicine. 1978;**89**(5_Part_1):589-593

[55] Pfau PR, Pleskow DK, Banerjee S, Barth BA, Bhat YM, Desilets DJ, et al. Pancreatic and biliary stents. Gastrointestinal Endoscopy. 2013;**77**(3):319-327

[56] Moole H, Jaeger A, Cashman M, Volmar FH, Dhillon S, Bechtold ML, et al. Are self-expandable metal stents superior to plastic stents in palliating malignant distal biliary strictures? A meta-analysis and systematic review. Medical Journal Armed Forces India. 2017;**73**(1):42-48

[57] Bruno MJ, Maluf-Filho F. Palliation of malignant pancreaticobiliary obstruction. In: Clinical Gastrointestinal Endoscopy. Amsterdam, The Netherlands: Elsevier; 2019. pp. 734-747

[58] Moss AC, Morris E, Leyden J, MacMathuna P. Do the benefits of metal stents justify the costs? A systematic review and meta-analysis of trials comparing endoscopic stents for malignant biliary obstruction. European Journal of Gastroenterology and Hepatology. 2007;**19**(12):1119-1124

[59] Dumonceau JM, Tringali A, Blero D, Devière J, Laugiers R, Heresbach D, et al. Biliary stenting: Indications, choice of stents and results: European Society of Gastrointestinal Endoscopy (ESGE) clinical guideline. Endoscopy. 2012;**44**(03):277-298

[60] Doria C, Rogart J. Hepato-Pancreato-Biliary Malignancies: Diagnosis and Treatment in the 21st Century. Switzerland: Springer Nature; 2022

[61] Lam R, Muniraj T. Fully covered metal biliary stents: A review of the literature. World Journal of Gastroenterology. 2021;**27**(38):6357

[62] Saleem A, Leggett CL, Murad MH, Baron TH. Meta-analysis of randomized trials comparing the patency of covered and uncovered self-expandable metal stents for palliation of distal malignant bile duct obstruction. Gastrointestinal Endoscopy. 2011;**74**(2):321-327

[63] Li J, Li T, Sun P, Yu Q, Wang K, Chang W, et al. Covered versus uncovered self-expandable metal stents for managing malignant distal biliary obstruction: A meta-analysis. PLoS One. 2016;**11**(2):e0149066

[64] Yoon WJ, Lee JK, Lee KH, Lee WJ, Ryu JK, Kim YT, et al. A comparison of covered and uncovered Wallstents for the management of distal malignant biliary obstruction. Gastrointestinal Endoscopy. 2006;**63**(7):996-1000

[65] Elmunzer BJ, Maranki JL, Gómez V, Tavakkoli A, Sauer BG, Limketkai BN, et al. ACG clinical guideline: Diagnosis and management of biliary strictures. The American Journal of Gastroenterology. 2023;**118**(3):405-426

[66] Sawas T, Al Halabi S, Parsi MA, Vargo JJ. Self-expandable metal stents versus plastic stents for malignant biliary obstruction: A meta-analysis. Gastrointestinal Endoscopy. 2015;**82**(2):256-267

[67] Seo DW, Sherman S, Dua KS, Slivka A, Roy A, Costamagna G, et al. Covered and uncovered biliary metal stents provide similar relief of biliary obstruction during neoadjuvant therapy in pancreatic cancer: A randomized trial. Gastrointestinal Endoscopy. 2019;**90**(4):602-612

[68] Tringali A, Hassan C, Rota M, Rossi M, Mutignani M, Aabakken L. Covered vs. uncovered self-expandable metal stents for malignant distal biliary strictures: A systematic review and meta-analysis. Endoscopy. 2018;**50**(06):631-641

[69] Park DH, Kim MH, Choi JS, Lee SS, Seo DW, Kim JH, et al. Covered versus uncovered wallstent for malignant extrahepatic biliary obstruction: A cohort comparative analysis. Clinical Gastroenterology and Hepatology. 2006;**4**(6):790-796

[70] Kullman E, Frozanpor F, Söderlund C, Linder S, Sandström P, Lindhoff-Larsson A, et al. Covered versus uncovered self-expandable nitinol stents in the palliative treatment of malignant distal biliary obstruction: Results from a randomized, multicenter study. Gastrointestinal Endoscopy. 2010;**72**(5):915-923

[71] Levy MJ, Baron TH, Gostout CJ, Petersen BT, Farnell MB. Palliation of malignant extrahepatic biliary obstruction with plastic versus expandable metal stents: An evidence-based approach. Clinical Gastroenterology and Hepatology. 2004;**2**(4):273-285

[72] Almadi MA, Barkun AN, Martel M. No benefit of covered vs uncovered self-expandable metal stents in patients with malignant distal biliary obstruction: A meta-analysis. Clinical Gastroenterology and Hepatology. 2013;**11**(1):27-37

[73] Bor R, Fábián A, Szűcs M, Bálint A, Rutka M, Tóth T, et al. Comparison of therapeutic efficacy and treatment costs of self-expandable metal stents and plastic stents for management of malignant biliary obstruction. BMC Gastroenterology. 2023;**23**(1):41

[74] Soderlund C, Linder S. Covered metal versus plastic stents for malignant common bile duct stenosis: A prospective, randomized, controlled trial. Gastrointestinal Endoscopy. 2006;**63**(7):986-995

[75] Kaassis M, Boyer J, Dumas R, Ponchon T, Coumaros D, Delcenserie R, et al. Plastic or metal stents for malignant stricture of the common bile duct? Results of a randomized prospective study. Gastrointestinal Endoscopy. 2003;**57**(2):178-182

[76] Walter D, van Boeckel PG, Groenen MJ, Weusten BL, Witteman BJ, Tan G, et al. Cost efficacy of metal stents for palliation of extrahepatic bile duct obstruction in a randomized controlled trial. Gastroenterology. 2015;**149**(1):130-138

[77] Inamdar S, Slattery E, Sejpal DV, Miller LS, Pleskow DK, Berzin TM, et al. Systematic review and meta-analysis of single-balloon enteroscopy–assisted ERCP in patients with surgically altered GI anatomy. Gastrointestinal Endoscopy. 2015;**82**(1):9-19

[78] Tarantino I, Barresi L, Fabbri C, Traina M. Endoscopic ultrasound guided biliary drainage. World Journal of Gastrointestinal Endoscopy. 2012;**4**(7):306

[79] Khan MA, Akbar A, Baron TH, Khan S, Kocak M, Alastal Y, et al. Endoscopic ultrasound-guided biliary drainage: A systematic review and meta-analysis. Digestive Diseases and Sciences. 2016;**61**:684-703

[80] Giovannini M, Bories E. EUS-guided biliary drainage. Gastroenterology Research and Practice. 2011;**2012**

[81] Wiersema MJ, Sandusky D, Carr R, Wiersema LM, Erdel WC, Frederick PK. Endosonography-guided cholangiopancreatography. Gastrointestinal Endoscopy. 1996;**43**(2):102-106

[82] Teoh AY, Dhir V, Kida M, Yasuda I, Jin ZD, Seo DW, et al. Consensus guidelines on the optimal management in interventional EUS procedures: Results from the Asian EUS group RAND/UCLA expert panel. Gut. 2018;**67**(7):1209-1228

[83] Kamal F, Khan MA, Lee-Smith W, Sharma S, Acharya A, Farooq U, et al. Efficacy and safety of EUS-guided biliary drainage for benign biliary obstruction–A systematic review and meta-analysis. Endoscopic Ultrasound. 2023;**12**(2):228

[84] Anderloni A, Fugazza A, Troncone E, Auriemma F, Carrara S, Semeraro R, et al. Single-stage EUS-guided choledochoduodenostomy using a lumen-apposing metal stent for malignant distal biliary obstruction. Gastrointestinal Endoscopy. 2019;**89**(1):69-76

[85] Nakai Y, Sato T, Hakuta R, Ishigaki K, Saito K, Saito T, et al. Long-term outcomes of a long, partially covered metal stent for EUS-guided hepaticogastrostomy in patients with malignant biliary obstruction (with video). Gastrointestinal Endoscopy. 2020;**92**(3):623-631

[86] Robles-Medranda C, Oleas R, Puga-Tejada M, Alcivar-Vasquez J, Del Valle R, Olmos J, et al. Prophylactic EUS-guided gallbladder drainage prevents acute cholecystitis in patients with malignant biliary obstruction and cystic duct orifice involvement: A randomized trial (with video). Gastrointestinal Endoscopy. 2023;**97**(3):445-453

[87] Lee TH, Choi JH, Park DH, Song TJ, Kim DU, Paik WH, et al. Similar

efficacies of endoscopic ultrasound–guided transmural and percutaneous drainage for malignant distal biliary obstruction. Clinical Gastroenterology and Hepatology. 2016;**14**(7):1011-1019

[88] Itoi T, Dhir V, Moon JH. EUS-guided biliary drainage: Moving into a new era of biliary drainage. Gastrointestinal Endoscopy. 2017;**85**(5):915-917

[89] Sharaiha RZ, Khan MA, Kamal F, Tyberg A, Tombazzi CR, Ali B, et al. Efficacy and safety of EUS-guided biliary drainage in comparison with percutaneous biliary drainage when ERCP fails: A systematic review and meta-analysis. Gastrointestinal Endoscopy. 2017;**85**(5):904-914

[90] Minaga K, Ogura T, Shiomi H, Imai H, Hoki N, Takenaka M, et al. Comparison of the efficacy and safety of endoscopic ultrasound-guided choledochoduodenostomy and hepaticogastrostomy for malignant distal biliary obstruction: Multicenter, randomized, clinical trial. Digestive Endoscopy. 2019;**31**(5):575-582

[91] Uemura RS, Khan MA, Otoch JP, Kahaleh M, Montero EF, Artifon EL. EUS-guided choledochoduodenostomy versus hepaticogastrostomy. Journal of Clinical Gastroenterology. 2018;**52**(2):123-130

[92] Steel AW, Postgate AJ, Khorsandi S, Nicholls J, Jiao L, Vlavianos P, et al. Endoscopically applied radiofrequency ablation appears to be safe in the treatment of malignant biliary obstruction. Gastrointestinal Endoscopy. 2011;**73**(1):149-153

[93] Yang J, Wang J, Zhou H, Zhou Y, Wang Y, Jin H, et al. Efficacy and safety of endoscopic radiofrequency ablation for unresectable extrahepatic cholangiocarcinoma: A randomized trial. Endoscopy. 2018;**50**(08):751-760

[94] Sofi AA, Khan MA, Das A, Sachdev M, Khuder S, Nawras A, et al. Radiofrequency ablation combined with biliary stent placement versus stent placement alone for malignant biliary strictures: A systematic review and meta-analysis. Gastrointestinal Endoscopy. 2018;**87**(4):944-951

[95] Zheng X, Bo ZY, Wan W, Wu YC, Wang TT, Wu J, et al. Endoscopic radiofrequency ablation may be preferable in the management of malignant biliary obstruction: A systematic review and meta-analysis. Journal of Digestive Diseases. 2016;**17**(11):716-724

[96] Kadayifci A, Atar M, Forcione DG, Casey BW, Kelsey PB, Brugge WR. Radiofrequency ablation for the management of occluded biliary metal stents. Endoscopy. 2016;**48**(12):1096-1101

[97] Nayar MK, Oppong KW, Bekkali NL, Leeds JS. Novel temperature-controlled RFA probe for treatment of blocked metal biliary stents in patients with pancreaticobiliary cancers: Initial experience. Endoscopy International Open. 2018;**6**(05):E513-E517

[98] Pereira P, Santos AL, Morais R, Vilas-Boas F, Rodrigues-Pinto E, Santos-Antunes J, et al. Endoscopic radiofrequency ablation for palliative treatment of hilar cholangiocarcinoma. VideoGIE. 2021;**6**(4):195-198

[99] Albers D, Schmidt A, Schiemer M, Caca K, Wannhoff A, Sauer P, et al. Impact of endobiliary radiofrequency ablation on biliary drainage in patients with malignant biliary strictures treated with uncovered self-expandable metal stents: A randomized controlled multicenter trial. Gastrointestinal Endoscopy. 2022;**96**(6):970-979

[100] Dolak W, Schreiber F, Schwaighofer H, Gschwantler M, Plieschnegger W, Ziachehabi A, et al. Endoscopic radiofrequency ablation for malignant biliary obstruction: A nationwide retrospective study of 84 consecutive applications. Surgical Endoscopy. 2014;**28**:854-860

[101] Tal AO, Vermehren J, Friedrich-Rust M, Bojunga J, Sarrazin C, Zeuzem S, et al. Intraductal endoscopic radiofrequency ablation for the treatment of hilar non-resectable malignant bile duct obstruction. World Journal of Gastrointestinal Endoscopy. 2014;**6**(1):13

[102] Auriemma F, De Luca L, Bianchetti M, Repici A, Mangiavillano B. Radiofrequency and malignant biliary strictures: An update. World Journal of Gastrointestinal Endoscopy. 2019;**11**(2):95

[103] Ortner ME, Caca K, Berr F, Liebetruth J, Mansmann U, Huster D, et al. Successful photodynamic therapy for nonresectable cholangiocarcinoma: A randomized prospective study. Gastroenterology. 2003;**125**(5):1355-1363

[104] Choi JH, Oh D, Lee JH, Park JH, Kim KP, Lee SS, et al. Initial human experience of endoscopic ultrasound-guided photodynamic therapy with a novel photosensitizer and a flexible laser-light catheter. Endoscopy. 2015;**47**(11):1035-1038

[105] Strand DS, Cosgrove ND, Patrie JT, Cox DG, Bauer TW, Adams RB, et al. ERCP-directed radiofrequency ablation and photodynamic therapy are associated with comparable survival in the treatment of unresectable cholangiocarcinoma. Gastrointestinal Endoscopy. 2014;**80**(5):794-804

[106] Talreja JP, DeGaetani M, Ellen K, Schmitt T, Gaidhane M, Kahaleh M. Photodynamic therapy in unresectable cholangiocarcinoma: Not for the uncommitted. Clinical Endoscopy. 2013;**46**(4):390-394

[107] Lu Y, Liu L, Wu JC, Bie LK, Gong B. Efficacy and safety of photodynamic therapy for unresectable cholangiocarcinoma: A meta-analysis. Clinics and Research in Hepatology and Gastroenterology. 2015;**39**(6):718-724

[108] Kahaleh M, Mishra R, Shami VM, Northup PG, Berg CL, Bashlor P, et al. Unresectable cholangiocarcinoma: Comparison of survival in biliary stenting alone versus stenting with photodynamic therapy. Clinical Gastroenterology and Hepatology. 2008;**6**(3):290-297

[109] Siegel RL, Miller KD, Jemal A. Cancer statistics, 2019. CA: A Cancer Journal for Clinicians. 2019;**69**(1):7-34

[110] Han CQ, Tang XL, Zhang Q, Nie C, Liu J, Ding Z. Predictors of pain response after endoscopic ultrasound-guided celiac plexus neurolysis for abdominal pain caused by pancreatic malignancy. World Journal of Gastroenterology. 2021;**27**(1):69

[111] WHO Guidelines for the Pharmacological and Radiotherapeutic Management of Cancer Pain in Adults and Adolescents. Geneva: World Health Organization; 2018

[112] Wiersema MJ, Wiersema LM. Endosonography-guided celiac plexus neurolysis. Gastrointestinal Endoscopy. 1996;**44**(6):656-662

[113] Yan BM, Myers RP. Neurolytic celiac plexus block for pain control in unresectable pancreatic cancer. Official Journal of the American College of Gastroenterology|ACG. 2007;**102**(2):430-438

[114] Wyse JM, Carone M, Paquin SC, Usatii M, Sahai AV. Randomized, double-blind, controlled trial of early endoscopic ultrasound–guided celiac plexus neurolysis to prevent pain progression in patients with newly diagnosed, painful, inoperable pancreatic cancer. Journal of Clinical Oncology. 2011;**29**(26):3541-3546

[115] Kanno Y, Koshita S, Masu K, Ogawa T, Kusunose H, Murabayashi T, et al. Efficacy of EUS-guided celiac plexus neurolysis compared with medication alone for unresectable pancreatic cancer in the oxycodone/fentanyl era: A prospective randomized control study. Gastrointestinal Endoscopy. 2020;**92**(1):120-130

[116] Fujii-Lau LL, Bamlet WR, Eldrige JS, Chari ST, Gleeson FC, Dayyeh BK, et al. Impact of celiac neurolysis on survival in patients with pancreatic cancer. Gastrointestinal Endoscopy. 2015;**82**(1):46-56

[117] Eisenberg E, Carr DB, Chalmers TC. Neurolytic celiac plexus block for treatment of cancer pain: A meta-analysis. Anesthesia & Analgesia. 1995;**80**(2):290-295

[118] Cornman-Homonoff J, Holzwanger DJ, Lee KS, Madoff DC, Li D. Celiac plexus block and neurolysis in the management of chronic upper abdominal pain. Seminars in Interventional Radiology. Vol. 34, No. 4. New York, NY: Thieme Medical Publishers; 2017. pp. 376-386

[119] Iwata K, Yasuda I, Enya M, Mukai T, Nakashima M, Doi S, et al. Predictive factors for pain relief after endoscopic ultrasound-guided celiac plexus neurolysis. Digestive Endoscopy. 2011;**23**(2):140-145

[120] Scotti GB, Sapienza P, Lapolla P, Crocetti D, Tarallo M, Brachini G, et al. Endoscopic stenting and palliative chemotherapy in advanced colorectal cancer: Friends or foes? An analysis of the current literature. In Vivo. 2022;**36**(3):1053-1058

[121] Sagar J. Colorectal stents for the management of malignant colonic obstructions. Cochrane Database of Systematic Reviews. 2011;**11**:1-32

[122] Van Hooft JE, Veld JV, Arnold D, Beets-Tan RG, Everett S, Götz M, et al. Self-expandable metal stents for obstructing colonic and extracolonic cancer: European Society of Gastrointestinal Endoscopy (ESGE) Guideline–Update 2020. Endoscopy. 2020;**52**(05):389-407

[123] Vandervoort J, Tham TC. Colonic stents for malignant obstruction—Not a bridge too far? Gastrointestinal Endoscopy. 2006;**64**(6):921-924

[124] Mashar M, Mashar R, Hajibandeh S. Uncovered versus covered stent in management of large bowel obstruction due to colorectal malignancy: A systematic review and meta-analysis. International Journal of Colorectal Disease. 2019;**34**:773-785

[125] Sano T, Nozawa Y, Iwanaga A, Azumi M, Imai M, Ishikawa T, et al. Comparison of the efficacy of self-expandable metallic stents in colorectal obstructions caused by extracolonic malignancy and colorectal cancer. Molecular and Clinical Oncology. 2021;**15**(2):1-7

[126] Van den Berg MW, Ledeboer M, Dijkgraaf MG, Fockens P, Ter Borg F, van Hooft JE. Long-term results of palliative stent placement for acute malignant colonic obstruction. Surgical Endoscopy. 2015;**29**:1580-1585

[127] Meisner S, González-Huix F, Vandervoort JG, Repici A, Xinopoulos D,

Grund KE, et al. Self-expanding metal stenting for palliation of patients with malignant colonic obstruction: Effectiveness and efficacy on 255 patients with 12-month's follow-up. Gastroenterology Research and Practice. 2012;**2012**

[128] Manes G, de Bellis M, Fuccio L, Repici A, Masci E, Ardizzone S, et al. Endoscopic palliation in patients with incurable malignant colorectal obstruction by means of self-expanding metal stent: Analysis of results and predictors of outcomes in a large multicenter series. Archives of Surgery. 2011;**146**(10):1157-1162

[129] Trompetas V, Saunders M, Gossage J, Anderson H. Shortcomings in colonic stenting to palliate large bowel obstruction from extracolonic malignancies. International Journal of Colorectal Disease. 2010;**25**:851-854

[130] Keswani RN, Azar RR, Edmundowicz SA, Zhang Q, Ammar T, Banerjee B, et al. Stenting for malignant colonic obstruction: A comparison of efficacy and complications in colonic versus extracolonic malignancy. Gastrointestinal Endoscopy. 2009;**69**(3):675-680

[131] Donnellan F, Cullen G, Cagney D, O'Halloran P, Harewood GC, Murray FE, et al. Efficacy and safety of colonic stenting for malignant disease in the elderly. International Journal of Colorectal Disease. 2010;**25**:747-750

[132] Sebastian S, Johnston S, Geoghegan T, Torreggiani W, Buckley M. Pooled analysis of the efficacy and safety of self-expanding metal stenting in malignant colorectal obstruction. Official Journal of the American College of Gastroenterology|ACG. 2004;**99**(10):2051-2057

[133] Harrison ME, Anderson MA, Appalaneni V, Banerjee S, Ben-Menachem T, Cash BD, et al. The role of endoscopy in the management of patients with known and suspected colonic obstruction and pseudo-obstruction. Gastrointestinal Endoscopy. 2010;**71**(4):669-679

[134] Van Halsema EE, Van Hooft JE, Small AJ, Baron TH, García-Cano J, Cheon JH, et al. Perforation in colorectal stenting: A meta-analysis and a search for risk factors. Gastrointestinal Endoscopy. 2014;**79**(6):970-982

[135] Kabbinavar FF, Flynn PJ, Kozloff M, Ashby MA, Sing A, Barr CE, et al. Gastrointestinal perforation associated with bevacizumab use in metastatic colorectal cancer: Results from a large treatment observational cohort study. European Journal of Cancer. 2012;**48**(8):1126-1132

[136] Soota K, Rustagi T. EUS-guided colocolostomy by use of a lumen-apposing metal stent for malignant sigmoid colon obstruction. Gastrointestinal Endoscopy. 2021;**94**(2):430-431

[137] Emmanuel J, Kollanthavelu S, Henry F, See LT. Endoscopic ultrasound-guided colo-colostomy in a case of acute large bowel obstruction. Endoscopy International Open. 2021;**9**(03):E289-E291

Chapter 15

Advanced Esophageal Cancer Palliative Surgical Therapy Using Isoperistaltic Gastric Tube

Jose Luis Braga De Aquino and Vania Aparecida Leandro-Merhi

Abstract

Although malignant neoplasms of the esophagus remain a very common disease, their diagnosis might often come late, which explains why 50% of patients require palliative treatment. The ideal scenario would be the performance of procedures that provided an adequate quality of life and satisfactorily restored swallowing. This chapter aims to describe the results of palliative methods, discussed with emphasis on the technique of the isoperistaltic greater curvature gastric tube (IGCGT). About 143 patients with unresectable squamous cell carcinoma of the esophagus (T4b) were evaluated at this facility. In the early postoperative evaluation, 64 patients (44.7%) presented systemic complications, with pulmonary infection being the most frequent; 51 patients (35.6%) presented local complications, with cervical esophagogastric anastomosis leak being the most frequent. Thirteen patients (9.1%) died as a result of postoperative complications. Out of 112 patients who were adequately followed up, 91 (81.2%) achieved good palliation with this procedure, as they had adequate restoration of swallowing function, with a median survival of 3 years in 63 patients (69.2%). With these results, it is possible to conclude that despite showing non-negligible morbidity, IGCGT can be performed quickly and safely, offering adequate palliation and survival rate.

Keywords: esophageal neoplasms, palliative surgery, isoperistaltic gastric tube, esophagectomy, surgical therapy

1. Introduction

Malignant esophagus neoplasia continues to be a very frequent condition, ranking third among the most frequent tumors of the gastrointestinal tract and the eighth most prevalent in the world [1–4]. Recent studies have demonstrated that these tumors have increased approximately 10% per year, causing an estimated 400,000 deaths per year and being the sixth leading cause of cancer patients' death [5–7].

In Brazil, it is the seventh most common malignant neoplasm with an estimate of 13,550 new cases in 2018; its higher incidence occurs in the south and southeast regions of the country [8, 9].

Diagnosis is almost always delayed because dysphagia, its main symptom, only occurs when 50% or more of the esophageal lumen is clogged by the tumor. Delayed diagnosis, excessive weight loss due to dysphagia, and the association of cardiopulmonary diseases resulting from tobacco abuse make clinical control of patients with this disease rather difficult, leaving the doctor with few therapeutic options [3, 4, 10, 11].

This reflects in the indication of esophagectomy, because although this surgical procedure continues to be the best therapeutic indication for the potential cure of this condition, in most cases, due to the advanced stage of the disease and to the great nutritional clinical impairment in those patients, only 30–40% of the patients are able to undergo this treatment, which causes the prognosis to be quite unfavorable [1, 5, 11–13].

Thus, a palliative treatment is required in more than 50% of patients plagued with this neoplasm. Ideally, we should have procedures available that would provide a more adequate quality of life and satisfactorily restore swallowing, without further hospitalizations and with lower complications rates [14–17].

Choosing the best therapeutic options while trying to fulfill these requirements is a difficult task, since all methods have limitations and often contraindications due to the high potential for disease morbidity.

2. Palliation methods

In practice, the palliative therapy can be classified into two groups:

2.1 Nonsurgical

The current recommended methods are endoscopic techniques that are indicated for:

- Patients who have an indication for final chemoradiation, but who present severe dysphagia in the initial evaluation, thus requiring such previous intervention [5, 18].
- Failure to resolve dysphagia palliation with the initial therapy [5, 18].
- Recurrent dysphagia due to locoregional failure [5, 18].
- Recurrent dysphagia due to benign stenosis in patients who experienced successful chemoradiation [5, 18].
- Patients with clinical comorbidities, particularly cardiovascular and pulmonary diseases, which contraindicate surgical treatment and/or chemoradiation [5, 18].

Among the recommended endoscopic methods, the self-expandable metallic endoprosthesis stands out, which, although expensive, has shown adequate results, with satisfactory recovery of swallowing, low morbidity rate, and 6–10 months median survival in most of the series that have used this method [19, 20]. On the other hand, the use of endoscopic dilation, alcoholization, and laser has little application nowadays, because it, in addition to the poor resolution outcome, must be performed several times, increasing the morbidity potential [18, 20, 21].

2.2 Surgical

Palliative surgical therapy is mainly indicated for patients with satisfactory clinical conditions, but with unresectable tumors. Surgery can be performed using the following procedures:

2.2.1 Gastrostomy and jejunostomy

This type of procedure performed alone should be discarded as a palliative method of choice in the treatment of advanced esophageal neoplasia. Although easy to perform, including with local anesthesia, it does not bring any relief of the symptoms exhibited by those patients; in addition, patients must endure the presence of a probe inserted into the abdominal wall, which invariably presents leaks of digestive fluid around the tube, as well as exuberant growth of granulation tissue. The patient still does not intake food by mouth and is predisposed to saliva aspiration into the tracheobronchial tree, due to the permanence of esophageal obstruction. Thus, the method does not favor quality of life and fails to comply with the principles of an adequate palliative therapy. In addition, complications are frequently associated such as bronchopneumonia invariably due to aspiration, abdominal wall dehiscence, bleeding, and digestive fistula with consequent mortality potential and low survival [5, 22, 23].

Thus, the works reported in the literature serve only as a background review, since they date from the 1960s, 1970s, and early 1980s, when the endoscopic methods available today were not well-known. Meniconi [22], in a review of the literature involving 967 patients submitted to this type of procedure, reports complications ranging from 15 to 50%, with a mortality rate of up to 33% with survival time usually not exceeding 90 days in most of the patients studied and without having achieved a satisfactory quality of life.

Thus, gastrostomy/jejunostomy are exceptional procedures nowadays and are restricted only to cases of unresectable cervical esophageal cancer or as the first stage of another palliative or non-palliative procedure.

2.2.2 Resection

For several years now, it has been demonstrated that the best form of palliation for patients with unresectable advanced esophageal neoplasia, but with low clinical comorbidity, is the esophageal resection, because in addition to preventing the course of the esophageal disease, tumor hemorrhage, aspiration pneumonia, fistula in the respiratory tree, and mediastinitis, it also provides adequate dysphagia relief, a fact rarely observed with any other palliative method [1, 2, 4, 5, 24]. It also allows an increase in survival with an improved quality of life [11, 15, 25].

Over the years, a number of literature series have shown that palliative resections have caused higher morbidity and mortality than curative resections. In this connection, the work by Muller et al. [26] stands out. In an extensive review, these authors were able to review 13,061 curative and 16,024 palliative resection cases and demonstrated that the mortality associated with the curative and the palliative procedure was 11% and 18%, respectively. This finding was statistically significant and was confirmed by Law et al. [24] who reported 9% mortality for curative resections and 20% for palliative ones.

However, in recent years, with more appropriate postoperative care, with teams trained and accustomed to esophageal surgical procedures, a decrease in morbidity and mortality has ensued [14, 15, 19, 23].

Furthermore, with the evolution of radiotherapy and chemotherapy, it has been possible to enhance the survival to those patients, on average 24 months, compared to those who did not undergo any kind of treatment [2, 5, 11, 13].

As a result, palliative resection has a well-established position despite yielding suboptimal survival. It provides, however, an adequate quality of life by making the patient swallow naturally.

2.2.3 Bypass surgeries

This method is indicated for patients who have advanced cancer with extensive mediastinal invasion.

However, as it is a medium-major surgery, patients should have satisfactory clinical and nutritional conditions, which is quite uncommon in advanced stages of the disease.

This fact has been well demonstrated in the experience of Aquino et al. [27] where, out of 318 inoperable/unresectable patients from a series of 789, only 34.9% were able to undergo some kind of bypass surgery. In the other 2/3, another type of nonsurgical palliative treatment or even no procedure at all was undertaken due to the patients' poor clinical conditions.

The most used viscera include:

2.2.3.1 Jejunum

This reconstruction was designed by Wullstein [28] and Roux [29] and was used in isolated cases for more than one hundred years and is not used routinely today. The biggest obstacle to its use is the difficulty for the jejunum to reach the cervical region without tension or ischemia.

However, patients with tumors in the distal third of the esophagus that present spreading to the aorta and/or spine due to contiguity can have their swallowing rescued by the latero-lateral esophago-jejunal shunt, above the tumor area, through the abdomen with median frenotomy [30].

The literature is scarce in relation to this type of procedure, with the exception of the review by Meniconi [22], which, in 93 patients who had unresectable cancer of the distal third of the esophagus and submitted to this type of procedure, showed 30% morbidity, with 25% death in the immediate postoperative period and median survival of 6 months.

2.2.3.2 Colon

Based on past reports, palliative colonic interposition is quite an old technique, since it was used already in 1911 by Keeling and Vullet who recommended this type of reconstruction in patients with advanced unresectable esophageal tumor. In the few cases reported, the patients died also due to the limited resources available at that time [22].

Even today, with more resources, that procedure is not widely used, because it is a major surgery, with extensive mobilization of the colon, multiple anastomoses, and many complications.

Meniconi [22] demonstrated the experience that the Esophageal Surgery Service of the Hospital das Clínicas of the University of São Paulo School of Medicine (USP) has by operating 13 patients with palliative intent; the surgery outcome included a high incidence of complications with 23% deaths, 38% anastomotic fistulas, and 15% pulmonary complications. Thus, Meniconi [22] concluded that such a procedure should no longer be performed, due to the high morbidity rate. Postlethwait [31] also had the same opinion after assessing the high rate of complications in 690 patients who underwent this type of reconstruction.

Thus, the use of coloplasty for the palliative treatment of patients with advanced esophageal neoplasia should be viewed today with great caution and used with parsimony; it should be indicated only as an exception, when there are no technical conditions to perform other types of reconstruction.

2.2.3.3 Stomach

In this type of procedure, several authors recommend burial of the cervical and abdominal esophagus, with transposition of the stomach *via* a retrosternal route, seeking to shorten the time of the surgical procedure [5, 22, 25, 31, 32].

However, as this surgery is most often performed on patients with poor nutritional conditions and clinical morbidities, this procedure presents a number of local or systemic complications, such as dehiscence of the proximal and distal esophagus stump, fistula of the cervical esophagogastric anastomosis, and pulmonary infection.

Meniconi [22], in a review of the literature, found that in 483 patients submitted to this procedure, morbidity varied from 27 to 63.3% and mortality from 4 to 37%, with a median 7.5 months survival, but most patients obtained a satisfactory swallowing.

Another fact that has been always discussed is the possibility of this procedure producing mucocele, with potential mediastinitis due to the complete exclusion of the esophagus; however, the studies reviewed do not present any consistent casuistry that evidences this fact [14, 22, 31–33]. To prevent this complication, some authors indicated drainage of the thoracic esophagus with a tubular probe, which is also not free of complications, such as the tube escaping from its insertion site with consequent mediastinitis and peritonitis and fatal evolution in most patients [22, 27, 31].

Based on these facts, some authors, mainly from the Chinese school, led by Wong et al. [34], recommended the use of the surgery proposed by Kirschner, already back in 1920, for benign esophageal stenosis secondary to the ingestion of caustic agents. The procedure consists of transposing the stomach to the cervical region, anastomosing the cervical esophagus, and draining the abdominal esophagus through a jejunal loop (Billroth II or Roux Y), thereby allowing drainage of the esophageal content and thus preventing the potential development of mucoceles in the thoracic esophagus.

In Brazil, this type of procedure is undervalued. Only the work by Brandalise et al. [35] stands out, according to which, a total of 13 patients assessed presented a morbidity rate of 40%, mortality of 15.3%, and median survival of 8.5 months.

Aquino et al. [27] assessed 17 patients with unresectable esophageal cancer who underwent total gastric transposition; three of them with whom the Kirschner procedure was used also demonstrated that this procedure has a high morbidity rate. A total of 47% of all the patients experienced complications, mostly cardiopulmonary, and three patients died due to clinical and/or local complications. With regard to palliation, it was adequate in 70% of the patients, who reported satisfaction with the surgery because they managed to recover swallowing, although with a 7 months mean survival.

Considering the non-negligible morbidity rate and the new techniques available today, palliative total gastric transposition is not indicated as the first option for surgical treatment, being only an exception procedure aiming at those patients in whom other procedures cannot be used.

2.2.3.4 Greater curvature gastric tube

This technique was developed with the aim of resolving the dysphagia of patients with esophageal stenosis. Its principle is to minimize the complications that commonly affect surgical procedures on the esophagus, intending to be simple and causing low morbidity and mortality.

The great advantage is that it simultaneously drains both the esophagus and the stomach, thus avoiding potential esophageal mucoceles.

Historically, Beck and Carrel [36] demonstrated continent gastrostomy in cadavers and experimental animals, using a tube made from the greater gastric curvature irrigated by the left gastroepiploic artery. They also envisaged the possibility of esophagoplasty using this long, highly curved tube.

Subsequently, Carter et al. [37], in experimental animals, demonstrated the possibility of constructing the gastric tube with a greater curvature nourished by both the left and right gastroepiploic arteries. They named the gastric tube according to the direction of peristalsis: the part nourished by the right gastroepiploic artery and with a free end close to the gastric body-fundus junction, isoperistaltic gastric greater curvature tube, and the one nourished by the left gastro-epiploic artery and free end close to the antrum-pyloric gastric junction, anisoperistaltic gastric greater curvature tube.

In a clinical experience in 1951, Dan Graviliu reported having successfully constructed the first gastric tube with anisoperistaltic greater curvature in a cervical bypass in the treatment of esophageal stenosis [38].

At a later date, Heimlich [39] demonstrated his experience with gastric tube of greater anisoperistaltic curvature in cervical derivation in the treatment of esophagoplasties that failed with the use of stomach, colon, jejunum, or even prostheses. A total of 67 patients underwent this procedure with only 3 fatal cases.

Almost at the same time, Postlethwait [40], in the United States, referred to the use of the gastric tube with a greater curvature in an isoperistaltic direction in the treatment of a benign stenosis and in 29 unresectable malignant neoplasms of the esophagus with a 13% mortality rate.

In Brazil, Speranzini [41] reported the first national experience in the palliative treatment of esophageal neoplasia using an isoperistaltic greater curvature gastric tube in cervical bypass. Out of 13 patients who underwent this procedure, no death occurred.

From that time on, and especially with the advent of mechanical suturing, both linear and circular, several authors began to demonstrate greater experience with this procedure, as it is fast, simple, and yields acceptable morbidity rates [14, 19, 27, 42–44].

3. Surgical technique

The surgical technique involves the creation of a tube using the greater gastric curvature of about 2.5 cm in width, with preservation of the right gastroepiploic vessels.

To obtain this tube, the stomach is divided in a line parallel to the greater curvature, extending from the fundus to the gastric antrum, with the aid of a cutting linear mechanical suture (**Figure 1**).

The sectioned stomach resembles a "V," whose part corresponding to the lesser curvature drains the distal esophagus in relation to the tumor (**Figure 2**).

Transit reconstruction is performed by transposing the isoperistaltic tube *via* a retrosternal route, with manual anastomosis in two planes or circular mechanical performed in the cervical region (**Figure 3**).

In all patients, a jejunostomy is performed for enteral feeding, to be continued until the release of the enteral diet.

Aquino et al. [14], in a report of their experience with 112 patients submitted to palliative retrosternal transposition of the greater curvature gastric tube, demonstrated that such procedure was beneficial. This is because although this procedure was not free of complications, these were quite acceptable in view of the profile of the patient who was with advanced cancer, with 25.7% of systemic complications and

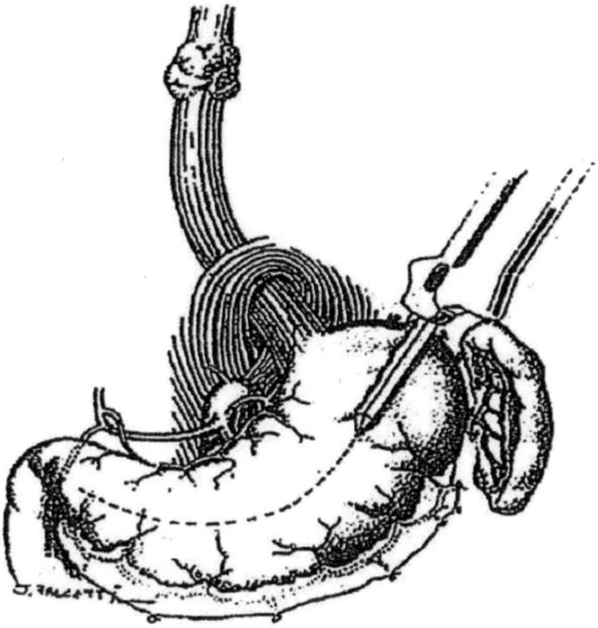

Figure 1.
Longitudinal incision approximately 2.5 cm from the greater gastric curvature. Source: Aquino et al. [23].

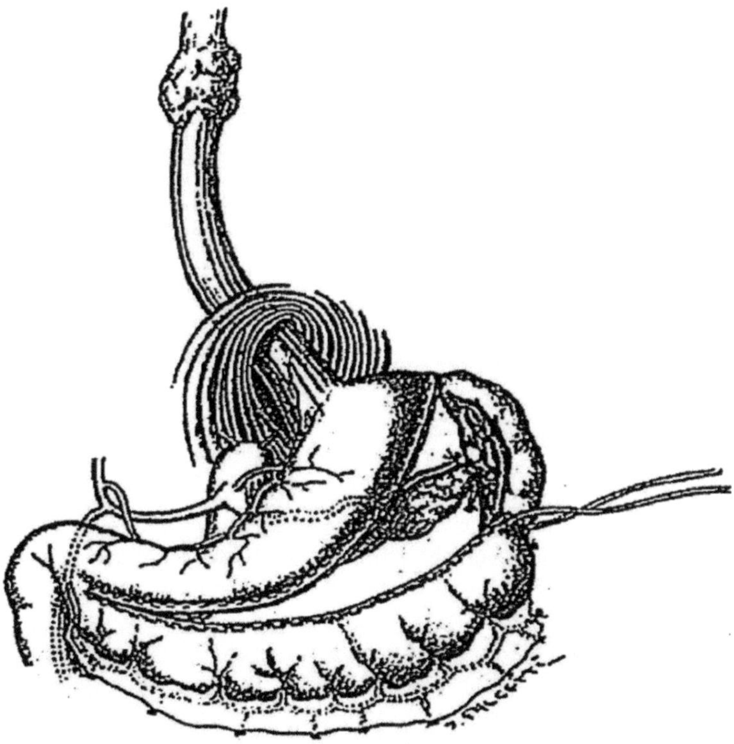

Figure 2.
Sectioned stomach resembling a "V," with preservation of the right gastroepiploic artery. Source: Aquino et al. [23].

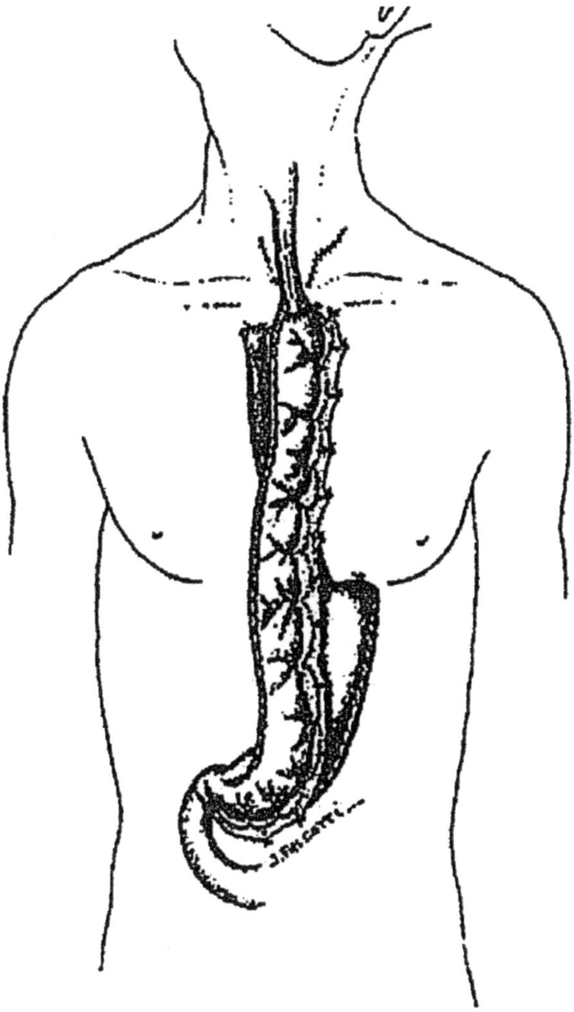

Figure 3.
Gastric tube transposed by retrosternal route. Source: Aquino et al. [23].

34% of local complications that were mainly related to dehiscences and stenoses of the cervical esophagogastric anastomosis. They also demonstrated that dehiscence was significantly more frequent with manual suture (p31/83 = 37.3%) than with mechanical suture (p4/29–13.8%).

In order to increase survival, the advantages of performing palliative surgery before radiotherapy and chemotherapy have recently been demonstrated, even using a minimally invasive technique, since patients who recover swallowing exhibit a better nutritional status, which helps preventing the drawbacks and complications of radiotherapy and chemotherapy [45–47].

This had already been demonstrated by Aquino et al. [27] who assessed 36 patients submitted to chemoradiation; 80.5% of those patients, after palliative transposition of the gastric tube, obtained a median 18 months survival; in patients who after the transposition were not submitted to chemoradiation, survival was 39.5%.

Some authors have also demonstrated in recent reports that in patients submitted to exclusive chemoradiation with a palliative purpose because they have advanced tumors, often a regression of the disease stage at the mediastinal level occurs, and therefore, it is possible to perform a rescue esophagectomy [3, 4, 13, 48, 49].

Aquino and Leandro-Merhi [50] also demonstrated the validity of rescue esophagectomy. Out of 82 patients who underwent radiotherapy and chemotherapy after prior creation of the palliative gastric tube, 37 experienced tumor regression, with rescue esophagectomy performed by thoracotomy. Although 2 patients eventually died due to postoperative complications, in the others, survival was quite adequate in relation to time: from 36 to 48 months in 26 patients and 3 patients died due to the metastatic disease within 9–15 months after rescue surgery.

4. Experience of the surgery service at the Hospital PUC-Campinas, Brazil

During the period from January 1993 to December 2022, 1614 patients were diagnosed with squamous cell carcinoma of the esophagus; a palliative large-curved isoperistaltic gastric tube was inserted in 143 of them because they had unresectable tumors (T4b) but with clinical conditions that allowed them to be subjected to this type of procedure. In the early postoperative evaluation, 64 patients (44.7%) had systemic complications, particularly cardiovascular and pulmonary; 51 patients (35.6%) developed local complications, the cervical esophagogastric anastomosis fistula being the most frequent, and 13 patients (9.1%) died due to complications.

Out of 112 patients, we were able to perform a follow-up in 91 patients (81%); the isoperistaltic gastric tube provided good palliation, as these patients restoration adequate swallowing, including the ingestion of solid foods.

Regarding the median survival, out of the 112 patients evaluated, all presented different evolution according to the association of complementary treatment or not:

In 30 patients in whom no complementary treatment was associated to the palliative surgical procedure, the median survival was 14 months.

In 45 patients treated with chemoradiation after the palliative surgical procedure, the median survival was 29 months, and in the 37 patients in whom palliative surgery was associated with rescue esophagectomy due to tumor regression, in addition to chemoradiation, the median survival was 42 months.

5. Final considerations

It is difficult to decide on the best palliative surgical therapy indication, due to the great impairment of the general conditions of patients with advanced esophageal neoplasia. Thus, some measures ought to be emphasized:

a. Careful patients' selection, since over 50% are unable to undergo any surgical procedure due to clinical comorbidities, particularly cardiopulmonary, besides an impaired nutritional status

b. Careful selection of the palliative surgical procedure, because although all of them can cause potential complications, the isoperistaltic gastric tube with greater curvature seems to be the technique that causes the lowest morbidity rate, besides being fast and safe to perform, particularly after the advent of the mechanical suture, offering palliation and quite adequate survival

c. Association of radiotherapy and chemotherapy after construction of the palliative gastric tube in well-selected patients, as those therapies seem to provide a higher survival rate, in addition to being able to allow the performance of rescue esophagectomy.

Acknowledgements

To hospital PUC-Campinas.

Conflict of interest

The authors declare no conflict of interest.

Author details

Jose Luis Braga De Aquino* and Vania Aparecida Leandro-Merhi
Graduate Program in Health Sciences, Pontifícia Universidade Católica de Campinas, Campinas, Brazil

*Address all correspondence to: jlaquino@sigmanet.com.br

References

[1] Kumagai K, Mariosa D, Tsai JÁ, Nilsson M, Ye W, Lundell L, et al. Systematic review and meta analysis on the significance of salvage esophagectomy for persistent or recurrent esophageal squamous cell after chemoradioterapy. Diseases of the Esophagus. 2016;**29**(7):734-739

[2] Swishwer SG, Marks J, Rice D. Salvage esophagectomy for persistent or recurrent disease after definitive chemoradiation. Annals of Cardiothoracic Surgery. 2017;**6**(2):144-151

[3] Fajardo R, Abbas AE, Petrov RU, Bakhos CT. Salvage esophagectomy. Surgical Clinics of North America. 2021;**101**(3):467-482

[4] Watanabe M. Salvage esophagectomy for residual tumor after definitive chemoradiotherapy for esophageal squamous cell carcinoma invading the neighboring organs. It is feasible choice? Annals of Surgical Oncology. 2020;**34**(5):123-129

[5] Sohda M, Kuwano H. Current status and future prospects for esophageal cancer treatment. Annals of Thoracic and Cardiovascular Surgery. 2017;**23**:1-11

[6] Watanabe M, Otake R, Kozuki R, Tochat T, Taka-Hashi K, Okamura A, et al. Recent progress in multidisciplinary treatment for patients with esophageal cancer. Surgery Today. 2020;**50**(1):12-20

[7] Swisher SG, Moughan J, Komari RU. Final results of NRG oncology RTOG 0246: In organ preserving selective resection strategy in esophageal cancer patient treated with definitive chemoradiation. Journal of Thoracic Oncology. 2017;**12**:368-374

[8] Instituto Nacional de Câncer José Alencar Gomes da Silva. Incidência de câncer no Brasil: Estimativa 2017. Rio de Janeiro: INCA; 2017. Disponível em: http://www.inca.gov.br/estimativa2017. Portuguese [Acesso: 23 abril, 2017]

[9] Tustmi F, Kimura CMS, Takeda FR, Sallum RAA, Ribeiro Junior U, Ceconello I. Avaliação da disseminação linfonodal, metástases à distância e invasão local do carcinoma esofágico. ABCD Arquivos Brasileiros de Cirurgia Digestiva. 2016;**29**(4):215-217. Portuguese

[10] Yuan X, Jiahua LV, Dong H, Wang J. Does cervical lymph node recurrence after oesophagectomy or definitive chemoradiotherapy for thoracic esophageal squamous cell carcinoma benefit from salvage treatment? Interactive Cardiovascular and Thoracic Surgery. 2017;(5):24, 792-795

[11] Kiyozumi Y, Yoshida N, Ishimoto T, Yagi T, Koga Y, Uchihara T, et al. Prognostic factors of salvage esophagectomy for residual or recurrent esophageal squamous cell carcinoma after definitive chemoradiotherapy. World Journal of Surgery. 2018;**42**(9):2887-2893

[12] Lerbutsayanukul C, Tharavej C, Klaikea WN, Prayongrat A, Lowanitchai C, Sriuranpong V. High dose radiation with chemotherapy followed by salvage esophagectomy among patients with locally advanced esophageal squamous cell carcinoma. Thoracic Cancer. 2017;**8**:219-228

[13] Yagi K, Toriu T, Aikou S, Yamashita H, Seto Y. Salvage treatment after definitive chemoradiotherapy for esophageal squamous cell carcinoma.

Annals of Gastroenterological Surgery. 2021;**5**:436-445

[14] Aquino JLB, Said MM, Brandi LA, Oliveira JMVP, Maziero D, Merhi VL. Tubo gástrico isoperistáltico de grande curvatura gástrica com sutura mecânica no trata-mento cirúrgico do câncer de esôfago irressecável. Arquivos Brasileiros de Cirurgia Digestiva. 2009;**22**(3):147-152. Portuguese

[15] Morita M, Yoshida R, Ikeda K, Egashira A, Oki E, Sadanaga N. Advances in esophageal cancer surgery in Japan: An analysis of 1000 consecutive patients treated at as single institute. Surgery. 2008;**143**(4):499-508

[16] Cen P, Hofstetter WL, Lee JH, Ross WA, Wu T, Swisher SG. Value of endoscopic ultrasound staging in conjuction with evaluation of lymphovascular invasion, in identifying low-risk esophageal carcinoma. Cancer. 2008;**112**(3):503-510

[17] Patel AN, Buenaventura PO. Current staging of esophageal carcinoma. Surgical Clinics of North America. 2005;**85**(3):355-367

[18] Wu H, Minamide T, Yano T. Role of photodynamic therapy in the treatment of esophageal cancer. Digestive Endoscopy. 2019;**31**:508-514

[19] Moura EGH. Tratamento paliativo do câncer de esôfago por endoprótese e tubo gástrico isoperistáltico [tese]. São Paulo: Universidade de São Paulo; 2000. Portuguese

[20] Sigounas DE, Krystallis C, Couper G. Argon plasma coagulation compared with stent placement in the palliative treatment of inoperable oesophageal cancer. United European Gastroenterology Journal. 2017;**5**:21-29

[21] Yano T, Kasai H, Horimatsu T, Yoshimura K, Teramukai S, Morita S, et al. A multicenter phase II study of salvage photodynamic therapy using talaporfin sodium (Me2906) and a diode laser (PLN6405EPG) for local failure after chemoradiotherapy or radiotherapy for esophageal cancer. Oncotarget. 2017;**8**(13):221-235

[22] Meniconi MTM. Estudo prospectivo da aplicação do tubo gástrico de grande curvatura isoperistáltico no tratamento da neoplasia avançada do esôfago: análise de 50 casos [tese]. São Paulo: Universidade de São Paulo; 1977. Portuguese

[23] Aquino JLB, Andreollo NA, Lopes LR. Terapêutica cirúrgica paliativa do câncer de esôfago. In: Fraga GP, JLB A, Andreollo NA, editors. Atualidades em clínica cirúrgica, intergastro e trauma. São Paulo: Editora Atheneu; 2010. pp. 283-284. Portuguese

[24] Law SYK, Fok M, Wong J. Risk analysis in resection of squamous cell carcinoma of the esophagus. World Journal of Surgery. 1994;**18**(3):339-346. DOI: 10.1007/BF00316812

[25] Fok M, Law SYK, Wong J. Operable esophageal carcinoma: Current results from Hong Kong. World Journal of Surgery. 1994;**18**(3):355-360. DOI: 10.1007/BF00316814

[26] Muller JM, Erasmi H, Stelner M, Zieren U, Pichmaier H. Surgical therapy of esophageal carcinoma. British Journal of Surgery. 1990;**77**(8):845-857

[27] Aquino JLB, Said MM, Brandi-Filho LA, Oliveira JMP, Maziero D, Lenharo G. Transposição visceral paliativa com tubo gástrico isoperistáltico de grande curvatura no câncer de esôfago irressecável: análise de 112 pacientes. In: Anais do Congresso

Brasileiro de Cirurgia, 28; São Paulo. São Paulo: Colégio Brasileiro de Cirurgiões; 2009. Portuguese

[28] Wullstein L. Ueber antethorakale Oesophago-Jejunostomie und operationen nach Gleichem Prinzip. Deutsch Med Wochenchr. 1904;**30**(20):734-744

[29] Roux L. Oesophago-jejuno-gastrostomie, nouvelle operation pour retrecissement infranchisable de l'oesophage. Semaine Médicale. 1907;**27**:37-40

[30] Pinotti HW. Acesso extrapleural ao esôfago por frenolaparatomia. Revista da Associação Médica Brasileira. 1976;**22**:56-60. Portuguese

[31] Postletwaith RW. Colonic interposition for esophageal substitution. Surgery, Gynecology and Obstetrics. 1983;**156**(3):377-383

[32] Lerut T, Leyn P, Coosemans W, Van Raemdonck D. Die chrugies desoesophagus carcinons. Der Chirurg. 1992;**63**:722-729

[33] Bardini R, Asolati M, Roul A, Bonavina L, Bassggio S, Peracchia A. Anastomosis. World Journal of Surgery. 1994;**18**:373-378

[34] Wong J, Lam KH, Wei WI, Ong GB. Results of the Kirschner operation. World Journal of Surgery. 1981;5:547-452

[35] Brandalise NA, Andreollo NA, Leonardi LS, Callejas-Neto F, Nagase Y. Utilizaçãodotubogástriconareconstrução do transito digestivo em neoplasias do esôfago e junção esofagogástrica. Revista do Colégio Brasileiro de Cirurgiões. 1985;**12**:152-155. Portuguese

[36] Beck C, Carrel A. Demonstration of specimens illustrating a method of formation of a prethoracic esopahgus. Illinois Medical Journal. 1905;7:463-468

[37] Carter BN, Abott OA, Hanlon CR. An experimental study of tubes made from the greater curvature of the stomach. Journal of Thoracic Surgery. 1941;**11**:494-509

[38] Heimlich HJ. The use of a gastric tube to replace the esophagus as performed by Dr. dan Gavriliu of Bucharest, Rumania: A preliminary report following a visit to Bucharest, Rumania. Surgery. 1957;**42**:693-695

[39] Heimlich HJ. Reversed gastric tube (RGT) esophagoplasty for failure of colon, jejunum and prosthetic interposition. Annals of Surgery. 1975;**182**(2):154-160

[40] Postlethwait RW. Technique for isoperistaltic gastric tube for esophageal by-pass. Annals of Surgery. 1979;**189**(6):673-676

[41] Speranzini MB, Fujimurai I, Pires PWA, Mittelstaed WEM, Deutsch CR, Bourroul-Filho RC, et al. Esofagoplastia com tubo gástrico isoperistáltico em derivação no tratamento do câncer de esofagotorácico: estudo de 13 casos. Revista da Associação Médica Brasileira. 1989;**35**(3):91-98. Portuguese

[42] Alcantara PS, Spencer-Netto FA, Silva Junior JF, Sores LA, Pollara WM, Bevilaqua RG. Gastroesophageal isoperistaltic by-pass in the palliation of irressectable esophageal cancer. International Surgery. 1997;**82**(3):249-253

[43] Meunier B, Spiopoulos Y, Stasik C, Lakéhal M, Malledant Y, Launois B. Retrosternal operation for unresectable squamous cell cancer of the esophagus.

Annals of Thoracic Surgery. 1996;**62**(2):373-377

[44] Chunwei F, Qingzeng N, Jianliang L, Weiji W. Cervical esophagogastric anastomosis with a new stapler in the surgery of esophageal carcinoma. European Journal of Cardio-Thoracic Surgery. 2005;**28**(2):291-295. DOI: 10.1016/j.ejcts.2005.04.019

[45] Zhou D, Wang Y, Tang F, Yang C, Duo D. Laparoscopically assisted tubular stomach constructive for the radical ressection of esophageal cancer. Alternative Therapies in Health and Medicine. 2023;**29**(2):200-205

[46] Knitter S, Andreou A, Hoffann T, Chopra S, Denecke C, Thuss-Patience PC, et al. Minimally invasive versus Ivor-Lewis esophagectomy for esophageal cancer or cancer of the gastroesophageal junction: Comparison of postoperative outcomes and long term survival using propensity score matching analysis. Anticancer Research. 2021;**41**:3499-3510

[47] Gupta V, Allen-Ayodobo C, Davis L, Zhao H, Hallet J, Mahar AL, et al. Patient reported symptoms for esophageal cancer patients undergoing curative intent treatment. Annals of Thoracic Surgery. 2020;**109**(2):367-374. DOI: 10.1016/j.athoracsur.2019.08.030. Epub 2019 Sep 21

[48] Zhou N, Hofstetter WL, Esophageal Squamous Cell Carcinoma Working Group, Mitchell KG, Bayley EM, Ajani JA, et al. Salvage esophagectomy definition influences comparative outcomes in esophageal squamous cell cancers. Annals of Thoracic Surgery. 2022;**114**(6):2032-2040. DOI: 10.1016/j.athoracsur.2021.10.046. Epub 2021 Dec 6

[49] Aquino JLB, Andreollo NA, Lopes LR. Esofagectomia de resgate no câncer de esôfago. In: Fraga GP, Pereira GS, Lopes LR, editors. Atualidades em clínica cirúrgica, intergastro e trauma. 2a. ed. Rio de Janeiro: Atheneu; 2011. p. 307-318. Portuguese

[50] Aquino JLB, Leandro Merhi VA. Salvage esophagectomy in treatment of advanced esophageal carcinoma. In: Sanna A, editor. Esophageal Surgery-Current Principles and Advances. London: IntechOpen; 2022. pp. 1-17. DOI: 10.5772/intechopen.106857

Chapter 16

Oral and Dental Care for Patients on Palliative Care

Firoozeh Samim, Ali Abdolrahmani, Elahe Akbari and Aia Naksho

Abstract

Therapeutic improvements and epidemiologic changes over the last three decades have led to increased numbers of survivors and aged population, resulting in greater need for continuing management of oral and dental health in this population. Generally, the palliative care patient oral health needs are complex, requiring multidisciplinary collaboration among medical and dental professionals with special knowledge and training in the field of oral medicine and oncology. This chapter offers clinical protocols and information for medical providers to assist in understanding oral complications and their management in these patients and survivors, and their oral and dental health care needs. Oral and dental care is impacted by the patient's initial oral and dental status, as well as the specific disorder for cancer location, type, and its treatment; thus, close communication between the dental professional and the medical team is required for appropriate therapy. Patients undergoing palliative care are at high risk of oral complications with the potential of causing significant morbidity and mortality. Dental professionals should play a fundamental role in the prevention and treatment of oral sequelae in thesis patients. However, the dental and medical community is not well informed/experienced in managing the oral complications of these vulnerable group.

Keywords: oral and dental health, oral manifestations, oral mucositis, oral infections, temporomandibular disorders

1. Introduction

Palliative care dentistry can be described as the examination and treatment of individuals who are suffering from advanced, progressive diseases, where the oral cavity has been compromised either due to the disease itself or its treatment. The primary focus of this form of care is to enhance the patient's quality of life. It encompasses not only addressing the patient's physical requirements but also providing support for their spiritual well-being and that of their family. This chapter aims to highlight common challenges encountered in palliative care dentistry, specifically in relation to adults with terminal cancer and proposes appropriate solutions for these issues. To better illustrate the oral problems associated with palliative care, we have summarized the most common one in **Figure 1**.

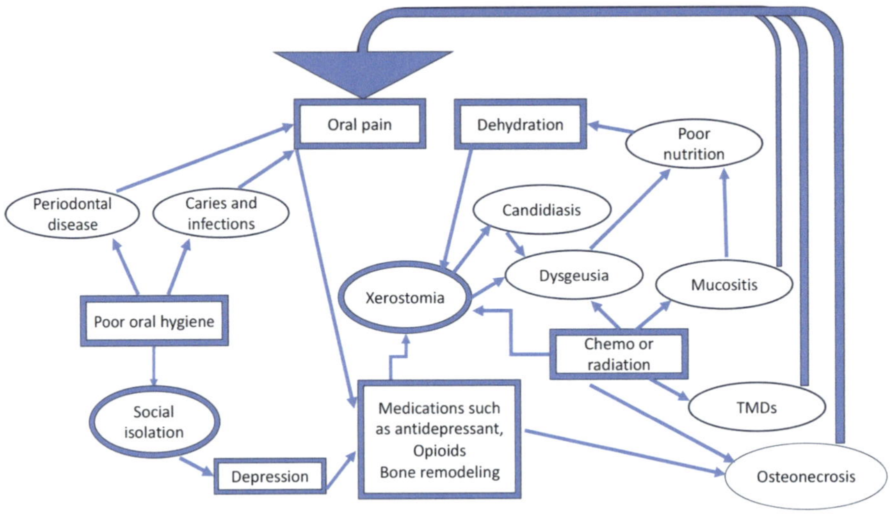

Figure 1.
Most common oral complications and its relations in patient in palliative care.

2. Oral pain in the cancer patient

Patients with cancer frequently experience orofacial and oropharyngeal pain, which can have underlying nociceptive, neuropathic, and psychosocial components. Oral pain in patients with advanced stages of cancer and other life-threating conditions in palliative care can be multifactorial, resulting from primary tumor or tumor-related pathology, mucositis, oral infections, TMJ problem and limitation in the mouth opening, xerostomia, dysgeusia and dysphagia, dental caries, periodontitis, and treatment-induced, complications such as ORN and MRONJ [1]. The impact of the oral pain can be profound, affecting essential functions such as eating, drinking, swallowing, and speaking and can lead to significant distress and diminish quality of life and patient overall well-being [2].

2.1 Oral mucositis

Oral mucositis is a common and distressing condition experienced by many palliative care patients and characterized by inflammation or/and ulceration of the oral mucosa, including buccal mucosa, tongue, and gingiva. Chemotherapy primarily affects rapidly dividing tissues, often impacting the oral cavity. It is estimated that approximately 40% of chemotherapy patients experience mucositis [3]. Diminished cell division leads to tissue atrophy, resulting in the formation of ulcers. This condition can be further complicated by microbial invasion [4]. Mucositis typically manifests within 5–7 days following chemotherapy administration which are known to have strong mucositis-inducing properties. In cases, where radiotherapy is employed to treat head and neck cancers, xerostomia (dry mouth) occurs due to the destruction of salivary tissues within the treatment area. The decrease in saliva's lubricating and protective properties renders the tissues more vulnerable to trauma and pathogenic invasion. Consequently, ulceration and erythema are observed in the affected tissues [5]. This condition can cause severe pain, difficulty in eating and swallowing, and increased risk of infections. In severe cases, intravenous or even total parenteral nutrition may be necessary to maintain adequate hydration and nutrition [6].

Several factors play a significant role in determining the extent and severity of mucositis. These factors encompass the particular drug used, dosage, method and frequency of administration, individual patient tolerance, genetic variations in drug-metabolizing pathways, immune signaling and cellular injury/repair mechanisms, and smoking history [7]. The following table (**Table 1**) provides a comprehensive list of cancer treatment drugs that have the potential to cause oral mucositis and summarizes the risk factors.

In palliative care, where the focus is on improving the quality of life for patients with advanced illness, effective management of oral mucositis is crucial. The management of these patients focuses on addressing symptoms and providing supportive care to ensure patient comfort and education. The goals include maintaining proper nutrition and oral hygiene while preventing opportunistic infections. It is crucial to closely monitor the patients and collaborate closely with their physicians. To prevent any potential sources of infection, all patients should undergo a thorough oral evaluation before undergoing radiation therapy. Whenever feasible, it is recommended to allow a healing period of 14 days after oral surgical procedures before initiating chemo or radiation therapy. Emphasizing oral hygiene is crucial both before, during, and after cancer therapy. To alleviate oral discomfort, topical anesthetics such as viscous lidocaine HCl (Xylocaine), diphenhydramine elixir (Benadryl), and throat lozenges containing dyclonine HCl can be used. Artificial saliva products such as Sage Moist Plus, Moi-Stir, and salivary can help reduce oral dryness. Laclede oral balance gel is a useful mouth moisturizing gel. Fungal overgrowth can be controlled with Nystatin and clotrimazole preparations. Chlorhexidine rinses are effective in managing plaque and candidiasis. Additionally, fluoride products, such as dentifrices, gels, and rinses, are applied to control dental caries. In **Table 2**, the recommendations and suggestions have been summarized:

2.2 Oral infection

During palliative care, patients often face the risk of acquiring secondary infections as a result of weakened immune systems and dysfunction in their salivary glands. One prevalent oral infection is candidiasis, which is primarily caused by *Candida albicans*. This opportunistic infection develops due to the combined effects of immunosuppression (common in chemotherapy, certain targeted therapies, and the use of intraoral topical steroids) and reduced salivary gland activity. Symptoms may vary and include pain, a burning sensation, changes in taste perception, and difficulties in consuming food and beverages [18]. The most typical manifestation is pseudomembranous candidiasis, characterized by easily removable white plaques that may leave behind small petechial hemorrhages.

The erythematous or atrophic form of candidiasis can present subtly with red patches and a burning sensation. To effectively manage candidiasis and prevent its recurrence during or after cancer therapy, antifungal treatment (both topical and systemic) is recommended, especially for individuals undergoing highly immunosuppressive chemotherapy regimens, such as allogeneic hematopoietic cell transplantation.

During palliative care or chemotherapy and other cancer therapies, herpes simplex virus infections can reoccur due to immunosuppression and stress. These irregular and painful ulcerations commonly affect the lips and tongue but can occur in any

Potential risk factors			
Specific anticancer agents			
Alkylating agents:	Busulfan, carboplatin, cisplatin, cyclophosphamide, and melphalan procarbazine	Prevent cell division primarily by cross-linking strands of DNA	Mild to moderate mucositis
Cytotoxic chemotherapy agents	Bleomycin, fluorouracil [FU], and methotrexate	Specific DNA cell cycle	Associated with higher rate of oral mucositis
	NOTE: Methotrexate, etoposide	Excreted through saliva	More damaging
Molecularly targeted agents: The occurrence of stomatitis varies across different molecularly targeted agents and depends on their class	Sunitinib, sorafenib, lenvatinib, and regorafenib	Tyrosine kinase inhibitors and vascular endothelial growth factor receptors	In 30–40% of patients
	Afatinib	Blocks signaling from the EGFR1 (erbB1), EGFR2 (HER2/erbB2), and erbB4	72%
	Erdafitinib and infigratinib	Oral fibroblast growth factor receptor inhibitors	56%
	Palbociclib	Cyclin-dependent kinase 4/6 inhibitor	25%
	Niraparib	Poly (ADP-ribose) polymerase (PARP) inhibitor	20%
	Cetuximab, erlotinib, dacomitinib, and mobocertinib	Epidermal growth factor receptor (EGFR)	10–46%
	Temsirolimus and everolimus	Target of rapamycin (mTOR) inhibitors	Aphthous like lesion in up to 75% of patient
	Note: A review found that mTOR inhibitor-associated stomatitis was the most frequent adverse event overall associated with these drugs (73%) and accounted for almost 30% of dose reductions, making it the most common dose-limiting toxicity (53%) [11]		
Immune checkpoint inhibitors	Mucosal toxicities related to immune checkpoint inhibitors include periodontal disease, stomatitis, oral lichen planus, xerostomia, and, rarely, a condition resembling Sjögren's disease that affects the salivary glands, as well as mucous membrane pemphigoid-like lesions [12, 13]		
Preexisting oral disease [14]	Chronic periodontal disease: Dental caries, poor oral hygiene, and periapical pathology		

Potential risk factors		
Age of patient	Younger patient at higher risk	Due to a faster epithelial mitotic rate
Additional factors	Nutritional status, the specific treatment protocol, the quality of oral care during treatment, pre-treatment neutrophil counts, the use of hematopoietic growth factor support during therapy, and variations in the oral microbiome [15, 16]	
	Genetic susceptibility [17]	Inherited variations in drug-metabolizing enzymes and proinflammatory cytokines

Table 1.
Factors associated with the development of oral mucositis [8–10].

intraoral site. They tend to be more extensive and take longer to heal compared to non-immunocompromised patients. Confirming the diagnosis can be done through PCR, direct fluorescent antibody test, culture, and cytology. Antiviral resistance and drug susceptibility can only be evaluated through culture. The management involves systemic antiviral therapy with medications, such as acyclovir or valacyclovir. For patients with unresolved infections despite antiviral therapy, considering antiviral susceptibility testing is recommended [19].

In immunosuppressed cancer patients, odontogenic infections may not present with typical signs such as swelling, erythema, and purulence. Fever or pain may be the only symptoms. It is crucial to promptly manage odontogenic infections in these cases by administering antibiotics and providing definitive care, such as tooth extraction. Patients with jaw osteonecrosis may also experience bacterial infections characterized by a mixture of oral flora [20]. The management of the oral infections has been summarized in **Table 3**.

2.3 Temporomandibular joint disorders (TMDS)

Palliative care is a specialized medical approach that focuses on providing relief and support to individuals facing serious illnesses, aiming to improve their quality of life. It is typically provided to patients with life-limiting conditions such as cancer, advanced heart disease, or neurodegenerative disorders. While palliative care primarily addresses pain management, symptom control, and emotional well-being, it also encompasses a holistic approach that considers the patient's overall health, including the management of specific conditions, such as temporomandibular dysfunction (TMD).

Temporomandibular dysfunction, also known as temporomandibular joint disorder (TMJ), refers to a group of conditions affecting the jaw joint and the surrounding muscles. It can cause pain, discomfort, restricted jaw movement, clicking or popping sounds, and even difficulties in eating or speaking. TMD can be caused by various factors, including jaw injuries, bruxism (teeth grinding or clenching), arthritis, or stress or cancer treatment [21].

When patients on palliative care experience TMD, managing their symptoms becomes an essential aspect of their overall care plan. Here are some considerations in addressing TMD in palliative care patients:

1. Pain management: TMD often causes significant pain and discomfort. Palliative care teams work closely with healthcare professionals, such as dentists, oral

General dental care	• Make available resources and support for individuals who wish to quit smoking. • Conduct an initial assessment of new patients to establish a baseline. • Instruct nurses or caregivers to actively screen for potential oral complications. • Provide both verbal and written guidance on maintaining oral hygiene from the beginning of the treatment. • Emphasize the importance of maintaining oral health throughout the treatment phase for the following reasons. a. Ensuring sufficient hydration and nutrition. b. Decreasing the occurrence, severity, and duration of oral mucositis. c. Preventing or minimizing the impact of oral complications. • It is recommended that a dental examination and any necessary interventions be carried out by a dentist or an oral oncology specialist prior to initiating radiation or chemotherapy • Emphasize and provide resources for smoking cessation.
Oral hygiene	• Floss at least once daily. • Brush 2–4 times daily within 30 minutes of eating and for at least 2 minutes with a small, extra soft nylon bristled manual toothbrush. • Use nonabrasive, fluoride toothpaste with a neutral taste. • Rinse toothbrush well with hot water after each use, allow to air dry. • Replace toothbrush when bristles are no longer standing up straight. • If unable to brush, clean teeth with clean, moist gauze or foam swab accompanied with vigorous rinsing using recommended oral rinse solution or use lollipop cleaning sponge. • If there has been an oral infection, use a new toothbrush after infection has resolved. • Patients should be assessed for the use of daily fluoride tray. • Use oral rinses to keep your mouth moist and clean. • After brushing, rinse mouth with the below recopies for minimum of four times daily or after each brushing. • Recipe #1: Normal saline (NS)—1/2 teaspoon (2.5 ml) of salt in 8 oz. (240 ml) of water • Recipe #2: NS/sodium bicarbonate mixture — 1/4 teaspoon (1.25 ml) of salt and 1/4 teaspoon (1.25 ml) baking soda in 8 oz. (240 ml) of water • Recipe #3: Sodium bicarbonate—1/4 to 1/2 teaspoon (1.25–2.5 ml) baking soda in 8 oz. (240 ml) of water • Multi-agent rinses—"Magic Mouthwash" (may include a topical analgesic, a steroid, an antifungal agent, an antibacterial agent and/ or a mucosal coating agent) may be prescribed to help palliate pain, discuss with your dentist or health care provider. • Benzydamine Hydrochloride 0.15% (Tantum®) is an anti-inflammatory mouth rinse that is recommended for use to prevent and/or relieve the pain and inflammation associated with oral mucositis. • Increase frequency as needed for symptom severity increases. • AVOID using commercial mouthwashes, which contain alcohol as well as povidone-iodine, hydrogen peroxide, sucralfate, or lemon glycerin swabs.
Lip care	• Use water-soluble, lanolin, or oil-based lubricants to protect the lips and keep moist. • Use after oral care, at bedtime, or as often as required. NOTE: Oil-based lubricants (e.g., petroleum jelly) are generally not recommended due to increased risk of aspiration and occlusive nature may increase the growth of pathogens.

Dentures	• All dentures, plates, and/or prostheses should be removed before oral hygiene is performed. • Brush and rinse dentures after every meal and at bedtime. • Soak dentures in oral rinse solution, rinse before placing in mouth. • Avoid wearing tight- or loose-fitting dentures. • Give your oral cavity enough resting time without wearing dentures, at least 8 hours daily (e.g., overnight). • Ear the denture only during mealtime if mouth sensitive or in case of pain or oral mucositis.
Cryotherapy	• Patients should be instructed to hold ice chips in mouth five minutes prior, during, and for 30 minutes after the chemotherapy, such as bolus infusion of fluorouracil (5FU) to reduce the risk and severity of oral mucositis. • It is contraindicated if regimens includes oxaliplatin due to potential exacerbation of cold-induced. Pharyngolaryngeal dysesthesia
Dietary management	• Recommendation 1. Daily fluid intake of 8–12 cups (2–3 liters), unless contraindicated, to help keep oral mucosa moist (e.g., water, sugar-free popsicles, nonacidic juices, ice cubes, sports drinks, and broth). 2. Well-balanced diet high in protein, vitamins B and C. 3. The use of soft, moist, and bland foods as symptoms develop or progress. 4. Add nonacidic sauces, gravy, salad dressings, butter/margarine, broth, or another liquid to help moisten and thin foods. • Avoid 1. Dry or coarse foods (e.g., toast, crackers, and chips). 2. Spicy or hot temperature foods. 3. Highly acidic fluids and foods (e.g., lemon glycerin swabs, vitamin C lozenges). 4. Fluid or foods high in sugar (e.g., pop, some fruit juices). 5. Caffeine, alcohol, and tobacco.
Patient education and follow-up	It is important to discuss oral care and hygiene recommendations with the patient and their family. This includes explaining how to perform a daily oral assessment at home. It is crucial to provide both verbal and written information on how to maintain oral hygiene during the treatment. Additionally, it is essential to provide contact information and emphasize to the patient and their family when to seek immediate medical attention in case of certain emergent conditions, such as: • Fever with a temperature equal to or greater than 38°C, presence of white patches, redness, or foul odor, which may indicate a possible infection. • Difficulty breathing, which could be a sign of respiratory distress. • Bleeding that lasts longer than 2 minutes, which may indicate thrombocytopenia. • Inability to eat or drink fluids for more than 24 hours, putting the patient at risk of dehydration. • Difficulty swallowing, which reflects the severity of symptoms. • Uncontrolled pain, indicating a deteriorating patient status and severity of symptoms. Furthermore, it is important to instruct the patient and their family to reach out if mucositis worsens, does not improve, or if any other complications develop.

Table 2.
General recommendation for prevention and treatment of oral mucositis in palliative care patients.

Fungal	Oral candidiasis	• The goal is to reestablish a normal balance of oral flora and improve oral hygiene. • The disinfection of all removable oral prostheses with antifungal denture-soaking solutions and the application of antifungal agents on the tissue-contacting surfaces is necessary to remove a potential source of fungal reinfection.
	Topical antifungal agents Note: Creams and ointments are ideal for treating patients wearing complete or partial dentures	• Clotrimazole (Mycelex) troches 10 mg. • Mycostatin pastilles 200,000 U. • Nystatin vaginal suppositories 100,000 U. • Nystatin ointment. • Ketoconazole (Nizoral) cream 2%. • Clotrimazole (Gyne-Lotrimin, Mycelex-G vaginal cream 1% [OTC]). • Miconazole (Monistat 7) nitrate vaginal cream 2% (OTC). • Nystatin (Mycostatin, Nilstat) oral suspension 100,000 U/mL.
	Systemic antifungal agents	• Fluconazole (Diflucan) tablets 100 mg. • Note: It should be used with caution in patients with impaired liver function (a history of alcoholism or hepatitis).
	Angular cheilitis and cheilosis	• Nystatin-triamcinolone acetonide (Mycolog II, Mytrex) ointment. • Polymyxin B/Bacitracin (Polysporin) ointment (OTC). • Clotrimazole-betamethasone dipropionate (Lotrisone) cream • Hydrocortisone-iodoquinol (Vytone) cream 1%. • Ketoconazole (Nizoral) cream 2%. • Clotrimazole (Gyne-Lotrimin, Mycelex-G) vaginal cream 1% (OTC). • Miconazole (Monistat 7) nitrate vaginal cream 2% (OTC).
Viral	HSV	• Reactivation of herpes virus might cause intraoral or extraoral lesions. • The current recommendation from the food and drug Administration is using systemic acyclovir to treat oral herpes only for immunocompromised patients. • Valacyclovir has been approved for the prevention and management of oral recurrent herpes simplex infections.
	Varicella zoster (Shingles):	• Precipitating factors include thermal, inflammatory, radiologic, and mechanical trauma, stress, as well as immunosuppression, promptly initiate antiviral therapy to reduce the duration and symptoms of the lesions. Patients over 60 years of age are particularly prone to postherpetic neuralgia (PHN).
	Topical antiviral agents	• Penciclovir (Denavir) cream 1%. • Docosanol (Abreva) cream (OTC).Acyclovir and hydrocortisone cream (Xerese).
	Systemic antiviral agents	• Valacyclovir (Valtrex) caplets 500 mg. • Acyclovir (Zovirax) capsules 800 mg.

Table 3.
Management of oral infections in patients on palliative care.

medicine, and pain specialists, to develop individualized pain management strategies. This may involve a combination of medications, physical therapy, heat or cold therapy, and relaxation techniques [22].

2. Oral health assessment: It is crucial to assess the patient's oral health status regularly. Dental professionals can examine the jaw joint, teeth, and surrounding tissues to identify any oral issues contributing to TMD symptoms. They may also provide recommendations for dental appliances, such as splints or mouthguards to alleviate jaw pressure and facilitate proper jaw alignment [23].

3. Patient education: Palliative care teams and dental professionals play a vital role in educating patients and their caregivers about TMD. They can explain the condition, its causes, and potential triggers to help patients understand and manage their symptoms effectively. Patient education may include guidance on stress reduction techniques, relaxation exercises, and lifestyle modifications to minimize TMD-related discomfort [24].

4. Nutritional support: TMD can affect a patient's ability to eat and speak, potentially impacting their nutrition and overall well-being. Palliative care teams collaborate with dieticians or nutritionists to ensure patients receive adequate nutrition while considering their specific TMD-related limitations. Soft food options or modifications to food textures may be recommended to accommodate their needs [25].

5. Emotional support: Palliative care recognizes the importance of addressing patients' emotional and psychological well-being. Living with a life-limiting illness and experiencing chronic pain can be emotionally challenging. Supportive services, such as counseling, support groups, or complementary therapies, such as music or art therapy, can help patients cope with the emotional impact of TMD and the overall palliative care journey [26].

6. Collaborative care: Palliative care involves a multidisciplinary approach, where different healthcare professionals work together to provide comprehensive support. In the case of TMD, this may involve collaboration between palliative care specialists, dentists, oral surgeons, physical therapists, and pain management experts. Regular communication and coordination among the care team ensure that all aspects of the patient's care, including TMD management, are addressed effectively.

It is important to note that the management of TMD in palliative care patients should be individualized and consider the patient's specific condition, overall health status, and personal goals of care. Open communication and collaboration among the patient, their caregivers, and the healthcare team are essential for providing optimal palliative care and addressing the challenges posed by TMD.

2.4 Xerostomia

Saliva plays a crucial role in various oral functions, including taste perception, swallowing, and speech. It also acts as a protective mechanism against infection and tooth decay by effectively cleansing the teeth and gums and maintaining an optimal oral pH level. However, patients with cancer particularly head and neck cancer (HNC) who undergo cytotoxic chemotherapy and radiotherapy often experience persistent dry mouth or xerostomia due to reduced saliva production (hyposalivation). This reduction is a result of radiation-induced damage to the salivary glands or effects of chemotherapy [27, 28]. It is worth noting that a significant proportion of patients (up to 64%) who undergo conventional radiotherapy continue to suffer from moderate to severe permanent xerostomia, with some cases persisting for as long as 22 years after treatment. Xerostomia manifests with symptoms such as thick and stringy saliva, increased thirst, changes in taste perception, difficulties in swallowing or speaking, a sore or burning sensation, and the occurrence of cuts or cracks in the lips or corners of the mouth. Additionally, changes in the texture of the tongue's surface may also be observed [27, 29, 30]. The alterations in salivary composition, characterized by increased viscosity and lower pH levels, can have a detrimental impact on oral health. They can lead to a reduction in tooth remineralization, increased tooth sensitivity, and an elevated risk of dental caries. Moreover, these changes can also contribute to the development of candidiasis and lead to psychological complications associated with challenges in nutrition and social interaction [31, 32]. Therefore, the compromised saliva quality associated with xerostomia further contributes to the oral health challenges faced by patients.

2.4.1 Prevention & treatment

The management of hyposalivation involves a comprehensive approach that assesses saliva production and employs various treatment strategies to stimulate residual salivary function. One effective approach is to stimulate chewing and taste, along with the use of systemic sialagogues such as pilocarpine (Salagen), cevimeline (Evoxac), or bethanechol (Urecholine). These systemic sialagogues have demonstrated their potential in enhancing saliva production from functioning salivary glands. However, it is important to acknowledge that when acinar of the salivary glands is destroyed, the medical approach is ineffective [27, 28, 31]. To alleviate the symptoms associated with hyposalivation, patients should be advised to adopt certain practices. These include regularly sipping water, chewing sugar-free gum or candies, and avoiding substances such as caffeine, tobacco, alcohol, and hard or dry foods. Increasing fluid intake is also crucial to prevent dehydration [30]. Creams and ointments containing wax or lanolin have demonstrated effectiveness in moisturizing and safeguarding the lips. However, it is advisable to avoid products based on petrolatum [33]. Additionally, maintaining a cool and moist mouth can be achieved by using sugar-free popsicles, plain ice cubes, or ice water. It is important to note that individuals with teeth should avoid consuming foods high in acidity as this can further irritate oral tissues and contribute to tooth demineralization [27, 28]. In conjunction with these self-care measures, promoting regular oral hygiene practices and scheduling frequent dental visits are essential. Fluoride toothpaste or rinse and remineralization supplementation should also be considered to counteract the effects of insufficient saliva. For patients experiencing persistent hyposalivation, additional interventions such as moistening oral surfaces, enhancing saliva substitutes with inorganic substances such as calcium and phosphate, and utilizing antimicrobial mouth rinses have proven to be safe and effective in relieving dry mouth symptoms and reducing the risk of infections [6, 30, 34]. By adopting a comprehensive approach to manage hyposalivation, individuals can significantly improve their oral health and overall well-being (**Table 4**).

2.5 Dental caries

Various factors contribute to an increased risk of dental caries. These include a shift in the oral microflora toward a cariogenic flora, a decrease in the concentration

Management strategies	Description
Saliva substitutes	• Glandosane: A saliva substitute that contains carboxymethylcellulose as a thickening agent. It is designed to provide moistening and lubricating properties to alleviate xerostomia symptoms. • Orthana: A saliva substitute that incorporates natural mucins, specifically porcine gastric mucin and bovine submandibular mucin. These natural mucins aim to replicate the viscoelastic properties of human saliva, providing enhanced moistening and lubrication for xerostomia patients. • Xialine: A saliva substitute based on the natural biopolymer xanthan gum. It can Improve speech and sense perception.
Systemic sialogogues	• pilocarpine (Salagen) 5 mg: 3–6 tabs daily. Note: Contradiction with asthma, glaucoma, and liver dysfunction. • Cevimeline (Evoxac) 30 mg: 1 table 3 times daily Note: Contradiction with asthma, glaucoma, liver dysfunction, and cardiovascular disease. • Bethanechol (Urecholine) 25 mg: 1 table 3 times daily. Note: Contradiction with asthma, peptic ulcer, and bladder inflammation.
Mouthwash	• Home-made mouthwashes: Saline solution (0.9% NaCl), bicarbonate solution. • Commercial mouthwashes: Biotène, oral balance, and Zendium. They contain antimicrobial proteins, have a gentle flavor, and are free from detergents, such as sodium lauryl sulfate (SLS).
Oral hygiene	• Emphasize meticulous oral hygiene practices, including regular brushing and flossing, to prevent oral infections. • Provide proper education on denture cleaning for denture patients, particularly emphasizing the importance of removing the appliance before going to sleep.
Dietary modifications	• Maintain regular water intake, chew sugar-free gum, consume sugar-free candy, avoid caffeine, tobacco, alcohol, and hard, dry, spicy, or acidic foods, and increase their fluid intake.
Moisture retention	• Suggest the application of creams and ointments containing wax or lanolin for moisturizing and protecting the lips. Caution against using products based on petrolatum due to an increased risk of aspiration and the potential for promoting pathogen growth due to their occlusive nature.
Humidifiers	• Recommend the use of humidifiers in the bedroom or throughout the home to increase moisture in the air.

Table 4.
Management of xerostomia associated with head and neck radiotherapy in palliative care patients.

of salivary antimicrobial proteins, and the loss of mineralizing components. In the case of conventional radiotherapy, significant changes occur in the oral microflora, leading to dominance of acidogenic bacteria, notably Streptococcus mutans and Lactobacilli [27, 34]. Unlike typical caries, radiation-associated caries can progress rapidly, and become evident as early as 3 months after treatment completion. They tend to affect nontraditional tooth surfaces, such as cusp tips and cavities at the gum line. Furthermore, radiation-associated caries have a higher recurrence rate and pose an increased risk of treatment failure, often requiring additional dental procedures. This condition can cause pain, infections, and functional impairments within the oral cavity. Additionally, the extraction of affected teeth after radiation therapy increases the risk of osteoradionecrosis (ORN), which is a complex complication that often requires extensive surgical intervention [34, 35].

2.5.1 Prevention & treatment

Radiation caries, a common complication of radiotherapy, can be prevented through proactive oral health management strategies. To address this issue, it is recommended that patients undergoing or planning to undergo radiotherapy or chemotherapy adopt a comprehensive approach to oral care. This involves thorough dental examinations, diagnoses, and necessary treatments, such as restorations and extractions, prior to starting cancer treatment. Additionally, scheduling regular dental check-ups is crucial for early detection of demineralization and carious lesions, enabling timely intervention [35]. To prevent severe dental demineralization and cavities, it is advised to apply 1.1% neutral sodium fluoride gel daily for at least 5 minutes. Ideally, a custom-fitted vinyl tray should be made for this purpose, starting from the first day of radiation therapy and continuing throughout the period of reduced salivary flow and dry mouth. In cases where fluoride trays are not feasible or preferred, high-potency fluoride brush-on gels and dentifrices can serve as suitable alternatives [28, 34]. For patients exhibiting signs of tooth demineralization and reduced saliva production, the use of remineralizing products containing calcium and phosphate is essential. These products provide the necessary building blocks for teeth and should be used in conjunction with topical fluoride treatments [35]. In addition to these preventive measures, dietary guidance and oral hygiene counseling play a crucial role in managing patients undergoing cancer therapy particularly radiotherapy for head and neck cancer. By implementing the proactive dental management plan outlined above and focusing on preserving salivary function and stimulating residual gland function, it is possible to enhance caries control and achieve improved overall oral health outcomes. Regular follow-up appointments and adherence to these recommendations will contribute to the success of the oral health management plan [32, 34].

2.6 Periodontitis

Periodontitis, a chronic disease characterized by the loss of tooth-supporting tissue, presents significant risks for patients with head and neck cancer (HNC) or patients on bone remodeling medications such as bisphosphonate or denosumab as part of their cancer treatment, including the development of osteoradionecrosis (ORN) and other complications. Cancer patients undergoing radiation therapy particularly to the head and neck area are more susceptible to periodontal disease due to factors such as hyposalivation, changes in the bone turnover, osteoporosis, and alterations in the oral microbiome. Research has shown substantial loss of periodontal attachment and gingival recession following radiation therapy. The severity of these effects depends on the location and radiation dose as well as type of the chemotherapy, and preexisting periodontal disease can worsen with cancer treatment. This is concerning because periodontal disease has been linked to an increased risk of ORN and oral mucositis. Accurate diagnosis and effectively management of periodontitis in cancer patients are crucial to mitigate its adverse impact on oral health and treatment outcomes as well as patient general well-being [28, 34–36].

2.6.1 Prevention & treatment

Comprehensive dental examination and treatment are crucial before, during, and after cancer therapy, with a specific focus on periodontal disease. Prior to cancer treatment, a thorough evaluation of oral health, including clinical and radiographic assessments should be done to address any preexisting conditions. Patients should be educated about oral hygiene, nutrition, and the risks associated with smoking and alcohol consumption. They should also receive instructions on effective oral care techniques. Treatment for periodontal diseases prior to cancer therapy may involve scaling, root planning, extractions, and antimicrobial therapy. It is important to schedule tooth extractions at least 14 days before cancer treatment to prevent osteoradionecrosis or delayed wound healing. During cancer therapy or palliative care, emphasize should be placed on oral hygiene and preventive measures such as using chlorhexidine and fluoride mouthwashes. Urgent dental procedures can be performed based on blood counts and patient overall health and minimize long-term complications Mechanical plaque control and chemical plaque control through mouthwashes are essential. Conservative approaches are recommended for periodontal care, and tooth extractions should be carefully planned. In certain cases, Periodontal surgery may be considered as an alternative to extraction, with decisions made in consultation with the medical team [35, 36].

2.7 Apical lesions

The high prevalence and rapid development of caries following radiotherapy based on the region suggest increased pulpal involvement in the caries process and the subsequent bacterial intrusion into the pulpal space. Moreover, radiation-exposed pulp experiences a decrease in cellularity, rendering it more susceptible to necrosis triggered by uncontrolled caries. Consequently, an increase in the occurrence of apical periodontitis is expected among patients who have undergone radiation therapy [6, 36]. In a study, apical periodontitis was observed in 7.8% of teeth among patients who received radiation therapy in the head and neck area [37].

2.7.1 Prevention & treatment

A comprehensive radiographic assessment is essential in conjunction with clinical evaluation to identify periapical abnormalities, assess periodontal health, detect dental conditions, and determine tumor invasion in the bone. Prior to cancer treatment, dental assessments should encompass panoramic radiographs in addition to selective periapical or bitewing films to ensure a thorough evaluation [27, 34]. Focal infections, such as periapical or periodontal pathologies, and mucosal trauma from ill-fitting dentures, significantly increase the risk of osteonecrosis in individuals who have undergone cancer therapy. Therefore, an interdisciplinary approach involving a comprehensive dental examination before cancer therapy, coupled with ongoing monitoring during the palliative care by a specialized dental team, is crucial. It is important to pay close attention to the periodontal condition throughout and after cancer therapy while strictly adhering to mechanical oral hygiene practices. Maintaining optimal oral and periodontal hygiene, including personalized fluoride carriers, is essential for long-term care due to the compromised healing ability of the periodontium following cancer therapy [34].

2.8 Jaw osteonecrosis

Osteonecrosis of the jaw (ONJ) is a debilitating condition and can develop after radiation therapy to the head and neck (osteoradionecrosis) or after treatment with antiresorptive therapies, or rarely antiangiogenic targeted therapies called medication-related osteonecrosis of the jaw or (MRONJ); Osteoradionecrosis results from radiation-induced changes due to hypocellularity, hypovascularity, and ischemia in the jaws. MRONJ results from an imbalance in bone homeostasis due to osteoclast inhibition. Osteonecrosis of the jaw is defined as the presence of exposed dental bone for longer than 8 weeks, which can be probed through an intraoral or extraoral fistula. While dental surgery, including tooth extraction, in setting of chronic dental infections for example periodontal disorders, or following any trauma such as trauma from ill-fitting denture, are common trigger for ONJ, this condition can also develop spontaneously. Secondary soft tissue infection is a prevalent occurrence and represents the leading cause of symptoms in this context. In more severe cases, advanced infection can result in the formation of an extraoral fistula. Additionally, symptoms may arise due to the compression of the inferior alveolar nerve or as a consequence of pathologic fractures.

The risk of developing these complications is particularly high in posterior mandibular areas. Moreover, patients who have received radiation doses exceeding 6500 cGy to the jaw, individuals with higher cumulative doses of antiresorptive therapy, smokers, and those who have undergone traumatic procedures, such as extractions with the use of local anesthetics containing epinephrine are also at an increased risk [38].

2.8.1 Prevention & treatment

The prevention of osteonecrosis of the jaw (ONJ) is a crucial concept that highlights the importance of dental stabilization before cancer therapy and maintaining good oral and dental health in survivors. Therefore, it is vital for palliative care patient who are scheduled to receive bone-modifying agents or radiation to head and neck area to undergo a comprehensive oral care assessment and necessary dental procedures before starting these medications. It is recommended to avoid elective invasive dental procedures that involve manipulation of the alveolar bone in patients using these medications or have history of head and neck radiation.

Protocols to reduce the risk of jaw osteonecrosis include selecting endodontic therapy over extraction, employing an atraumatic surgical technique if surgery is necessary. Additionally, prophylactic antibiotics should be initiated on the day of surgery and continued during the week of healing, typically penicillin VK for 7 days. While there is limited evidence supporting the use of local anesthetic without epinephrine or hyperbaric oxygen therapy as preventive measures for patients at risk of osteoradionecrosis (ORN), these approaches may be considered. It is important to note that hyperbaric oxygen therapy involves daily "dives" in a chamber under two atmospheres of oxygen pressure and carries certain risks such as middle ear injury, myopia, and seizures. When jaw osteonecrosis does occur, conservative management is generally effective in controlling symptoms and stabilizing the condition [39, 40].

To promote healing, it is important to brush the exposed bone thoroughly, and patients should rinse their mouths with chlorhexidine twice a day. If there is a bony sequestrum present, it should be removed to facilitate epithelialization. Debridement procedures can help reduce the risk of secondary infection and improve symptoms. In cases, where there is swelling and suppuration, broad-spectrum antibiotics are recommended.

Pathologic fractures should be managed by a surgeon, although not all fractures require surgery. If conservative measures fail to produce the desired outcome, surgical resection of the affected bone may be necessary. In the specific management of ORN, there is limited evidence supporting the use of hyperbaric oxygen treatment, involving 60- to 90-minute dives, 5 days per week, for a total of 20–30 dives. Additionally, the combination of pentoxifylline and tocopherol has shown some potential in the treatment of ORN [41].

Currently, there is insufficient evidence to support the temporary discontinuation of antiangiogenic or antiresorptive drugs (drug holiday) before dentoalveolar surgery in patients receiving an oncologic dose of these medications. Limited literature suggests that some adjunctive therapies, such as pentoxifylline and alpha-tocopherol (Pent-E) and photobiomodulation (PBM) with or without photodynamic therapy (PDT), have shown promising results in managing MRONJ. However, recent guidelines from the International Association of Oral and Maxillofacial Surgeons (IAOMS), as well as guidelines from the Multinational Association of Supportive Care in Cancer/International Society of Oral Oncology (MASCC/ISOO) and the American Society of Clinical Oncology (ASCO), only recommend topical antimicrobial rinses, antibiotics, effective oral hygiene, and surgical interventions [39, 42]. Insufficient evidence exists to support the discontinuation of antiangiogenic or antiresorptive drugs after the diagnosis of MRONJ.

2.9 Neuropathic pain and chemosensory changes such as taste change (dysgeusia)

Dysgeusia can refer to an abnormal or impaired sense of taste, where the ability to taste is affected. It can also describe an unpleasant alteration of taste sensation, where tastes may be distorted or altered in an unpleasant way. Additionally, dysgeusia can refer to a distortion or perversion of the sense of taste, where the perception of taste is not accurate or is perceived differently than normal [43].

Dysgeusia is closely linked to changes in olfaction as both taste and smell play a role in producing the sense of flavor. Taste and smell work together to create our perception of flavors, and alterations in either of these senses can affect the overall sensory experience of food or beverages. Therefore, when dysgeusia occurs, it is often accompanied by changes in the sense of smell, leading to a disruption in the overall perception of flavor. Several mechanisms contribute to taste alterations in patients on palliative care particularly cancer patients such as cancer-related inflammation, adverse effects of chemotherapy and other drugs used to treat complications, nutritional status, and the lifestyle habits of the patients. Chemotherapy is associated with dysgeusia through multiple mechanisms, such as damage to taste buds and olfactory receptors, impairment to neurotransmission, and other physical (i.e., xerostomia) or psychological effects [44, 45].

Dysgeusia can become a chronic issue and negatively influence patients' quality of life, worsening their dysphagia and their nutritional status. The management of dysgeusia includes using zinc supplementation, self-care management of dry mouth, and dietary counseling [46].

Patient on palliative care, particularly cancer patients may also experience long-term persistent orofacial neuropathic pain. While symptoms may vary, the most frequently reported experience is a strong burning sensation, particularly aggravated by movement and activity. In rare instances, individuals with a history of severe and extensive ulcerations (such as mucositis), as well as those who have experienced shingles or severe herpes simplex virus reactivation, may develop post-inflammatory dysesthesias. These dysesthesias are typically characterized by a burning feeling, sometimes accompanied by reduced or altered taste perception. Addressing these symptoms poses a challenge, but patients can potentially benefit from the use of topical and systemic anticonvulsant medications [47].

2.10 Bleeding

Almost 6–10% of palliative care patients present with clinically significant bleeding [48]. It has been described that 74% of this population experienced bleeding during their final month of life in the head and neck region including the oral cavity [49].

The risk of oral bleeding is much higher in patient undergo high-dose chemotherapy or with end-stage renal and liver disease or any medications or treatment that affects bone marrow. Gingival bleeding and submucosal hemorrhage may arise due to minor incidents such as tongue biting, toothbrushing, or swallowing, particularly when the platelet count decreases to less than 50,000 (especially below 20,000) cells/mm3. Notable observations in clinical practice involve the presence of palatal petechiae, purpura along the sides of the tongue, and instances of gingival bleeding or seepage. Gingival bleeding can be worsened by inadequate oral hygiene. To address this issue, individuals experiencing easy gingival bleeding should consider using gentler cleaning tools like sponge Toothettes. If gingival bleeding cannot be controlled, certain local approaches can be employed. These may include applying pressure using a gelatin sponge infused with thrombin or microfibrillar collagen on the affected area. Another option is to use gauze soaked in an oral antifibrinolytic solution, such as aminocaproic acid [Amicar] syrup 250 mg/mL. If local measures prove ineffective, platelet transfusion might be necessary.

3. Systemic management of the oral pain

The primary objective of palliative care is to alleviate the suffering and burden of illness experienced by both patients and caregivers during the progression of a chronic condition. This approach aims to minimize the physical, emotional, and psychological distress from the moment of diagnosis until the end of life. A comprehensive palliative care approach recognizes the importance of supporting not only the patient but also their caregivers, treating them as a cohesive unit of care. Moreover, it acknowledges and attends to the grief process before death and during the subsequent bereavement period [50].

To decrease nociceptive pain, opioid analgesics are included in current pharmacologic treatment recommendations [1, 51]. In addition, intrathecal opioid delivery has been shown to provide effective pain relief with reduced adverse effects for chronic persistent/intractable cancer pain [52]. However, opioids are limited in efficacy in the treatment of neuropathic pain, use of anticonvulsant medications, centrally-acting antidepressants, and biopsychosocial treatments are often indicated in cancer patients [2].

Transnasal fentanyl (a rapidly acting opioid) may be used for the treatment of breakthrough pain in patients with head and neck cancer, especially because of increased likelihood of mucosal damage leading to difficulties with the administration of transoral or transmucosal preparations. In addition to baseline systemic analgesics, topical oropharyngeal preparations may be applied [53].

As for the management of mucositis-related pain, a study reviewed use of oral rinses and systemic analgesics that include opioids and introduced investigation of novel use of methylene blue oral rinse in management [54]. A systematic review of topical anesthetics and analgesics for oral mucositis pain in 2020, provided a suggestion for use of morphine 0.2% solution, other agents discussed included topical coating agents, topical anesthetics, and topical doxepin [55]. A randomized trial studied the difference between a single dose of doxepin rinse or diphenhydramine-lidocaine-antacid mouthwash versus placebo for oral mucositis-related pain. Pain reduction was similar for both, more drowsiness was observed with doxepin [56]. Pregabalin and doxepin rinse were found effective for neuropathic pain and pain associated with oral mucositis respectively in HNC patients [57]. Application of photobiomodulation (PBM) has been described for prevention of oral mucositis associated with radiotherapy to the head and neck and has been shown to provide pain reduction and reduced analgesic use during and following cancer therapy [58].

Relief of cancer pain has been reported with tetrahydrocannabinol (THC) and cannabidiol combination [59]. A study found a direct role of cannabinoid receptor agonists in the reduction of mechanical allodynia and discussed potential positive effects upon cancer cell viability, suggesting the potential of antitumor effect [60].

A literature review identified positioning stents during RT for HNC to avoid unwanted radiation to the jaw and salivary glands [61]. Chemical neurolysis was found to provide significant pain relief to patients with refractory cancer-related pain, with minimal risk of manageable adverse effects [62]. Spheno-palantine nerve block with bupivacaine for pain in the maxillary division of the trigeminal nerve and transcutaneous electrical nerve stimulation (TENS) during the last 2 weeks of RT caused a decrease in head and neck cancer-related neuropathic pain scores [63, 64].

4. Conclusions

Patients nearing the end of life often experience a range of oral complications that can significantly impact their quality of life. These complications include pain, dysfunction of the salivary glands, difficulty swallowing (dysphagia), and infections affecting the mouth and mucous membranes. These issues may arise either as a result of treatments administered during the terminal phase or due to the progressive nature of the underlying disease. The oral well-being plays a crucial role in various aspects of our lives, such as effective communication, proper eating, clear speech, and efficient swallowing. Any compromises in this area can significantly impact one's quality of life, potentially leading to functional decline and a failure to thrive. Therefore, it becomes imperative to integrate oral health care as an essential component of palliative care. The primary objectives of such care include preventing oral complications, preserving optimal oral function, and enhancing overall quality of life and comfort. In the context of palliative care, it is recommended to uphold regular oral hygiene practices whenever feasible. Additionally, addressing the need for treating dental issues such as decay, fractures, or missing teeth should be considered if it aligns with the patient's desires and is in accordance with their care objectives.

The overall concerns include:

- Difficulties in eating can result in reduced food consumption, inadequate nutrition, weight loss, and changes in facial structure.
- Speech and communication challenges can cause significant stress and frustration for both patients and their caregivers/families.
- Patients' concerns about their facial and oral appearance may stem from their desire for dignity and respect at the end of life.
- Neglecting regular oral hygiene practices toward the end of life can contribute to problems such as gingivitis, periodontitis, tooth decay, tooth loss, and bad breath. These issues can impact self-esteem, and loved ones may avoid close contact due to halitosis, exacerbating the patient's feelings of isolation and depression.
- Decayed, broken, or missing teeth can impair chewing abilities and increase the risk of oral tissue injuries, leading to further disability.
- Dysfunction of salivary glands, primarily not only resulting in dry mouth (xerostomia) but also affecting taste (dysgeusia), can affect appetite, formation of food boluses, swallowing, and speech and communication.
- Oral pain and poorly fitting dentures can hinder oral intake and further limit a patient's ability to communicate, especially in cases where cachexia is associated with a terminal illness.

Maintaining optimal oral hygiene plays a crucial role in reducing the risk of various oral health issues such as gingivitis, periodontitis, oral infections, and caries. To ensure proper oral hygiene, the following practices should be performed at least twice a day:

1. Brushing: Utilize a soft-bristled toothbrush along with either an over-the-counter fluoride toothpaste or a prescription-strength fluoride toothpaste containing 1.1% sodium fluoride. Begin by placing the brush at the gum line and using a circular motion to cover all tooth surfaces. Patients with limited mobility, coordination, or dexterity may find electric toothbrushes more effective.

2. Rinsing: Thoroughly rinse your mouth with water or an alcohol-free mouthwash. This helps reduce bacterial load and improves halitosis (bad breath).

3. Denture care: If you wear dentures, remove them and meticulously brush them with a denture brush and warm water. In the case of candidiasis (oral fungal infection), dentures may require soaking in a prescribed solution.

4. Lip care: To address dry or chapped lips, consider using over-the-counter lip care moisturizers such as lanolin, oral balance, unflavored Chapstick, or cocoa butter.

5. Alternative options: For individuals who cannot rinse or spit due to physical limitations or swallowing difficulties, gently swab the mouth and teeth twice daily with a sponge Toothette soaked in alcohol-free 0.12% chlorhexidine gluconate.

6. High caries risk: Individuals with increased caries risk, particularly due to functional or cognitive impairment, may benefit from additional measures. These include applying fluoride gels (1.1% sodium fluoride gel) with a brush daily, using topical fluoride varnish (5% sodium fluoride varnish, 0.4 mL dose) at 3-month intervals, or applying silver diamine fluoride (38% silver diamine fluoride) at 3-month intervals.

By incorporating these practices into your daily routine, you can maintain excellent oral hygiene and reduce the likelihood of oral health problems.

Conflict of interest

The authors declare no conflict of interest.

Author details

Firoozeh Samim[1*], Ali Abdolrahmani[2], Elahe Akbari[1] and Aia Naksho[2]

1 Faculty of Dental Medicine and Oral Health, McGill University, Montreal, QC, Canada

2 Oral Medicine and Oral Pathology Clinic, Montreal General Hospital, Montreal, QC, Canada

*Address all correspondence to: firoozeh.samim@mcgill.ca

References

[1] Bossi P, Giusti R, Tarsitano A, Airoldi M, De Sanctis V, Caspiani O, et al. The point of pain in head and neck cancer. Critical Reviews in Oncology/ Hematology. 2019;**138**:51-59

[2] Epstein JB, Elad S, Eliav E, Jurevic R, Benoliel R. Orofacial pain in cancer: Part II--Clinical perspectives and management. Journal of Dental Research. 2007;**86**(6):506-518

[3] Singh V, Singh AK. Oral mucositis. National Journal of Maxillofacial Surgery. 2020;**11**(2):159-168

[4] Nash AA, Dalziel RG, Fitzgerald JR. Mechanisms of cell and tissue damage. Mims' Pathogenesis of Infectious Disease. 2015;**2015**:171-231

[5] Naidu MU, Ramana GV, Rani PU, Mohan IK, Suman A, Roy P. Chemotherapy-induced and/or radiation therapy-induced oral mucositis--complicating the treatment of cancer. Neoplasia. 2004;**6**(5):423-431

[6] Samim F, Epstein JB, Zumsteg ZS, Ho AS, Barasch A. Oral and dental health in head and neck cancer survivors. Cancers Head Neck. 2016;**1**:14

[7] Sonis S, Haddad R, Posner M, Watkins B, Fey E, Morgan TV, et al. Gene expression changes in peripheral blood cells provide insight into the biological mechanisms associated with regimen-related toxicities in patients being treated for head and neck cancers. Oral Oncology. 2007;**43**(3):289-300

[8] Boers-Doets CB, Epstein JB, Raber-Durlacher JE, Ouwerkerk J, Logan RM, Brakenhoff JA, et al. Oral adverse events associated with tyrosine kinase and mammalian target of rapamycin inhibitors in renal cell carcinoma: A structured literature review. The Oncologist. 2012;**17**(1):135-144

[9] Watters AL, Epstein JB, Agulnik M. Oral complications of targeted cancer therapies: A narrative literature review. Oral Oncology. 2011;**47**(6):441-448

[10] Wu YL, Cheng Y, Zhou X, Lee KH, Nakagawa K, Niho S, et al. Dacomitinib versus gefitinib as first-line treatment for patients with EGFR-mutation-positive non-small-cell lung cancer (ARCHER 1050): A randomised, open-label, phase 3 trial. The Lancet Oncology. 2017;**18**(11):1454-1466

[11] Kwitkowski VE, Prowell TM, Ibrahim A, Farrell AT, Justice R, Mitchell SS, et al. FDA approval summary: Temsirolimus as treatment for advanced renal cell carcinoma. The Oncologist. 2010;**15**(4):428-435

[12] Shazib MA, Woo SB, Sroussi H, Carvo I, Treister N, Farag A, et al. Oral immune-related adverse events associated with PD-1 inhibitor therapy: A case series. Oral Diseases. 2020;**26**(2):325-333

[13] Jacob JS, Dutra BE, Garcia-Rodriguez V, Panneerselvam K, Abraham FO, Zou F, et al. Clinical characteristics and outcomes of oral mucositis associated with immune checkpoint inhibitors in patients with cancer. Journal of the National Comprehensive Cancer Network. 2021;**19**(12):1415-1424

[14] Barasch A, Peterson DE. Risk factors for ulcerative oral mucositis in cancer patients: Unanswered questions. Oral Oncology. 2003;**39**(2):91-100

[15] Bowen J, Al-Dasooqi N, Bossi P, Wardill H, Van Sebille Y, Al-Azri A, et al. The pathogenesis of mucositis: Updated perspectives and emerging targets. Supportive Care in Cancer. 2019;**27**(10):4023-4033

[16] Mougeot JC, Stevens CB, Morton DS, Brennan MT, Mougeot FB. Oral microbiome and cancer therapy-induced oral mucositis. Journal of the National Cancer Institute. Monographs. 2019;**2019**(53):lgz002

[17] Pratesi N, Mangoni M, Mancini I, Paiar F, Simi L, Livi L, et al. Association between single nucleotide polymorphisms in the XRCC1 and RAD51 genes and clinical radiosensitivity in head and neck cancer. Radiotherapy and Oncology. 2011;**99**(3):356-361

[18] Chitapanarux I, Wongsrita S, Sripan P, Kongsupapsiri P, Phakoetsuk P, Chachvarat S, et al. An underestimated pitfall of oral candidiasis in head and neck cancer patients undergoing radiotherapy: An observation study. BMC Oral Health. 2021;**21**(1):353

[19] Tayyar R, Ho D. Herpes simplex virus and varicella zoster virus infections in cancer patients. Viruses. 2023;**15**(2):439

[20] Garcia-Cuesta C, Sarrion-Pérez MG, Bagán JV. Current treatment of oral candidiasis: A literature review. Journal of Clinical and Experimental Dentistry. 2014;**6**(5):e576-e582

[21] Pauli N, Mejersjö C, Fagerberg-Mohlin B, Finizia C. Temporomandibular disorder in head and neck cancer patients undergoing radiotherapy: Clinical findings and patient-reported symptoms. Head & Neck. 2019;**41**(10):3570-3576

[22] Butts R, Dunning J, Pavkovich R, Mettille J, Mourad F. Conservative management of temporomandibular dysfunction: A literature review with implications for clinical practice guidelines (narrative review part 2). Journal of Bodywork and Movement Therapies. 2017;**21**(3):541-548

[23] Shaffer SM, Brismée JM, Sizer PS, Courtney CA. Temporomandibular disorders. Part 1: Anatomy and examination/diagnosis. The Journal of Manual & Manipulative Therapy. 2014;**22**(1):2-12

[24] Gauer RL, Semidey MJ. Diagnosis and treatment of temporomandibular disorders. American Family Physician. 2015;**91**(6):378-386

[25] Nasri-Heir C, Epstein JB, Touger-Decker R, Benoliel R. What should we tell patients with painful temporomandibular disorders about what to eat? Journal of the American Dental Association (1939). 2016;**147**(8):667-671

[26] Penlington C, Bowes C, Taylor G, Otemade AA, Waterhouse P, Durham J, et al. Psychological therapies for temporomandibular disorders (TMDs). Cochrane Database of Systematic Reviews. 2022;**8**(8):Cd013515

[27] Devi S, Singh N. Dental care during and after radiotherapy in head and neck cancer. National Journal of Maxillofacial Surgery. 2014;**5**(2):117-125

[28] Hancock PJ, Epstein JB, Sadler GR. Oral and dental management related to radiation therapy for head and neck cancer. Journal of the Canadian Dental Association. 2003;**69**(9):585-590

[29] Riantiningtyas RR, Carrouel F, Bruyas A, Bredie WLP, Kwiecien C, Giboreau A, et al. Oral somatosensory alterations in head and neck cancer

patients—An overview of the evidence and causes. Cancers (Basel). 2023;**15**(3):718

[30] Arya L, Brizuela M. Oral Management of Patients Undergoing Radiation Therapy. StatPearls, Treasure Island (FL): StatPearls Publishing Copyright © 2023, StatPearls Publishing LLC; 2023

[31] Epstein JB, Thariat J, Bensadoun RJ, Barasch A, Murphy BA, Kolnick L, et al. Oral complications of cancer and cancer therapy: From cancer treatment to survivorship. CA: A Cancer Journal for Clinicians. 2012;**62**(6):400-422

[32] Buglione M, Cavagnini R, Di Rosario F, Maddalo M, Vassalli L, Grisanti S, et al. Oral toxicity management in head and neck cancer patients treated with chemotherapy and radiation: Xerostomia and trismus (part 2). Literature review and consensus statement. Critical Reviews in Oncology/Hematology. 2016;**102**:47-54

[33] Santos PS, Tinôco-Araújo JE, Souza LM, Ferreira R, Ikoma MR, Razera AP, et al. Efficacy of HPA Lanolin® in treatment of lip alterations related to chemotherapy. Journal of Applied Oral Science. 2013;**21**(2):163-166

[34] Kielbassa AM, Hinkelbein W, Hellwig E, Meyer-Lückel H. Radiation-related damage to dentition. The Lancet Oncology. 2006;7(4):326-335

[35] Sroussi HY, Epstein JB, Bensadoun RJ, Saunders DP, Lalla RV, Migliorati CA, et al. Common oral complications of head and neck cancer radiation therapy: Mucositis, infections, saliva change, fibrosis, sensory dysfunctions, dental caries, periodontal disease, and osteoradionecrosis. Cancer Medicine. 2017;**6**(12):2918-2931

[36] Irie MS, Mendes EM, Borges JS, Osuna LG, Rabelo GD, Soares PB. Periodontal therapy for patients before and after radiotherapy: A review of the literature and topics of interest for clinicians. Medicina Oral, Patología Oral y Cirugía Bucal. 2018;**23**(5):e524-ee30

[37] Hommez GM, De Meerleer GO, De Neve WJ, De Moor RJ. Effect of radiation dose on the prevalence of apical periodontitis--A dosimetric analysis. Clinical Oral Investigations. 2012;**16**(6):1543-1547

[38] Nadella KR, Kodali RM, Guttikonda LK, Jonnalagadda A. Osteoradionecrosis of the jaws: Clinico-therapeutic management: A literature review and update. Journal of Oral and Maxillofacial Surgery. 2015;**14**(4):891-901

[39] Ruggiero SL, Dodson TB, Aghaloo T, Carlson ER, Ward BB, Kademani D. American Association of Oral and Maxillofacial Surgeons' position paper on medication-related osteonecrosis of the Jaws-2022 update. Journal of Oral and Maxillofacial Surgery. 2022;**80**(5):920-943

[40] Ruggiero SL, Dodson TB, Fantasia J, Goodday R, Aghaloo T, Mehrotra B, et al. American Association of Oral and Maxillofacial Surgeons position paper on medication-related osteonecrosis of the jaw—2014 update. Journal of Oral and Maxillofacial Surgery. 2014;**72**(10):1938-1956

[41] Watanabe T, Asai K, Fukuhara S, Uozumi R, Bessho K. Effectiveness of surgery and hyperbaric oxygen for antiresorptive agent-related osteonecrosis of the jaw: A subgroup analysis by disease stage. PLoS One. 2021;**16**(1):e0244859

[42] Yarom N, Shapiro CL, Peterson DE, Van Poznak CH, Bohlke K, Ruggiero SL,

et al. Medication-related osteonecrosis of the jaw: MASCC/ISOO/ASCO clinical practice guideline. Journal of Clinical Oncology. 2019;**37**(25):2270-2290

[43] Hovan AJ, Williams PM, Stevenson-Moore P, Wahlin YB, Ohrn KE, Elting LS, et al. A systematic review of dysgeusia induced by cancer therapies. Supportive Care in Cancer. 2010;**18**(8):1081-1087

[44] Murtaza B, Hichami A, Khan AS, Ghiringhelli F, Khan NA. Alteration in taste perception in cancer: Causes and strategies of treatment. Frontiers in Physiology. 2017;**8**:134

[45] Kinjo T, Kanda K, Fujimoto K. Effects of a self-monitoring intervention in breast cancer patients suffering from taste alterations induced by chemotherapy: A randomized, parallel-group controlled trial. European Journal of Oncology Nursing. 2021;**52**:101956

[46] Togni L, Mascitti M, Vignigni A, Alia S, Sartini D, Barlattani A, et al. Treatment-related dysgeusia in oral and oropharyngeal cancer: A comprehensive review. Nutrients. 2021;**13**(10):3325

[47] Mendlik MT, Uritsky TJ. Treatment of neuropathic pain. Current Treatment Options in Neurology. 2015;**17**(12):50

[48] Prommer E. Management of bleeding in the terminally ill patient. Hematology. 2005;**10**(3):167-175

[49] Shuman AG, Yang Y, Taylor JM, Prince ME. End-of-life care among head and neck cancer patients. Otolaryngology and Head and Neck Surgery. 2011;**144**(5):733-739

[50] Kelley AS, Morrison RS. Palliative care for the seriously ill. The New England Journal of Medicine. 2015;**373**(8):747-755

[51] McDermott JD, Eguchi M, Stokes WA, Amini A, Hararah M, Ding D, et al. Short- and long-term opioid use in patients with oral and oropharynx cancer. Otolaryngology and Head and Neck Surgery. 2019;**160**(3):409-419

[52] Bruel BM, Burton AW. Intrathecal therapy for cancer-related pain. Pain Medicine. 2016;**17**(12):2404-2421

[53] Mercadante S, Masedu F, Valenti M, Aielli F. Breakthrough pain in patients with head & neck cancer. A secondary analysis of IOPS MS study. Oral Oncology. 2019;**95**:87-90

[54] Roldan CJ, Chai T, Erian J, Welker J. Oral pain associated with cancer therapy, a pain medicine perspective. Pain Management. 2018;**8**(6):487-493

[55] Saunders DP, Rouleau T, Cheng K, Yarom N, Kandwal A, Joy J, et al. Systematic review of antimicrobials, mucosal coating agents, anesthetics, and analgesics for the management of oral mucositis in cancer patients and clinical practice guidelines. Supportive Care in Cancer. 2020;**28**(5):2473-2484

[56] Sio TT, Le-Rademacher JG, Leenstra JL, Loprinzi CL, Rine G, Curtis A, et al. Effect of doxepin mouthwash or diphenhydramine-lidocaine-antacid mouthwash vs placebo on radiotherapy-related oral mucositis pain: The Alliance A221304 randomized clinical trial. Journal of the American Medical Association. 2019;**321**(15):1481-1490

[57] Lefebvre T, Tack L, Lycke M, Duprez F, Goethals L, Rottey S, et al. Effectiveness of adjunctive analgesics in head and neck cancer patients receiving curative (chemo-) radiotherapy: A systematic review. Pain Medicine. 2021;**22**(1):152-164

[58] de Pauli PM, Alves CGB, Fontes EK, Lopes MA, Ribeiro ACP, Brandão TB, et al. Is photobiomodulation therapy effective in reducing pain caused by toxicities related to head and neck cancer treatment? A systematic review. Support Care Cancer. 2019;**27**(11):4043-4054

[59] Bar-Sela G, Avisar A, Batash R, Schaffer M. Is the clinical use of cannabis by oncology patients advisable? Current Medicinal Chemistry. 2014;**21**(17):1923-1930

[60] Saghafi N, Lam DK, Schmidt BL. Cannabinoids attenuate cancer pain and proliferation in a mouse model. Neuroscience Letters. 2011;**488**(3):247-251

[61] Chen D, Chen X, Chen X, Jiang N, Jiang L. The efficacy of positioning stents in preventing oral complications after head and neck radiotherapy: A systematic literature review. Radiation Oncology. 2020;**15**(1):90

[62] Khawaja SN, Scrivani SJ. Utilization of neurolysis in management of refractory head and neck cancer-related pain in palliative patients: A retrospective review. Journal of Oral Pathology & Medicine. 2020;**49**(6):484-489

[63] Pena I, Knoepfler ML, Irwin A, Zhu X, Kohan LR. Sphenopalatine ganglion blocks in the management of head and neck cancer-related pain: A case series. A&A Practice. 2019;**13**(12):450-453

[64] Lee JE, Anderson CM, Perkhounkova Y, Sleeuwenhoek BM, Louison RR. Transcutaneous electrical nerve stimulation reduces resting pain in head and neck cancer patients: A randomized and placebo-controlled double-blind pilot study. Cancer Nursing. 2019;**42**(3):218-228

Section 4

Wellbeing and Spirituality

Chapter 17

Attitudes and Values of Three Monotheistic Religions Regarding Ethical Dilemmas in Palliative Care: Qualitative Study

Rok Mihelič and Erika Zelko

Abstract

Palliative care, aimed at improving the quality of life for individuals with life-limiting illnesses, often raises complex ethical questions. This research explores the viewpoints of monotheistic faiths, namely Christianity, Islam, and Judaism, and on this matter examines how religious beliefs and values impact decision-making in the provision of palliative care, particularly when faced with difficulies. Christianity, for instance, emphasizes the sanctity of life, encouraging compassionate care while respecting patient autonomy. Islam, on the other hand, underscores the importance of relieving suffering and allowing for a natural death while upholding key principles of faith. Judaism places great value on preserving life, but this can be balanced with the consideration of human dignity and quality of life. Understanding the religious perspectives on ethical dilemmas within palliative care is vital for healthcare professionals and policymakers. It enables them to respect patients' religious beliefs while providing appropriate care. By considering these perspectives, it is possible to find common ground and develop guidelines that ensure ethical and culturally sensitive palliative care for a diverse range of patients. This study aims to contribute to the ongoing dialog and cooperation between religious and medical communities in delivering compassionate and ethically sound palliative care.

Keywords: palliative care, ethical dilemmas, monotheistic religions, patients, religious beliefs

1. Introduction

The challenges in our society, armed conflicts, and economic crises require numerous adjustments in an individual's way of life. These changes affect not only society but also the approach to end-of-life care. Efforts to uphold the principle of respecting human life are continuously strengthening, even though we are aware that this fundamental principle is severely threatened in altered circumstances, and its respect is facing a significant test. From a medical perspective, the health crisis of coronavirus disease has increased the importance and urgency of palliative care for patients suffering from incurable diseases, their families, and all involved healthcare workers. This significance of care is most prominently exemplified in the field of intensive care, which deals with the most complex treatment goals: enabling critically ill patients to survive life-threatening conditions, improving current and future health quality, or early efforts to enhance the quality of dying and death [1, 2]. In this context, the global pandemic highlights the advantages and drawbacks of providing quality palliative care while also offering an opportunity to contemplate the capacities and opportunities that quality palliative care demands. Ethical dilemmas arise daily, many of which are related to decisions about continuing, limiting, or discontinuing life-sustaining treatment [3]. The poor prognosis of critical illness, appropriate ongoing care for these patients, and end-of-life care require a comprehensive and multidisciplinary approach [4–6]. A holistic approach in palliative care is essential as it ensures healthcare for the multidimensional needs of patients and their families [7]. Palliative care, therefore, requires a wide range of competencies, not only clinical but also relational, communicative, and ethical [8]. Interdisciplinary clinical collaboration between different professional fields signifies the realization of the standard of the highest quality of end-of-life care [9]. An essential and integral part of this approach is spiritual care. The fields of ethics, spiritual care, and treatment in palliative care often overlap, especially when making decisions about the cessation of treatment and the withdrawal of life-sustaining measures. Therefore, the role of religion and spirituality becomes increasingly important in questions related to the end of life [10–12]. Despite emerging evidence and the status of spiritual care as a central dimension of palliative care, it remains the least developed and most neglected part of care, primarily due to complications in standardizing and conceptualizing religion and spirituality and their definition within the palliative care process [13, 14]. Discussions about the end of life, which involve distinguishing the moral significance between actions and omissions, are raised in various bioethical contexts [15]. Most moral theories believe that allowing a patient to die from an ethical perspective is ethically acceptable in certain cases and fundamentally different from actively ending human life [16, 17]. On the other hand, the concept of the sanctity of life, which represents the foundation of Christian, Jewish, and Islamic ethics, emphasizes the importance of recognizing the moral equivalence between killing and letting die [18]. The intensity of the discussion increases in the context of euthanasia [19–21]. However, most ethical systems take the position that preserving human life is the highest moral duty, so intentionally causing a patient's death cannot be ethically justified in any case [16, 22]. In today's postmodern and secularized era, the use of the word "spirituality" is not always entirely clear, especially because it is increasingly detached from religious traditions and institutions. The relationship between spirituality and religion seems unclear due to the collective nature of religion and the individualized/subjective nature of spirituality [23]. On one hand, spirituality is an overtly religious concept, while on the other, an interest in spirituality may not necessarily arise from religious pursuits. Spirituality touches upon the meaning and purpose of life, which may not necessarily involve religious beliefs [24]. Many people today prefer to use the term "spirituality" rather than "religion," also because it is broader, less concrete, and less tied to an institution [25]. The term "religion" (from Latin "religare") is commonly used to denote a system of beliefs, ethical values, and actions through which a person expresses their relationship with the sacred and holy reality. On a subjective level, it signifies belief, while on an objective level, it represents a religious institution that connects a person to the supernatural and the sacred through a specific system of knowledge and practice, theology, and ethics. These two levels are complementary but can occasionally be contradictory or even mutually exclusive. Meanwhile, "spirituality" (from Latin "spiritualitas") means the way a believer internalizes the spiritual and moral principles of faith, often referred to as prayer, asceticism, religious practice, meditation, or spiritual reading, or it signifies the dynamics of inner life, the whole lived faith at a personal and communal level (General Religious Lexicon 2007, s.v. "religion"; "spirituality"). Questions about spiritual care are particularly relevant for seriously ill and dying patients. The fulfillment of spiritual needs significantly affects patients' health and well-being [26]. For many patients, faith in the supernatural (spirituality) is important in both health and illness. Faith gives meaning to their lives, provides security when not everything is going well, and remains even when other options are exhausted [27]. As Teoli and Kalish [28] state, it is a common misconception that healthcare and palliative care focus only on physical needs. Numerous issues related to psychological, cultural, ethical, legal, psychiatric, religious, and social needs must be considered. This is especially important when religious questions arise in the context of ethical dilemmas. The World Health Organization recognizes the significance of spiritual care in its definition of palliative care as being equally important as other activities in palliative care [29]. The European Association for Palliative Care (EAPC) defines spirituality as "a dynamic dimension of human life relating to the way individuals (individually and in community) experience, express, and seek meaning, purpose, and transcendence, and the way they connect to the moment, to self, to others, to nature, and to the significant and/or sacred" [30]. Many authors within palliative care define the concept of spirituality in the broadest sense of the word, as an intuitive, interpersonal, altruistic, and integrative expression that includes fundamental existential questions, life principles, values, beliefs, moral values, as well as the relationship with God or a higher power, or as religiously lived spirituality [30, 31]. In palliative care or at the end of life, religion and religious traditions serve two primary functions: providing a set of fundamental life beliefs and establishing an ethical foundation for clinical decision-making [32]. Both religion and spirituality support a person's sense of security and belonging, which can be vital in end-of-life care, as they offer individuals a way to find meaning in both dying and living [32, 33]. They help patients and their families to cope with hope, the search for meaning, and purpose amidst all the adjustments and life changes required by life-threatening medical conditions [34]. On the other hand, the impact of diseases and life-threatening medical conditions on religion and spirituality can be negative due to experiences that include negative confrontations with the illness, anger, even toward God, and the loss of religious beliefs [12, 35]. The diversity of religions and religious beliefs in the modern world creates challenges in recognizing the culture of sensitivity, allowing an understanding of how patients in palliative care will comprehend their illness or ultimately their death. Religion and spirituality, in their highest form, have a significant impact on the development of human culture [25]. The broader cultural context is not only determined by nationality and ethnicity but also influenced by specific spirituality, religion, education level, gender, age, sexual orientation, country of origin, and immigrant status. Culture is an essential concept in palliative care alongside religion and spirituality since an individual's culture also influences how they will make decisions about end-of-life treatment [36, 37].

1.1 Judaism

The term "Judaism" originates from the word "Iudaismus," a Latinized form of the Greek word "Ioudaismos." The Greek word is derived from the noun "Ioudaios," which is typically translated as "Jew," "Jewish," or from the verb "ioudaizein," meaning "to live as a Jew." The Hebrew equivalent of "Judaism" is "Yahadut." Judaism is the religion of the Jewish people, the oldest monotheistic religion upon which both Christianity and Islam are built. In the broadest sense, it encompasses the faith of the Jewish people from the Babylonian exile onwards, including shared history, formed mentality, and culture. When searching for a deeper answer to who a Jew is, it is crucial to understand that there is no simple response. The identity of a Jew is determined by three elements: the Torah (Law), the chosen people (collectiveness), and the promised land. These elements have developed over time and began shaping Judaism. Various forms and branches of Judaism exist due to different relationships among these three elements. Modern Judaism, despite an awareness of common Jewish culture and faith, is highly plural. The emergence of numerous denominations and divisions was influenced by several factors. Judaism has never been uniform, showing exceptional adaptability to various circumstances and societal challenges throughout the centuries. Consequently, there are three forms of Judaism: Reform, Orthodox, and Conservative Judaism. Traditional Jewish legal and ethical thinking is grounded in the interpretation and understanding of three main sources, each of which is extensive, diverse, and complex. Jewish medical ethics as a related field did not exist until modern times. Discussions on medical ethics were scattered throughout Jewish law, professional manuals, and commentaries on religious texts. With the advancement of medicine, challenges emerged in the Jewish community to consolidate existing works on medical ethics and create new ones that remain rooted in religious tradition. Patients and physicians can find works that help them explore the Jewish perspective on various medical and healthcare issues, from abortion to organ transplantation. All these works are based on the rich tradition of Jewish law. In Judaism, bioethical research and the study of halakha (Jewish law) draw their principles from other Jewish texts and their commentaries and use a developed system for explaining halakha. Among the three streams of Judaism, there is no difference in having their own legal system (halakha), but rather the level of respect for it [38]. Halakha (from the Hebrew verb "halak," meaning "to walk") signifies the path one should follow; that is, the legislation to be adhered to in life. Halakha represents the corpus of Jewish law, customs, and tradition [39]. Fundamental to the understanding of halakhic interpretation and the sources of Jewish law is an integral part of the discussion on Jewish medical ethics [38]. There are three sources of Jewish legal and ethical thinking: Hebrew scriptures of ancient Israel, the Talmud, and Responsa [1]. Hebrew scriptures encompass written tradition (the written Torah, also known as the Pentateuch or the Five Books, and the traditional sense of the Pentateuch) and oral tradition (the oral Torah), which dates back to Moses and was transmitted from generation to generation until it finally received its written form in Midrash, the Mishnah, and the Talmud. Jewish interpretation uses the Midrash (from the Hebrew verb "darash," meaning "to seek, investigate, examine") as the oldest way to pass on the oral tradition. It represents an explanation of the Holy Scriptures, aiming to delve deep into its content and extract as many shades of meaning as possible. There are two types of Midrash: Halakha (normative way, rules) and Hagada (homiletic and explanatory narrative). If Halakha explains what a devout Jew must do, Hagada tells why one must do it. Halakha and Hagada reflect the great pluralism within Judaism as they are written based on discussions and reflect contrasting opinions among different schools. The Pentateuch holds the highest level of law in Judaism. The Mishnah was enhanced with commentaries that became known as the Gemara (two versions exist: Palestinian and Babylonian). Together, the Mishnah and the Gemara constitute [2] the Talmud, the second source of law, but its influence on Jewish law and moral codes is even greater than that of Hebrew writings. The Talmud

DOI: http://dx.doi.org/10.5772/intechopen.1004552

(from the Hebrew word "talmud," meaning "study, teaching") is a collection of laws, religious tradition provisions, discussions of legal scholars, and interpretations of the Torah. It is especially important because it sheds light on the process and structure of halakhic reasoning, which involves reasoned analysis, logic, and analogy. The Talmud is religious literature that is more extensive compared to the Holy Scripture and the Quran [3]. The third source of legal authority is Responsa literature. In Judaism, it represents a collection of responses (in Hebrew, "she'elot u-teshuvot," meaning "questions and answers") to complex issues related to religious law, philosophy, and related fields, which have become the most significant source of Halakha. It is actually a collection of opinions on modern matters, interpreted by Hebrew writings and the Talmud. The literature spans centuries of thought and content of opinions and represents a continuation of a 2000-year-old interpretation tradition that creates an intellectual connection with the past.

1.2 Catholicism

Catholicism, in a general sense, emphasizes the universality of the Christian gospel message, which is intended for every individual, nation, language, culture, civilization, and society. In a narrower sense, it represents the shared dignity of all Christians based on equality among believers, in both communal and hierarchical (ministerial) or sacramental service context. The foundation of the Catholic Church, as referred to in the following paragraphs, is the primacy of the pope, who holds leadership and jurisdictional primacy over the entire Church. The Catholic Church is organized as a visible Christian community with hierarchies and laypeople. There are three hierarchies: the clergy, the canon law, and the honorary hierarchy. The Catholic Church does not represent a monarchy, an oligarchy, or a democracy, but it is a hierarchically organized community, where each member has a role and a task for the benefit of the whole. According to Catholic doctrine, nature and the supernatural, human free will, and God's grace presuppose and complement each other. Therefore, in Catholic morality, three theological virtues (faith, hope, and love) and four natural virtues (prudence, justice, temperance, and fortitude) are complementary. The sources of Catholic morality are the Old Testament (the Ten Commandments, personal responsibility), the New Testament (love for God and neighbor), and natural ethics. It is systematically studied by moral theology, and within the community, it is carefully regulated by canon law. Pope John Paul II officially expressed the Church's position on the value and inviolability of human life in 1995 in the encyclical Evangelium vitae – The Gospel of Life. Likewise, the document titled "Samaritanus bonus" by the Congregation for the Doctrine of the Faith, published in September 2020, provides doctrinal foundations and pastoral guidelines for the care of people in critical and final phases of life. These documents are among the most important ones addressing ethical issues, including end-of-life ethical decisions. Within Catholic ethics, moral theology, or Catholic bioethics, two fundamental values exist: human dignity and the interconnectedness of every individual in terms of responsibility toward one another. All other values stem from these two. It is minimalistic to define human dignity, which is protected in democratic legal systems and is legally enforceable, as it does not encompass.

According to German moral theologian Schockenhoff [40], the core of human dignity is directed toward what makes a person human, their capacity for free action, and responsibility for self-determined autonomy. In other words, it means discovering a common living space that allows people to mutually respect each other as rational beings.

1.3 Islam

Islam is a monotheistic religion founded in the seventh century in Arabia by the Prophet Muhammad. It encompasses the belief in one God (Allah) and a comprehensive way of life, including religious, moral, and legal guidance. The primary sources of Islam are the Quran, the teachings, and practices of the Prophet Muhammad (Sunnah), consensus among Islamic scholars (Ijma), and reasoning by analogy (Qiyas). These sources provide the basis for Islamic jurisprudence and ethics [41]. Islamic belief is based on the concept of Tawhid, the absolute oneness of God, and the acknowledgment of Muhammad as the final prophet. The five pillars of Islam include the Shahada (declaration of faith), Salat (prayer), Sawm (fasting), Zakat (almsgiving), and Hajj (pilgrimage to Mecca). Islamic law, known as Sharia, is derived from the Quran and Sunnah, and it governs various aspects of life, including personal morality, family law, and criminal law. Islamic ethics emphasize justice, compassion, and mercy, and these principles have significant implications for end-of-life care. In Islam, the preservation of life is considered one of the highest values. Taking a human life is strictly prohibited, and euthanasia is not allowed. However, the alleviation of suffering is encouraged, and palliative care is seen as an important aspect of medical ethics in Islam. The decision to withdraw or withhold treatment must be made with a focus on relieving suffering rather than hastening death. There are differing opinions within the Islamic community on specific issues related to end-of-life care, and these differences can be influenced by cultural and regional factors. Despite these differences, the fundamental principles of compassion, justice, and the preservation of life remain core values in Islamic medical ethics [42, 43]. It's important to note that Islamic beliefs and practices can vary among different schools of thought within Islam, and individual interpretations may also play a role in end-of-life decisions. Islamic bioethics has its complexities, and the application of these principles may differ among individuals and communities. In Islamic ethics, guidance is found through idĵtihad, with fundamental principles, rules, and regulations from the main sources shaping the Islamic way of life. Together with idĵtihad, they provide a comprehensive moral and legal framework to address and adapt to human circumstances [44, 45]. Islamic jurisprudence, in its judicial practice, must consider five fundamental principles in resolving any issue: the preservation of life, the protection of individual freedoms or beliefs, the preservation of intellect, the protection of honor and integrity, and the safeguarding of property.

The purpose of our research was to assess the importance of ethics, religion, and spiritual care in palliative care, with an emphasis on religious perspectives on ethical dilemmas at the end of life and the importance of religious beliefs in medical care and healthcare at the end of life. We focused on three monotheistic religions, namely Judaism, Christianity, and Islam. We wanted to identify similarities and differences in the concept of understanding the importance of palliative care and ethical dilemmas in end-of-life treatment decisions.

2. Methods

In this study, we used qualitative methodology and employed a semi-structured open interview as the research instrument. Each interview was labeled as "IN," and a corresponding number was added to indicate the conducted interview, ranging from 1 to 9. The process of data acquisition was standardized among all participants in the study. We included six structured questions with sub-questions, as described below. We conducted interviews with nine participants, each representing one of three major religious communities: Catholic, Jewish, and Islamic. The research participants were purposefully selected after careful consideration by both researchers. The inclusion criterion was affiliation with a religious community and employment in healthcare for participants who were not spiritual leaders of the selected religious communities. A prerequisite was that they agreed to participate in the study and the recording of the conversation. Within each religious community, we ensured the inclusion of an official representative, such as a rabbi for the Jewish community, a priest for the Catholic community, and an imam for the Islamic community. We also considered that other participants from the religious communities involved in the study were employed in healthcare institutions, either as physicians, registered nurses, or pharmacists. This approach aimed to ensure the relevance of their professional and expert knowledge in the field of palliative care, impartiality, and an equal objective presentation of data. We also considered the criterion that the participants involved in the study were limited to the territory of the Republic of Slovenia. Due to the relevant sample size, we had to expand this criterion to the nearest Jewish community in the Zagreb area, based on the historical connection between the two communities before the establishment of the Jewish community in the Republic of Slovenia.

3. Results

In the conducted interviews and qualitative data analysis, we identified four main themes or content areas: (1) recognition of the significance of religion and spirituality in palliative care, (2) the provision of spiritual (religious) care in palliative care, (3) the importance of religion in ethical questions and dilemmas in palliative care, and (4) awareness of recognizing cultural and religious differences in palliative care. The main themes and their categories and codes are presented in **Table 1**.

3.1 Recognition of the significance of religion and spiritual care in palliative care

Based on the conducted interviews, it can be highlighted that the participants recognize the significance of religion and spirituality in palliative care primarily as guardians of the principles of (1) human dignity and the indispensable role of (2) spirituality in the comprehensive patient care. A participant from the Islamic faith said: "In Islam, life is sacred and must not be shortened in any way" (IN8). Some participants in the study also used the term human dignity: "Palliative care cares for the dignity of human life until the last moment" (IN1); similarly, we can observe that palliative care is "a reflection of care for the dignity and health of the individual" (IN5) or "the provision of palliative care significantly contributes to the preservation of human dignity" (IN6). One of the participants in the discussion emphasizes the important distinction when he says, "In the public discourse, we rarely talk about the sanctity of life but rather about the dignity of the human person and human life" (IN1). This means that even within our research, it is possible to determine the polemical use of the term or principle of "sanctity of life." Reconstructing the history of religious ideas to understand their original meaning is one thing, advocating fundamental religious arguments is quite another, as one of the participants notes when highlighting the necessity of recognizing and understanding religious traditions in ethical questions: "When it comes to ethical dilemmas, it is, of course, necessary

Theme	Categories	Kode
Recognition of the significance of religion and spirituality in palliative care.	Human dignity	Sanctity of life Quality of life Right and duty to treatment
	Spiritual care as part of comprehensive patient care in palliative care	Spirituality as a dimension of relationships Spirituality as a dimension of redemption Spirituality as an equal approach in comprehensive palliative care
The provision of spiritual (religious) care in palliative care.	Institutional provision of spiritual (religious) care in palliative care	Religious communities in public and private institutions
	Non-institutional provision of spiritual (religious) care in palliative care	Family, friends, relatives, and other institutions
The importance of religion in ethical questions and dilemmas in palliative care.	Palliative care without a religious perspective is insufficient	Multidisciplinary patient care Human and professional care
	Religion as a challenge for quality palliative care	Clash of values between religious and medical ethics Diverse cultural and value environments
Awareness of recognizing cultural and religious differences in palliative care.	Individual responsibility	Personal competencies Professional competencies
	Social responsibility	Importance of religious communities Importance of educational institutions

Table 1.
Main themes, categories, and codes.

to maintain a wide spectrum and view (Christian) ethics as something rational, often much more rational today than the ideology of unlimited freedom, which thinks that everything that is possible in medicine today is also right. If Christianity ever sets a limit to what is acceptable in ethical dilemmas, it is not ideological opposition but a rational argument against the ideology of misunderstood freedom that would sacrifice anything, even human life, just to confirm itself" (IN1).

In palliative care, religion recognizes the principle of human dignity in ensuring the principle of quality of life. A participant from the Catholic faith states, "In the Catholic Church, the absolute value is the sanctity of life, meaning the inviolability of life from conception to death" (IN2). Similarly, a participant from the Jewish faith says, "It seems to me incredibly important to provide people with a dignified life until the end" (IN6), and one from the Islamic faith adds, "Each religion has different views or rules that somehow influence the quality of palliative care" (IN9). It is important to note that participants in the interview, while recognizing the importance of maintaining the quality of life, oppose the contemporary anthropological utilitarian perspective, which is mainly linked to economic possibilities, well-being, beauty, and the enjoyment of physical life, and which deems life worthwhile only if it reaches an acceptable level of quality. Participants highlight that, from the perspective of monotheistic religious beliefs, the basis of human dignity, besides advocating the principle of the sanctity of life and ensuring the maximum quality of life, also includes the realization of the right and duty to treatment. Participants from the

Islamic faith mention that "[A] Quranic rule applies: 'Whoever kills one man, it is as if he killed the entire world, and whoever saves one man, it is as if he saved the entire world.' Therefore, it is necessary to fight for every life since it is God's gift we have received. Thus, as believers, we are obligated to care for our health" (IN7). They also emphasize that "In our religion, there are no specific instructions/rules that would specifically prescribe that a believer should renounce or refuse a specific medical procedure. On the contrary, a Muslim is obliged to seek treatment" (IN8). Similarly, a participant from the Jewish faith describes such an obligation as the task of providing spiritual care: "I come from my spirituality, religion, faith. 'In the suffering, let one brother give his hand to another.' Even when everything fails, even when all medicine fails, or all possibilities are exhausted, in fact, even professionally, there's nothing more to 'do,' you can always do that" (IN2). Participants recognize the importance of spirituality in palliative care as an indispensable part of comprehensive patient care.

The study found that spirituality in palliative care is expressed in three ways: as a dimension of the relationship, as a dimension of salvation, and as an equal approach within holistic palliative care. Participants understand the role of spirituality in palliative care in a way that it originates from religion itself, and religion provides fundamental identity. Therefore, the spirituality they describe represents not only fundamental existential questions, principles, values, and beliefs but also primarily the relationship with God and its eschatological dimension. A participant from the Catholic faith describes it as follows: "A sense of reconciliation with loved ones and God, a sincere review of one's own life from the perspective of eternity, deep spirituality that often accompanies the person at the end of life" (IN2).

"In their final moments, all of this and much more are elements of spirituality in palliative care" (IN1), and concludes: "For a Catholic, the reason human life has such great value is manifold, including the belief that life on this Earth continues in some other form in eternity" (IN1). A participant of the Jewish faith similarly states: "Spirituality is very important in the final stage of life. Judaism views life as a cycle, a beginning, and an end. At the end of life, it is important, especially for palliative patients, to have someone with them who will understand their religious and cultural needs" (IN6). Similarly, a participant of the Islamic faith adds: "Faith gives us a sense of hope, so for a believer in palliative care, it is important to have the opportunity to devote oneself to God or to have someone assist them in doing so. People in this condition can have only hope" (IN7). Participants in the study highlight spirituality as a concept rather than focusing on the characteristics of spirituality itself. Spirituality, often, is not integrated into palliative care due to the lack of training, time constraints, and a lack of vocabulary surrounding spiritual matters among healthcare professionals. As one participant notes, "we have not yet developed the field of palliative care units and experts, so talking about spirituality as an equal and professional approach to the dying is something that is seen from a distance" (IN3). While participants emphasize spirituality as an approach equal to all other aspects of palliative care, it is necessary from a professional standpoint for healthcare workers to differentiate between institutional, religious, and, ultimately, political influences of spirituality in all modern secularized societal sectors where complex spiritual issues are encountered.

3.2 The provision of spiritual (religious) care in palliative care

In the study, we formulated another highlighted topic as spiritual (religious) care in palliative care. Using categories, we identified as institutional and non-institutional arrangements for providing spiritual (religious) care in palliative care, we created three forms of delivering spiritual care: (1) religious communities in public and private institutions, (2) family, friends, and relatives, and (3) other institutions. Catholic, Jewish, and Islamic religious communities have developed ethical obligations, legal guidelines, and religious positions concerning individual ethical dilemmas, particularly those related to a patient's religious affiliation. On the other hand, the legal regulation of palliative care in Slovenia is still non-systemic, so the aspect of religiosity or spirituality in the broadest sense is inadequately incorporated into legal regulations and health codes. In Slovenia, Catholic, Jewish, and Islamic religious communities have different experiences, either positive or negative. For the Catholic religious community, spiritual care is primarily provided in practice by priests as (formal) representatives of the religious community: "In the Catholic Church, the largest religious community in Slovenia, I can proudly state that we have very well-organized spiritual care, not only for the seriously ill and dying in palliative care and the hospice, but also for all other patients. We have several chaplain priests who are responsible for visits, administering sacraments, and accompanying all patients in all hospitals" (IN3). On the other hand, the Islamic religious community, where a similar spiritual (religious) care is provided by an imam, a representative of the religious community, highlights a negative experience, with a participant stating, "We have never succeeded in securing a small space in the largest clinical centers or hospitals for prayer in the same way as a chapel is arranged. There was no understanding for addressing this issue" (IN7). The Jewish religious community emphasizes that, being numerically smaller than other religious communities, the extent of such care depends primarily on the size of the community and the scope of assistance: "The Chief Rabbi of Slovenia is authorized to address these issues within the public healthcare in the Republic of Slovenia. The level of addressing these issues usually reflects the population density of any Jewish community" (IN4). A positive example in one of the hospice institutions is provided by a participant of the Catholic faith when they say, "In 2016, at the initiative of the director, five religious communities - the Catholic Church, the Islamic religious community, the Serbian Orthodox Church, the Protestant religious community, the Macedonian Orthodox Church - signed an agreement committing to always have their religious representatives available if the dying need them" (IN2). It is recognized that this form of providing spiritual (religious) care is carried out within the framework of individual initiatives of certain institutions, meaning that the current palliative care in Slovenia does not ensure uninterrupted comprehensive palliative care, also because there are no systematically established connections between different healthcare and other institutions. Study participants emphasized the importance of family, friends, and other forms that come into play in this context to provide spiritual (religious) care because "in Judaism, it is crucial."

"It is not necessary that a rabbi is always present at the end of a person's life. Representatives of religious communities, family members, or others can also be present and perform the final rites. In Judaism, there is a specific organization called 'Chevra Kadisha' that plays this role" (IN 6). Similarly, another participant states, "There are various groups of mourners that anyone in need can join during this difficult time" (IN 3).

3.3 The importance of religion in ethical questions and dilemmas in palliative care

As the third major theme in the study, we emphasize the significance of religion in ethical questions and dilemmas in palliative care. We identify two distinct approaches that raise the question of whether palliative care can be of sufficient quality without including a religious perspective. They also address how religion, spirituality, or spiritual care as part of an equitable approach to comprehensive palliative care can present a significant challenge. The religious perspective undoubtedly brings quality multidisciplinary teamwork and humane, professional end-of-life care. One participant notes, "If we take a holistic view of the patient, if we address them on all levels, then the team can find the best solution collectively" (IN 3). They continue, "If a physician in palliative care approaches the patient not only as a professional but as someone who wants to offer help... if we are all humans first, if the patient is at the centre of our team, then religion is not an obstacle to working in palliative care" (IN 3). On the other hand, there can be clashes between religious and medical ethics, especially when doubts arise about the correctness or incorrectness of individual decisions, and when legally sanctioned procedures and interventions are in conflict with the principles of a particular religious or ethical system. Legislation in Slovenia is framed in a way that, in general, religious communities do not see contradictions with official medicine, especially when it comes to euthanasia. A Catholic participant states, "In our country, there are no issues because our legislation aligns with ethical standards. If euthanasia were legalized, for example, this would change, and religious beliefs would play a significant role, but not because of the faith itself, but because of reasonable arguments against ethically questionable medical practices" (IN1). Similarly, a participant from the Islamic faith mentions, "Ethical concerns regarding Islam are never in conflict with official medicine, at least not in our Slovenian context and the legislation in this area, such as euthanasia" (IN 7). However, a participant from the Jewish community highlights that during the treatment of a patient, doctors may encounter doubts about the justifiability of administering certain medications to an individual. "In such cases," they say, "doctors should always discuss these issues with a rabbi" (IN 4). All monotheistic faiths have clear positions against euthanasia. "The Catholic Church is against euthanasia in any form, but it does not oppose the withholding of treatment, which varies from case to case" (IN 2). "Judaism considers human life and its preservation an absolute value, and patients must be kept alive" (IN 4). "In Islam, we must fight for every life, as it is a gift from God that we have received. Therefore, as believers, we are obligated to take care of our health" (IN 7). Misunderstanding the concept of compassion can raise ethical questions that are theoretical but significant in understanding a particular religious perspective. One participant reflects on this in relation to Christian compassion: "Due to Christ's example, His teaching of love, and my personal experience of this love in my life, I want to be like Christ in my relationship with people, especially the most suffering. He shapes my life, my work, my behavior. The patient may not necessarily emphasize spirituality in their life. If they are open to it and express specific questions, we can have direct conversations (with them or their family). However, many questions, answers, and conversations remain unspoken" (IN 2).

3.4 Awareness of recognizing cultural and religious differences in palliative care

As the final theme, we emphasize the importance of awareness when recognizing cultural and religious differences in palliative care. We divided this theme based on interviews into two parts: individual and societal responsibility in recognizing cultural and religious differences in palliative care. On one hand, recognizing these differences reflects personal orientation and individual engagement in understanding or recognizing the religious, spiritual, or cultural aspects. On the other hand, this question is raised as a matter of social responsibility both within religious communities and other educational institutions. Within individual responsibility, participants first highlight the importance of personal competencies. A Catholic participant emphasizes that "a priest or another spiritual collaborator should not view the patient merely as a person of faith but as a human being in need of assistance" (IN 3). Similarly, a participant from the Jewish community states, "Providing palliative care requires an exceptional commitment from the person providing it, provided that they want to do their work honorably" (IN 5). An Islamic participant also stresses the need for healthcare professionals to be more open to religion, as the quality of palliative care depends on it (IN 9). However, participants also note the importance of professional competencies in recognizing the spiritual and religious needs of patients. Participants from all three faiths agree that there is a lack of practical knowledge in the field of cultural and religious issues. A Catholic participant argues, "I believe that, in general, there is a lack of cultural and religious education in Slovenia. This is a broad framework that goes beyond the specific topic, but it is a fact that we know too little about our country, our culture, and are, therefore, less receptive to any profound understanding of culture, let alone religion" (IN 1). Similarly, a participant from the Jewish community adds, "In my opinion, healthcare workers are not well-informed about individual religious beliefs, and some of them are very resistant to this information" (IN 9). Therefore, the need for adequate education and regulation on this subject is evident. A participant from the Jewish community points out, "Patients expect to be treated with respect, including respect for their religious beliefs and other beliefs and opinions. Generally, a Jewish healthcare worker who is also a believer always treats the patient with due respect… while considering the absolute value of human life and its consequences. It is necessary to promote it in every way through appropriate education and legislation" (IN 4). In the Slovenian professional literature, there is a lack of published material that would systematically profile the profession's fundamental competencies or competencies based on training programs specific to specialized spiritual care in palliative care, for both healthcare workers and other pastoral workers and collaborators in providing spiritual care. Therefore, for the professional community, it is a clear challenge to focus and unite national guidelines and clinical and professional standards in a framework that encourages the discussion and development of the competence framework for spiritual care in palliative care, including religious practices as performed by certain pastoral workers from specific religious communities under the current conditions. In addition to individual engagement, the development of a competence model or standards for recognizing people's religious or faith orientation in palliative care is essential. Participants in the research emphasize the significance of religious communities and educational institutions and their role in shaping a framework for recognizing cultural, religious, and spiritual diversity in the context of a pluralistic and global setting. The Healthcare professionals work in different healthcare settings. Recognizing one's own cultural and spiritual foundations is the first step toward open exploration, as one of the participants states: "In Slovenia, due to its sad recent history, this is not obvious, but worldwide, it's clear that one of the fundamental parts of faith is also life in charity and diakonia, which means benevolence. These are the oldest Christian principles. Therefore, as we know from history, the Church has always cared for the poor, established schools, hospitals, alms-houses, and all kinds of institutions for the weakest. After what happened in our local history, the Church is somewhat hindered in this respect, but fortunately, this only applies to the (un)normality of our region. Nevertheless, despite everything, the Slovenian Church has greatly increased the number of elderly homes in recent decades. This is a typical measure that is usually overlooked when faith compels Christians to care for the poorest" (IN1). On another note, it is worth mentioning the guidelines of the EAPC, which specifically address the issue of education on spiritual care for all professionals involved in palliative care. Educational competencies in spiritual care for all providers of palliative care are guided by models of best practice and research evidence, which also encompass various developmental stages of palliative care services in the European region. Education on religious, spiritual, or cultural diversity can help healthcare professionals to avoid their own biases or reservations. In this way, the EAPC encourages high-quality, multidisciplinary, and academic education on spiritual care for all stakeholders in palliative care [30].

4. Discussion

The research illustrates the importance of ethics, religion, and spirituality in palliative care, with an emphasis on religious perspectives on ethical dilemmas at the end of life. Participants in our study recognize the significance of religion in palliative care, especially in providing spiritual care as part of comprehensive patient care. They emphasize that religion perceives palliative care as a means of ensuring and preserving the inalienable dignity of patients. This is consistent with the understanding of the sanctity of life upheld by all selected religious communities, which recognizes the importance of a dignified death in relation to ensuring the highest quality of life. The study further identifies that despite various legal mechanisms protecting fundamental rights and freedoms, including religious freedom, in the Republic of Slovenia, the provision of specific spaces for prayer and other religious rituals in various public healthcare and hospital institutions is inadequately regulated, for instance, for the Jewish (even though they are a small community) and Islamic religious communities. In the study, it is found that religious communities define their positions on specific ethical dilemmas through their ethical codes, a point also affirmed by participants. The study does not highlight any instances where religious beliefs conflict with the practice of medical professionalism, as Slovenian legislation does not oppose the ethical standards advocated by religious communities. Participants point out that religious ethical foundations are not arbitrary, capricious, or random, but they introduce ethical dilemmas to the progress of medicine and science that do not have simple right or wrong answers. Participants in the research identify that awareness among healthcare professionals in Slovenia regarding cultural and religious differences is insufficient. The reasons cited for this lack of awareness are numerous, encompassing both societal and individual factors. The challenge of understanding different value systems and beliefs of patients, sensitivity to cultural and religious differences, demands greater awareness from both religious communities and the state, as well as the broader social community. The theoretical overviews and research results presented provide a basis for further development in this field—in recognizing the interconnection of ethics and religion and in fostering a more inclusive and holistic practice of assuming responsibility for people. In healthcare, this process can be partially facilitated by introducing appropriate educational content into the curriculum, offering the opportunity to acquire specialist knowledge in ethics, religion, and spirituality, and conducting professional assessments of individual spiritual needs. It is nearly impossible to provide a comprehensive overview of the monotheistic view on end-of-life decisions, especially because there exist different theological and philosophical methodologies that intersect at various points on specific questions. In our discussion, we have highlighted important stances that characterize the Jewish, Catholic, and Islamic faiths.

Some methodological limitations of our study may relate to our open research question, and the explanatory character of the study may have been hampered by the inductive creation of codes and categories [46]. In the context of the latter, a potential criticism would be that the study was subjective, which is the most frequent criticism of qualitative research [46, 47]. However, all co-authors relied on a careful, deliberate research strategy, and respect for the basic characteristics of qualitative research during the data collection and analysis stages.

4.1 Judaism

In modern Jewish medical ethics, particularly in the 1960s and 1970s, the emphasis was predominantly from Orthodox Judaism, where divine authority expressed through the Torah and Talmud forms the foundation of the consultative process [38]. Much of Jewish bioethical literature is based on this perspective, assuming that with the appropriate interpretation of Talmudic texts and commentaries, answers to the most challenging questions can be found. In practice, a rabbi, whose opinion is sought for ethical guidance, serves as a "professional advisor" who interprets halakhic law for the specific situation, assisting both the doctor and the patient. In complex cases, a local rabbi or chaplain may consult more learned halakhic authorities. While traditional Jewish texts express numerous ethical principles worthy of consideration, there are a few fundamental principles that underpin a significant part of the Jewish bioethical tradition. These include:

1. Human life has infinite value.

2. Aging, illness, and death are natural parts of life.

3. Improving a patient's quality of life is a constant commitment.

4. People are "responsible caretakers" in preserving their bodies, which ultimately belong to God.

5. Individuals are obligated to violate any other law to save a human life, except for murder, incest, or idolatry.

Compared to secular values, these principles indicate a lesser role for patient autonomy. The duty to treat illness or preserve health takes precedence over any perceived right to refuse treatment or commit suicide. The principle of sanctity of life means that any decision that could indirectly or directly hasten death is prohibited. Traditional Judaism generally forbids suicide, euthanasia, withholding or withdrawing treatment, and abortion when the mother's life or health is not at risk, as well as many traditional "rights" associated with a strong concept of autonomy. The challenge Jews face in end-of-life decisions is typically not in determining appropriate halakha; the greater challenge is deciding the moment when hope for further life is lost, and the process of dying begins. Jewish law is relatively clear that one should not take life before the natural time of death. Regarding the issue of withholding and withdrawing life-sustaining treatment, Jewish law allows such actions only if the treatment is futile and repetitive, and provided the patient has given clear consent. This includes refraining from any activities that prolong life, such as intubation, surgery, chemotherapy, or dialysis, even after the treatment has begun because such an action is considered an omission rather than a withdrawal. For continuous forms of maintenance treatment, such as a respirator or a pacemaker, removal is prohibited. The strictest position in Judaism limits permission for withdrawal or discontinuation of treatment to cases where physicians anticipate the patient will die within 72 hours. Patients and physicians can discontinue clinical treatment in cases where the patient has a diagnosis of an incurable chronic illness if it is in the patient's best interest. Furthermore, halakha defines oxygen, food, and fluids as essential components of life, which every individual is entitled to. Therefore, a dying patient cannot be denied these basic necessities, and the withdrawal of artificial nutrition and hydration is not permitted as it constitutes an action leading to death. In cases where the continued provision of artificial nutrition and hydration causes suffering and complications to a patient approaching death, such support can be withdrawn upon the patient's request or if it is determined to have been the patient's wish. As for palliative sedation, there is a consensus in Jewish law that it is permitted, despite the risk that such medications may shorten life based on the principle of double effect (Padella).

4.2 Catholicism

In line with this, Christianity primarily emphasizes the importance of autonomy and the patient's presence in ethical decision-making or treatment [43]. The question of withholding or withdrawing treatment is permitted if it is burdensome, dangerous, extraordinary, and disproportionate to the expected results of medical procedures [48]. This is the so-called "refusal of therapeutic obstinacy," which means that the responsible person does not want to hold back death but rather accepts the fact that they cannot prevent it. The decision should be made by the patient if they are competent or capable of making it. If not, those who have the legal right to do so make this decision, always respecting the patient's reasonable will and their legitimate interests. In 1980, the Declaration on Euthanasia allowed pain relief with medication or the use of analgesia and sedation in dying patients, including the shortening of life as an unintended side effect (the principle of double effect). However, it is important to emphasize that the issue of pain and suffering holds special significance for Catholic bioethics, as it also represents an opportunity and the meaning of participating in Christ's suffering [48, 49]. In Catholic tradition, pain and suffering are not seen as goods in themselves. At this point, we recall the statement of Pope Pius XII when a group of anesthetists asked him whether pain relief medication should be offered to a patient, even if this unintentionally shortened the patient's life. The Pope replied that pain relief should be offered if no other means exist, even if it leads to unconsciousness and an inability to fulfill the patient's moral duties and family obligations. This judgment reflects the principle of double effect, which plays a crucial role in end-of-life care. It establishes that an act with a double effect, one good and one bad, is morally permissible if the act: 1) is not intrinsically evil, 2) is done with the intention of achieving a possible good effect, without intending the possible bad effect, although foreseeing that it is possible, 3) does not bring about a good effect through a bad effect, and 4) is done for a proportionate reason [48].

4.3 Islam

Ethical considerations regarding end-of-life issues in Islamic bioethics revolve around the sanctity of human life. This judgment is defined in the Quran with the following verses: "Do not take life, which God has made sacred, except in the course of justice" [50]. In line with this, it is forbidden for anyone to intentionally end their own life: "If anyone kills a person, it is as if he kills all of humanity, except those who commit murder or spread corruption in the land" [50]. Preserving life is one of the greatest merits and imperatives in Islam. Doctors are obliged to do everything in their power to prevent premature death. However, this imperative no longer applies when death is inevitable and clinical treatment is clearly futile. Islam acknowledges that people must sometimes recognize their limitations and allow nature to take its course [50]. Resorting to unwarranted treatment to avert death is unacceptable in Islam [49]. Muslim jurists agree that a doctor, patient, and family members can make a collective decision, based on informed consent, to reject medical interventions and discontinue treatment if these procedures in no way improve the patient's condition or quality of life [48]. If invasive treatment has been initiated to save a patient's life, Muslim jurists have determined that the medical equipment maintaining the patient's life should not be switched off unless the doctor is certain of the inevitability of death [51]. Islam advocates the stance that even at the end of life, patients should not be deprived of their right to nutrition and hydration. This is due to the fact that withholding such necessities would hasten death, which is prohibited in Islam [48]. However, the use of palliative sedation to alleviate end-of-life suffering is permitted, even if it expedites death. Islam teaches that "actions are to be judged by their intentions" [48, 51]. In Islam, pain is regarded as a test of faith and spirituality [50]. Therefore, Muslims should endure it patiently.

To endure pain patiently, this does not mean they are prohibited from seeking means to alleviate suffering. The Quran states that "good deeds will surely drive away evil deeds [that cause suffering]" [50]. This means that an individual should strive to overcome pain [51]. In Islamic ethics, an individual's well-being is closely tied to their family and community [51]. Therefore, neither autonomy nor paternalism are decisive factors in deciding on the course of end-of-life care; instead, it is a collective decision involving all parties connected to the patient, which may also require the involvement of religious authorities if necessary [48, 51]. It is worth noting that the two main branches of Islam, Sunni and Shia, may have some differences in interpretations, methodologies, and authoritative systems but not significantly in bioethical judgments. However, it should be noted that most Islamic communities will follow the views of their recognized religious scholars because the Islamic faith is not monolithic and encompasses diverse viewpoints [48].

Importance for everyday practice

1. We recognize the need for adequate regulation of specific spaces for prayer and other religious rituals in various public healthcare and hospital institutions for all religious groups.

2. Participants in the research identify that awareness among healthcare professionals in Slovenia regarding cultural and religious differences is insufficient and recognize the need of improving the curriculum in education regarding this topic.

3. Religion is not the common basis for ethics, but rather a rational reflection on human life, its value, and dignity.

5. Conclusion

The question of how to understand the place of religion between the patient and healthcare personnel is not straightforward. In contemporary Europe, there are various religious affiliations in every country and community. Within each religious community, divisions exist, such as between Shiite and Sunni Muslims, Orthodox and Reformed Jews, as well as Catholic, Orthodox, and Protestant Christians. In addition to these divisions, there is also diversity in the degree of religious affiliation, beliefs, and religious practices. The complex context reveals the space in which healthcare professionals work; each patient is unique in terms of their religious beliefs, and each healthcare professional is unique in terms of their religious affiliation. Every interaction between a patient and a healthcare professional takes place in the light of profound and evolving religious diversity [52]. Different ethnic, racial, and religious identities within the patient population lead to countless value systems present in clinical practice [38, 53]. Religious values shape ethical codes present not only in every religion but also often expressed in various cultural norms in society. Therefore, it is important to understand the religious values that can shape such a cultural encounter [28]. The fact is that no religion in the Western world can serve as a common basis for ethical reflection. Religion is not the common basis for ethics, but rather rational reflection on human life, its value, and dignity. However, the fact that religion is not a common foundation for ethics does not mean that religion cannot contribute to ethical discourse in a pluralistic society. A pluralistic society, religious pluralism, encourages us all involved in healthcare to be more aware and understand the different value systems and beliefs of patients entering the healthcare system. Sensitivity to cultural and religious differences leads to increased trust between medical staff and patients, resulting in a compassionate and high-quality environment for providing healthcare or end-of-life palliative care. Many ethical dilemmas require a structured approach through the various value systems of each individual or patient. One of the main ethical issues in the world today—how to provide palliative care to all patients regardless of their background and location—is a challenge that surpasses all ethical dilemmas and requires us to consider how to provide a structure of high-quality palliative care that will be accessible to as many patients as possible. The future research should focus on the possibility how to integrate the knowledge about the religiosity and spirituality in the curriculum of medical health staff and emphasize the young generation of healthcare providers for a culturally sensitive work, especially in palliative care.

Author details

Rok Mihelič[1] and Erika Zelko[2,3]*

1 Hospital Barmherzige Brüder Graz, Graz, AT, Austria

2 Medical Faculty, Institute for Palliative and Hopis Medicine, University Maribor, Maribor, SI, Slovenia

3 Medical Faculty, Institut for General Medicine, JKU Linz, Altenbergerstrasse, Linz, AT, Austria

*Address all correspondence to: erikazelko@gmail.com

References

[1] Bishop JP, Eberl JT. POINT: Is it ethically permissible to unilaterally withdraw life-sustaining treatments during crisis standards of care? Yes. Chest. 2021;**159**(6):2165-2166. DOI: 10.1016/j.chest.2021.01.029

[2] Ferrell BR, Handzo G, Picchi T, Puchalski C, Rosa WE. The urgency of spiritual care: COVID-19 and the critical need for whole-person palliation. Journal of Pain and Symptom Management. 2020;**60**(3):e7-e11. DOI: 10.1016/j.jpainsymman.2020.06.034

[3] Wiegand D, MacMillan J, Santos M, Bousso R. Palliative and end-of-life ethical dilemmas in the intensive care unit. AACN Advanced Critical Care. 2015;**26**:142-150. DOI: 10.1097/NCI.0000000000000085

[4] Andres SC, Machado LB, Franco FP, Santos D, dos Santos R, Torres F, et al. Nursing care for patients in palliative care. Research, Society and Development. 2021;**10**(6):e55910616140. DOI: 10.33448/rsd-v10i6.16140

[5] Ećimović P, Lahajnar-Čavlović S, Kompan L. Paliativna oskrba v intenzivni medicini – Prikaz primera in pregled literature. Zdravniški Vestnik. 2009;**78**(5):255-259

[6] Picollo DP, Fachini M. A atenção do enfermeiro ao pacien-te em cuidado paliativo. Revista de Ciências Médicas. 2018;**27**(2):85-92. DOI: 10.24220/2318-0897v27n2a3855

[7] Rochmawati E, Wiechula R, Cameron K. Centrality of spirituality/religion in the culture of palliative care service in Indonesia: An ethnographic study. Nursing & Health Sciences. 2018;**20**(2):231-237. DOI: 10.1111/nhs.12407

[8] Sepulveda C, Marlin A, Yoshida T, Ullrich A. Palliative care: The World Health Organization's global perspective. Journal of Pain and Symptom Management. 2002;**24**(2):91-96. DOI: 10.1016/s0885-3924(02)00440-2

[9] Snyder SH, Sederstrom N, Keith Mansel J, Groninger H. Palliative care, spiritual care, and clinical ethics: Widely available, but underused. Chest. 2017;**151**(6):1404-1406. DOI: 10.1016/j.chest.2017.03.034

[10] McCormick T, Hopp F, Becker HN, Ai AL, Schlueter in Jessica K. Camp. Ethical and spiritual concerns near the end of life. Journal of Religion, Spirituality, and Aging. 2012;**24**:301313. DOI: 10.1080/15528030.20 12.698385

[11] Nelson-Becker HB. Voices of resilience: Older adults in hospice care. Journal of Social Work in End-of-Life & Palliative Care. 2006;**2**(3):87-106. DOI: 10.1300/J457v02n03_07

[12] Puchalski C, Ferrell B, Virani R, Otis-Green S, Baird P, Bull J, et al. Improving the quality of spiritual care as a dimension of palliative care: The report of the consensus conference. Journal of Palliative Medicine. 2009;**12**(10):885-904. DOI: 10.1089/jpm.2009.0142

[13] Rogers M, Wattis J. Spirituality in nursing practice. Nursing Standard. 2015;**29**(39):51-57. DOI: 10.7748/ns.29.39.51.e9726

[14] Harrad R, Cosentino C, Keasley R, Sulla F. Spiritual care in nursing: An overview of the measures used to assess spiritual care provision and related factors amongst nurses. Acta bio-medica: AteneiParmensis. 2019;**90**(4-S):44-55. DOI: 10.23750/abm.v90i4-S.8300

[15] Rodríguez-Arias D, López BR, Monasterio-Astobiza A, Ivar R. Hannikainen. How do people use 'killing', 'letting die' and related bioethical concepts? Contrasting descriptive and normative hypotheses. Bioethics. 2020;**34**(5):509-518. DOI: 10.1111/bioe.12707

[16] Grošelj U, Oražem M, Trontelj J, Grosek Š. EtiČne dileme ob koncu življenja v intenzivnimedicini [End-of-life ethical dilemmas in intensive care unit]. Zdravniški vestnik. 2013;**82**(9):589-601

[17] Asscher J. The moral distinction between killing and letting die in medical cases. Bioethics. 2008;**22**(5):278285. DOI: 10.1111/j.1467-8519.2008.00616.x

[18] Lanazi M, Alanzi M. Is there a moral difference between killing and letting die in healthcare? International Journal of Research in Medical Sciences. 2015;**3**(1):1-10. DOI: 10.5455/2320-6012.ijrms20150101

[19] Bishop JP. Euthanasia, efficiency, and the historical distinction between killing a patient and allowing a patient to die. Journal of Medical Ethics. 2006;**32**(4):220-224. DOI: 10.1136/jme.2005.013839

[20] McLachlan HV. The ethics of killing and letting die: Active and passive euthanasia. Journal of Medical Ethics. 2008;**34**(8):636-638. DOI: 10.1136/jme.2007.023382

[21] Sprung CL, Truog RD, Randall Curtis J, Joynt GM, Baras M, Michalsen A, et al. Seeking worldwide professional consensus on the principles of end-of-life care for the critically ill: The consensus for worldwide end-of-life practice for patients in intensive care units (WELPICUS) study. American Journal of Respiratory and CriticalCare Medicine. 2014;**190**(8):855-866. DOI: 10.1164/rccm.201403-0593CC

[22] Pellegrino ED. Decisions to withdraw life-sustaining treatment: A moral algorithm. JAMA. 2000;**283**(8):10651067. DOI: 10.1001/jama.283.8.1065

[23] Koenig HG. A commentary: The role of religion and spirituality at the end of life. The Gerontologist. 2002;**42**(3):20-23. DOI: 10.1093/geront/42. suppl_3.20

[24] Long C. Cultural and spiritual considerations in palliative care. Journal of Pediatric Hematology/Oncology. 2011;**33**:S96-S101. DOI: 10.1097/MPH.0b013e318230daf3

[25] Platovnjak I. The role of (Christian) spirituality in the economy in the light Laudato si. Synthesis Philosophica. 2019;**67**(1):73-86. DOI: 10.21464/sp34106

[26] Burkhart L, Schmidt L, Hogan N. Development and psychometric testing of the spiritual care inventory instrument. Journal of Advanced Nursing. 2011;**67**(11):2463-2472. DOI: 10.1111/j.13652648.2011.05654.x

[27] Fosarelli P. Medicine, spirituality, and patient care. JAMA. 2008;**300**(7):836-838. DOI: 10.1001/jama.300.7.836

[28] Teoli D, Kalish VB. Palliative Care. V: StatPearls. Treasure Island, FL: StatPearls Publishing; 2020. Available from: https://www.ncbi.nlm.nih.gov/books/NBK493216/ [Accessed: May 10, 2022]

[29] World Health Organization. Palliative Care – Solidfacts. Geneva: World Health Organization; 2004

[30] Nolan S, Saltmarsh P, Leget C. Spiritual care in palliative care: Working towards an EAPC taskforce. European Journal of Palliative Care. 2011;**18**(2):86-89

[31] Clarke J. A critical view of how nursing has defined spirituality. Journal of Clinical Nursing. 2009;**18**(12):16661673. DOI: 10.1111/j.1365-2702.2008.02707.x

[32] Daaleman T, VandeCreek L. Placing religion and spirituality in end-of-life care. JAMA. 2000;**284**(19):2514-2517. DOI: 10.1001/jama.284.19.2514

[33] Chater K, Tsai C. Palliative care in a multicultural society: A challenge for western ethics. Australian Journal of Advanced Nursing. 2008;**26**:95-100

[34] Ferrell B, Munevar C. Domain of spiritual care. Progress in Palliative Care. 2012;**20**(2):66-71. DOI: 10.1179/1743291X12Y.0000000013

[35] Byrne M. Spirituality in palliative care: What language do we need? Learning from pastoral care. International Journal of Palliative Nursing. 2007;**13**(3):118-124. DOI: 10.12968/ijpn.2007.13.3.23273

[36] Mitchell BL, Mitchell LC. Review of the literature on cultural competence and end-of-life treatment decisions: The role of the hospitalist. Journal of the National Medical Association. 2009;**101**(9):920-926. DOI: 10.1016/s0027-9684(15)31040-3

[37] Diana SL, Yarrarapu SNS, Martin RL. Cultural Religious Competence in Clinical Practice. V. Statpearls. Treasure Island, FL: StatPearls Publishing; 2020. Available from: https://www.ncbi.nlm.nih.gov/books/NBK493216/ [Accessed: May 10, 2022]

[38] Padela A. Medical ethics in religious traditions: A study of Judaism, Catholicism, and Islam. Journal of the Islamic Medical Association of North America. 2006;**38**:106-117. DOI: 10.5915/38-3-5245

[39] Skralovnik S. Judovstvo: kršČanstvo in islam: Izvirnost in prepletenost. Ljubljana: Maribor; 2018

[40] Schockenhoff E. Etika življenja: temeljna naČela in konkretna vpraša- nja. Celje: Celjska Mohorjeva družba; 2013

[41] Splošni religijski leksikon. Ur. Drago Bajt in Marta Kocjan–Barle. In: Prev. Miro Bajt, Bogdan Gradišnik in MajaBreznik. Ljubljana: Modrijan; 2007

[42] Malik M. Islamic and Catholic bioethics of pain medication: A response to mercy argument. Journal of Islam in Asia. 2012;**9**(1):213-227. DOI: 10.31436/jia.v9i1.335

[43] Markwell H. End-of-life: A catholic view. The Lancet. 2005;**366**(9491):1132-1135. DOI: 10.1016/S01406736(05)67425-9

[44] Gatrad AR, Sheikh A. Medical ethics and Islam: Principles and practice. Archives of Disease in Childhood. 2001;**84**(1):72-75. DOI: 10.1136/adc.84.1.72

[45] JegliČ U, Mari Jože Osredkar. Pravni sistemi islama. Bogoslovni vestnik. 2018;**78**(4):1075-1086

[46] Flick U, Kardorff EV, Steinke I. Qualitative Interviews: An Overview. A Companion to Qualitative Research. London: Sage; 2004. pp. 203-208

[47] Flick U, Kardorff EV, Steinke I. Qualitative Content Analysis. A Companion to Qualitative Research. London: Sage; 2004. pp. 266-269

[48] Bülow H-H, Sprung CL, Reinhart K, Prayag S, Bin D, Armaganidis A, et al. The world's major religions' points of view on end-of-life decisions in the intensive care unit. Intensive Care Medicine. 2008;**34**(3):423-430. DOI: 10.1007/s00134-007-0973-8

[49] Kassim J, Nemie P, Alias F. Religious, ethical and legal considerations in end-of-life issues: Fundamental requisites for medical decision making. Journal of Religion and Health. 2016;**55**(1):119-134. DOI: 10.1007/s10943-014-9995-z

[50] Koran. Prevedel Erik Majaron. TržiČ: UČila International; 2004

[51] Sachedina A. End-of-life: The Islamic view. Lancet. 2005;**366**(9487):774-779. DOI: 10.1016/S01406736(05)67183-8

[52] Torry M. Ethical religion in primary care. London Journal of Primary Care (Abingdon). 2017;**9**(4):49-53. DOI: 10.1080/17571472.2017.1317407

[53] Khorfan R, Padela AI. The bioethical concept of life for life in Judaism, Catholicism, and Islam: Abortion when the Mother's life is in danger. Journal of Islamic Medical Association of North America. 2010;**42**(3):99-105. DOI: 10.5915/42-3-5351

Chapter 18

Spiritual Distress and Depression in Palliative Care

Teresa Velosa

Abstract

The Spirit is a movement that entails the five dimensions of the Human being—intellectual, physical, social, emotional, and spiritual. Spiritual distress (SD) and depression are related to spirituality and are most prevalent in palliative care (PC) settings. SD and depression have a deep connection to the inner energy of the Human being. Both can affect and be affected by all the five dimensions of the Human being and negatively impact the quality of these patients' lives. Men seek meaning in life (MIL), and a lack of this dimension is common in SD and depression. Nevertheless, although closely interrelated, SD and depression are distinct diagnoses. There seems to be evidence of having precise clinical indicators and different pharmacological and non-pharmacological therapeutic approaches. Patient-centred approaches should be the gold standard practice at this particularly vulnerable moment.

Keywords: spiritual distress, depression, spirituality, palliative care, person-centred care

1. Introduction

Patients facing chronic and life-threatening diseases have a high probability of having psychopathology. In PC settings, the prevalence of SD ranges from 10 to 63% [1–7] and depression from 5 to 50% [8–11].

SD and depression are closely interrelated and share some characteristics regardless of cultural traditions: at the bodily level, symptoms of insomnia, pain, and fatigue; at the emotional level, a sense of guilt, fear, anger, anxiety, loneliness, alienation, lack of confidence, and despair; at the existential level, experiencing a lack of hope, a lack of MIL, and a lack of serenity [12–14].

Notably, suffering is challenging for all health care teams caring for patients, and their families, with progressive diseases and impending death. This topic will provide an overview of the clinical indicators of SD and depression towards its differential diagnosis and the setting of proper treatment, whether pharmacological or non-pharmacological.

2. Background

2.1 The dimensions of the human being

Edith Stein's phenomenological-anthropological work describes the Human person as formed by a material part (*Körper*), a spiritual part (*Leib*) through which the empathy phenomenon occurs and a primordial metaphysical part. In this regard, the Human being is a 'body-soul-Spirit' conception [15].

Eastern's medicine holistic 'body-mind-Spirit' approach has a long tradition. It considers health a balance between individual and environmental dimensions. They take into account a multitude of conceptions, such as the *yin* and the *yang*, 'the five internal elements (metal, wood, water, fire, and earth), the six environmental conditions (dry, wet, hot, cold, wind, and flame), other external sources of harm (physical injury, insect bites, poison, overeat, and overwork), and the seven emotions (joy, sorrow, anger, worry, panic, anxiety, and fear)' ([16], pp. 261–2). They pay attention to the patient rather than to isolated symptoms, using exercise, meditation, benevolence, art, and bonding, beyond many specific therapies, to integrate the physical, emotional, and spiritual. They believe that letting go (excess emotions), the spirits (values, life philosophy, and beliefs) and the environment (diet, weather, exercise) are crucial in restoring harmony and health [16].

Western medicine traditionally focuses mainly on the disease. However, since 2013, the WHO Health construct considers the person's physical, mental, social, and spiritual dimensions [17]. PC, and Primary Health Care, are leaders in the holistic vision of care. Addressing the whole dimensions of the patients promotes joyful and healthy living and, ultimately, a peaceful, meaningful dying experience.

2.2 The spirit

The word spirit, in English, comes from the French '*esperit*', which comes from the Latin '*spiritus*', which means breath, vigor, and courage. It is the vital principle animating Humans and, in some views, all living creatures [18]. It differs from the Latin '*anima*', whose etymological meaning is also breathing but evolved to a concept named soul [18]. Some recognize the soul as the spiritual heart. It has the attributes of consciousness, affectivity, intellect, memory, will, and personality [19]. Some use the terms mind and soul interchangeably; others claim that the mind is part of the soul; to others, the soul does not exist, but only the mind is tangible [20].

We can describe Spirit as something real though immaterial that transcends the body-soul/body-mind dichotomy. Some call it Nature, Energy, God, Budahh, Allah and others just Consciousness or a Superior Being. It is within and beyond the person. Man's awareness of a spiritual world is millenary and a means of coping with the distress and tribulations of his life. It is a resource for strength, guidance, and courage in life's journey [21].

In 1988, Beck, Rawlins, and Williams conceptualized the Spirit as the core aspect of the person permeating its five dimensions (physical, social, emotional, intellectual, and their Spirituality) (**Figure 1**). The Spirit is perceptible in the thoughts, behaviors, and language [22, 23].

Viktor Frankl's extensive study, inclusive during the Second World War concentration camps, made him consider Man a spiritual being. He stated that despite the terrible surroundings, some sensitive people could reach high levels of spiritual life and spiritual freedom [24].

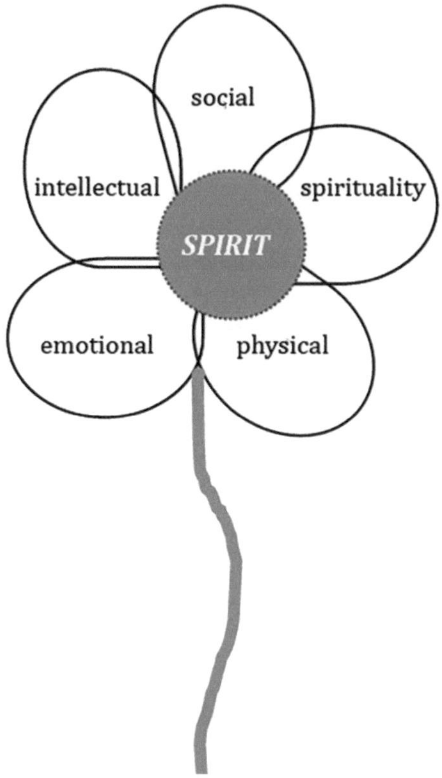

Figure 1.
A conceptualization of the dimensions of the Person as Beck, Rawlins, and Williams (adapted).

2.3 What is spirituality

A set of three health consensus conferences, held in 2009, 2012, and 2013, established the basis for defining spirituality as 'a dynamic and intrinsic aspect of humanity through which persons seek ultimate meaning, purpose, and transcendence, and experience relationship to self, family, others, community, society, nature, and the significant or sacred. Spirituality is expressed through beliefs, values, traditions, and practices' ([25], p. 646).

Spirituality has three axes: intrapersonal (with oneself), interpersonal (with others - persons, nature, arts), and transpersonal (with a superior transcendental dimension) [26]. It is a multidimensional construct that embraces all settings and cultures. Spirituality comprehends the search for purpose and meaning through religion or other paths. It may include arts, relationships with nature, others or the sacred, values, beliefs, prayer, faith, reason, and compassion [25, 27]. Therefore, as a universal human capacity, spirituality encompasses believers and agnostics [28].

In illness situations, questions such as 'Why me? What is the meaning of my suffering?' may arise. In these moments, the sense of connectedness with oneself, others or the sacred can be a means of positive or negative spiritual coping (SC). Positive SC gives a sense of a benevolent worldview and increases gratitude, hope, meaning, purpose, and peace [29]. Negative SC is related to higher levels of distress, anger, depression, uncontrollable pain, and other symptoms [30, 31]. Spirituality can significantly impact the individual's psychosocial and physical health and overall quality of life (QOL) [32].

2.4 PC

In the 1950s, PC began with the hospice movement, propelled by Dame Cicely Saunders's work and an increasing consciousness of unaddressed suffering and deprivation amongst cancer patients dying at home [33].

'PC is an approach that improves the QOL of patients and their families facing the problems associated with life-threatening illness, through the prevention and relief of suffering by means of early identification, impeccable assessment, and treatment of pain and suffering, including psychosocial, spiritual, and existential suffering as well as physical pain' [34]. Outcomes are optimized when PC begins early after the diagnosis, is delivered at the same time as curative or disease-modifying treatment, and is carried out until death [35].

PC is based on the patient's needs, not on the patient's prognosis. The World Health Organization advocates that PC should include assessing and managing pain, physical, cultural, social, psychological, and spiritual needs [34]. The gold standard is teamwork, dignity, compassionate, and person-centred care [27].

3. Definitions

3.1 Spiritual well-being (SWB)

Spirituality is one of the eight domains of quality supportive care for the dying [36], and SWB is a desired outcome for spiritual interventions in PC patients [25]. It comprises the positive aspects of spirituality, such as finding purpose and MIF (even though diseases and struggles might occur), a sense of connectedness (with ourselves or significant others), the capacity to bliss with art, music, literature, and nature, and a transcendent feeling that we are not alone, that we are nurtured and guided by a power greater than oneself [12, 21].

Although we might consider there are religious, existential, and non-spiritual individuals who can value or not the aspects of religion, faith, and a sense of peace and MIL [28, 37], they all experience spiritual cycles of development and depending on their spiritual growth, different levels of SWB [21].

SWB impacts health's physical and emotional aspects [38–40]. Research indicates a positive link between SWB, life expectancy, and QOL [41, 42]. SWB is a buffer to anxiety [43], depression [43, 44], hopelessness, suicidal ideation, and the desire for hastened death [45, 46]. Indeed, a crucial study found significant solid negative correlations between SWB and desire for hastened death, hopelessness, and suicidal ideation, being the most robust predictor and beyond that of depression [46].

3.2 SD

Distress results from potentially harmful psycho-biological changes in the human body (such as increased heartbeat, dyspnea, and elevated blood pressure) caused by stressors and unsuccessful coping mechanisms. Distress can be physical, social, emotional and spiritual [47, 48].

SD is 'a state of suffering related to the impaired ability to experience MIL through connectedness with self, others, world or a Superior Being. This definition contains the attributes of SD: suffering, impaired spirituality, contrary to SWB, and related to

MIL' ([12], p. 6). This SD definition is a North American Nursing Diagnosis Association-International (NANDA-I) nursing diagnosis [49], supported by the 2018 National Coalition for Hospice and PC guidelines [35], and is under the Puchalski et al., 2013 spirituality definition [25]. Subsequently, through a validation study in cancer patients, *'expresses suffering'* was the defining characteristic (DC) (**Table 1**) with the highest sensitivity value. Of all the reminder SD-DC, *'lack of MIL'* had the highest specificity value. We might conceptualize SD as a state of suffering related to a lack of MIL [2].

SD has been a nursing diagnosis since 1978. SD nursing diagnoses reported in PC patients [1, 2, 6] undertook three main steps: a clinical interview and identification of SD-DC by the health professional ('expresses lack of MIL' and 'expresses suffering' were necessary criteria); after the interview, the answer to the question 'Are you in SD?' (a positive response was a required condition); application of a SWB questionnaire (SD diagnosis required a score lower than the cutoff value defined for SWB). Some of the

- Anger behaviors
- Crying
- Decreased expression of creativity
- Disinterested in nature
- Dysomnias
- Excessive guilt
- Expresses alienation
- Expresses anger
- Expresses anger towards power greater than self
- Expresses concern about beliefs
- Expresses concern about the future
- Expresses concern about values system
- Expresses concerns about family
- Expresses feeling abandoned by power greater than self
- Expresses feeling of emptiness
- Expresses feeling unloved
- Expresses feeling worthless
- Expresses insufficient courage
- Expresses loss of confidence
- Expresses loss of control
- Expresses loss of hope
- Expresses loss of serenity
- Expresses need for forgiveness
- Expresses regret
- Expresses suffering
- Fatigue
- Fear
- Impaired ability for introspection
- Inability to experience transcendence
- Maladaptive grieving
- Perceived loss of MIL
- Questions identity
- Questions MIL
- Questions meaning of suffering
- Questions own dignity
- Refuses to interact with others

Source: *([49], p. 460).*

Table 1.
DCs of SD nursing diagnosis.

SWB questionnaires used are the Functional Assessment of Chronic Illness Therapy—SWB Scale (FACIT-Sp) [50] and the SWB Questionnaire (SWBQ) [51]. One study considered a practical resource in diagnosing SD scoring low (<3) in the SWBQ and the patient self-diagnosis as having SD [52]. Assessing SD should be cautious and patient-centred, respecting each one's values and beliefs. Therefore, health care professionals should be trained to be competent and compassionate in delivering spiritual care [27].

In times of serious illnesses, unmet spiritual needs [53], such as an impaired ability to pray, experience meaning and purpose, love and belonging, hope, peace, and gratitude [54], and inadequate SC strategies [53, 55–57] can lead to a state of SD [53]. Additionally, SD can lead to increased physical and emotional symptoms and health service utilization [53]. Patients with SD are more likely to be younger and have financial distress, pain, drowsiness, nausea, anxiety, and depression [4, 5]. In 2016, Velosa et al., in a study carried out in primary health care with PC patients, found an association between SD and alcoholism and between SD and traumatic life events [6]. Although there are literature references that link spirituality and alcoholism in the PC field [58], more research is necessary on this particular issue. As for traumatic life events, NANDA-I describes traumatic life events as risk populations to experience SD [49].

Unfortunately, some evidence shows that those with SD are less likely to ask for chaplaincy help [59]. Also, some patients may feel uncomfortable discussing this subject unless the health professional launches the issue [60]. As 'SD should be treated with the same intent and urgency as treatment for pain or any other medical or social problem' ([27], p. 891), PC professionals are urged to impeccably identify the patient's spiritual needs and screen for SD.

Assisting SD seems to allow spiritual/existential growth at the end of life [61, 62], improve the patient's cooperation with shared medical decisions [63], provide less aggressive care at the end of life [64], and have a role in pain control [65]. Addressing SD allows the patient to be regarded as a whole, not just a disease, and is a means to offer dignity and quality of care [21].

3.3 Depression

Mental health issues are frequent in the scope of those suffering from severe and life-threatening diseases, and depression is the most common [14]. Patients facing PC can be suffering from unrelieved pain, the burden of their symptoms, loneliness, and financial problems; they can be grieving the loss of their self-sufficiency, autonomy, self-image, or the shift of their roles within their family/ friends/community/work; they might be experiencing spiritual concerns, connectedness impairments, and unresolved complex psycho-social-spiritual issues. Many of them experience disease progression, treatment failure, and approaching death.

Sadness, fear, and distress are normal reactions in those with advanced diseases, but if the person has the necessary background, support, courage, and coping skills, depression may not occur. On the other hand, depression is more likely to occur if risk factors are present (**Table 2**). Amongst these, a history of depression is a significant risk factor [72], although de novo major depressive episodes occur in many cases [73].

Depression has devastating effects on the patient and their family QOL as it affects the capacity to interact with others, concentrate and resolve practical matters, and feel peace [13]. Also, there is a close bidirectional association between depression and physical symptoms [74], including pain [75], in PC patients. Suicidal ideation is associated with uncontrolled pain [76], meaning pain control is a primary concern when treating depression.

Physical: • Functional disability • Undermanaged pain control • Poor symptom control • Malnutrition, thiamine, vitamin B_{12}, and folate deficiencies • Cognitive decline	*Socioeconomic:* • Poor social support • Lack of intimate relationships, isolation • Financial distress
Medications and treatments: • Corticosteroids • Opioids • Interleukin-2 • Interferon • Amphotericin • Radiation therapy (to the brain or head and neck) • Chemotherapy agents (vincristine, vinblastine, asparaginase, intrathecal methotrexate, paclitaxel, docetaxel) • Hormonal agents (cyproterone, leuprolide, and tamoxifen) • Oral contraceptives • H2-blockers • Metoclopramide • Sedative-hypnotics • Antihypertensives (propranolol, reserpine, and methyldopa)	*Neoplasms:* • Head and neck cancer • Pancreatic cancer • Brain tumors • Brain metastasis • Carcinomatosis • Lung cancer • Lymphoma *Cancer-related:* • Hypercalcemia • Hypercortisolism (pituitary tumors) • Tumor-generated toxins • Neuroendocrine changes/ paraneoplastic syndromes • Immunologic reactions
Diseases: • Terminal or advanced illnesses • HIV/AIDS • Hypothyroidism • Alzheimer's disease • Parkinson's disease • Stroke • Huntington's disease • Multiple sclerosis *Miscellaneous:* • Non-compliance with treatments • Requests for assisted suicide • Denial (of a short life expectancy) • Loss of MIL • Race (less common in black men) • Female gender • Younger age	*Individual and family history:* • Past personal history of depression • Family history of depression • Alcoholism family history • Substance abuse • Recent negative life events • Pessimism, neuroticism, low self-esteem, worried, stress-sensitive, obsessive, unassertive, and dependent personality traits • Early loss, disturbing, hostile or negative environment during childhood
Sources: *Refs. [13, 14, 66–71].*	

Table 2.
Risk factors for depression in PC.

Additionally, depression is associated with incapacity [77], disfigurement [77], poorer prognosis, higher mortality [78, 79], increased costs [80], treatment withhold or withdrawal requests [14], higher requests to hasten death, and higher suicide rates in the terminally ill [81, 82]. Nevertheless, a critical study showed a strong correlation between depression and a desire for hastened death in participants low in SWB ($r = 0{\cdot}40$, $p < 0{\cdot}0001$) but not in those high in SWB ($r = 0{\cdot}20$, $p = 0{\cdot}06$) [46].

Self-transcendence seems to be directly and negatively related to depression [83]. Self-transcendence is a psycho-social-spiritual force that expands the self from its ego. When Humans transcend the limitations and boundaries of the ego, they release the entire manifestation of the Spirit sharing feelings, creating personal bounds, humor, laughter, enjoyment, and self-acceptance [15, 83].

Brief screening measures for depression in the terminally ill are easy to apply and avoid burdening these patients with extensive questionnaires, as they are already commonly distressed. The simple question 'Are you depressed?' or two questions (low mood and low interest) perform well in PC patients [84–86]. A full assessment and psychiatric clinical interview of the patient is then necessary.

Depression diagnostic criteria most widely accepted are the Diagnostic and Statistical Manual of Mental Disorders (DSM), presently in its fifth edition [87]. These include disruptive mood dysregulation disorder, major depressive disorder, persistent depressive disorder (dysthymia), substance/medication-induced depressive disorder, depressive disorder due to another medical condition, other specified depressive disorder (such as short duration or with incomplete criteria), and unspecified depressive disorder (such as that diagnosed in emergency room settings when incomplete data are available). These last two are sometimes named minor depression as they do not complete the criteria for major depression (just two to four items). However, in the settings of PC, receiving a severe diagnosis can lead to an adjustment disorder with depressive symptoms (onset of emotional or behavioral symptoms within 3 months from a stressor, if out of proportion towards the situation and not just a natural grieving) [85, 87].

The standard features of all depressive syndromes are sad, empty, or irritable mood with somatic or cognitive symptoms that disrupt everyday life [87]. Anhedonia and the absence of positive affect are specific to depression [76].

In diagnosing depression in PC patients, there is a need to rule out a substance/-medication-induced depressive disorder whose symptoms can occur after substance onset and withdrawal (included substances are: alcohol, phencyclidine, other hallucinogen, inhalant, opioid, sedative, hypnotic, or anxiolytic, amphetamine, or other stimulant and cocaine). Also, excluding a depressive disorder due to another medical condition is warranted, particularly in these severely ill patients with multiple comorbidities. Medical conditions possibly related to depression are stroke, Huntington's disease, Parkinson's disease, Cushing's disease, and hypothyroidism (**Table 1**). A detailed history of past depressive syndromes, family history, and time frames for the onset and remission of the depressive symptomatology is vital [87].

Disrupted mood dysregulation disorders present severe, persistent irritability with temper outbursts. The core features of persistent depressive disorder (dysthymia), which is chronic low-grade depression, are at least 2 years long, no more than two-month periods without depressed symptoms, and two or more of the six following symptoms: poor appetite or overeating, sleep disturbances, fatigue, low self-esteem, lack of concentration, and hopelessness [14, 87].

Major depression is the classical picture of depression. Criteria include loss of interest or pleasure (anhedonia) or depressed mood for at least 2 weeks and four additional symptoms of the following seven: significant weight loss or gain; insomnia or hypersomnia; psychomotor agitation or retardation; fatigue or loss of energy; feelings of worthlessness or inappropriate guilt; diminished ability to think or concentrate, or indecisiveness; recurrent thoughts of death or recurrent suicidal ideation (passive or active) [87].

However, the four somatic symptoms included in DSM criteria, fatigue, weight loss, sleep disturbances, and lack of concentration, can be caused by the underlying disease or the treatment side effects in those with cancer or chronic, severe illnesses. Therefore, Endicott replaced these four criteria with alternative cognitive symptoms:

brooding or self-pity or pessimism; tearful or depressed appearance in face or body posture; social withdrawal or decreased talkativeness; lack of reactivity or non-reactive mood or inability to be cheered [88]. Although the Endicott approach is used mainly in research, it is imperative in PC as it values signs of depression, sometimes only detected by relatives and close ones, as patients might be reluctant to show their emotional suffering and try to be positive in the presence of health care providers. Signs include irritability, flat affect, hunched shoulders, looking down, crestfallen appearance, slowed thought and movement, careless hygiene and clothing, negative expressions of sadness, and non-compliance with treatment [13, 88, 89].

Additionally, dysphoric mood, brooming/self-pity/pessimism, and loss of interest/pleasure are prominent features of depression in PC [8]. In the terminally ill, feelings of hopelessness, helplessness, worthlessness, guilt, lack of pleasure, and suicidal ideation (passive or active) strongly support depression diagnosis and are regarded as appropriate clinical hallmarks of depression [89, 90].

4. Prevalence of SD and depression in PC

4.1 Prevalence of SD in PC

The prevalence of SD is still a pursued goal, as research in this area is limited, and diagnostic criteria diverge within the research literature.

A scoping review in inpatient settings found a prevalence of SD between 10 and 63% [7]. Studies using questionnaires found a prevalence of depression of 44% in cancer PC patients [4, 5]. Studies using structured interviews showed SD prevalences of 28% in patients with end-stage renal disease undergoing hemodialysis [91] and 23% in cancer patients with ongoing oncologic treatment [3]. Other studies using a three-part methodology (clinical interview, the patient's opinion as having SD, and a SWB questionnaire) revealed SD prevalences of 23% in palliative patients followed in a primary care setting [6], 38.6% in women with breast cancer [1], and 40.8% in cancer patients undergoing chemotherapy [2].

4.2 Prevalence of depression in PC

As psychopathology is common in those facing serious and life-threatening diseases, depressive syndromes attain many PC patients. However, there are no valid, specific criteria for this population, and there may be marked differences depending on the diagnostic criteria.

The most standard method used in the research field to diagnose depression is the Structured Clinical Interview for DSM based on the DSM Diagnostic Criteria [87], followed by Endicott's Criteria [67, 88]. A study on a sample of PC patients found that 9.2% had depression according to the DSM-4 and 13.8% with Endicott's [8].

A meta-analysis based on studies using only psychiatric interviews provided a prevalence of all types of depression combined of 24.6% in PC settings and 20.7% in oncologic and hematologic settings [92].

Within a systematic review, 7 to 49% of a subgroup of PC cancer patients met depression diagnosis. This systematic review considered only studies that administered diagnostic interviews and met specific quality research criteria [11].

A median prevalence of depression of 29% (ranging from 16 to 50%) was revealed in a systematic analysis in inpatients with advanced diseases when all depressive disorders were included, such as major and minor depression, dysthymia, and depressive adjustment disorders, as measured by questionnaire. The Hospital Anxiety and Depression Scale (HADS) [93] was the most widely used assessment and accounted for the result. However, this systematic analysis also reported a median of 15% for major depression (ranging from 5 to 26%) when using psychiatric interviews [10].

4.3 Co-occurrence of SD and depression in PC

In two studies, 13% of adult PC patients followed at primary care had simultaneous SD and depression [6] and 15.1% in a study with patients admitted to a geriatric rehabilitation centre [92]. More research is desirable on this issue.

5. SD and depression differential diagnosis

Spirit, the core aspect of Humans [21, 23], affects all the Person dimensions (**Figure 1**). However, in this conceptualization, SD and depression, although interrelated, belong to different facets [94], the 'spirituality' and the 'emotional'.

Expressions such as 'Why me?', 'What is the point?', or 'Why can't I find a point in living?' were frequently mentioned in Swinton's qualitative work on depression [23]. Also, a sense of purposelessness and perceived loss of a relationship with God or a higher power were indicative of SD. He stated, 'Depression is a profound spiritual illness that digs into the heart of a person's spirit and forces them to face experiences of meaninglessness and hopelessness' ([23], p. 167).

MIF is a core aspect of Human life [24] and spirituality [12, 25, 95, 96]. PC research showed a negative correlation between MIF and depression, anxiety and the wish to hasten death and a positive correlation with life satisfaction [97]. Also, MIL is protective against psychological distress at the end of life [98]. In a study, women with breast cancer with higher levels of meaning and peace had significantly lower depressive symptoms at 6 months [99]. Another vital research with adults seeking treatment for mental illness revealed a 'significant negative association between depression symptom severity and MIF was observed at lower but not the highest levels of spirituality. In the presence of elevated depressive symptomatology, those participants who reported high levels of spirituality reported comparable levels of MIF to those without elevated depressive symptomatology' [100].

Spirituality can significantly impact the individual's psychosocial health [32]. However, depression relates to the emotional field, diverging from SD [94] and has precise medical diagnostic criteria [87, 88]. Depression can co-occur or mimic SD, as they share symptomatology.

SD is the opposite of SWB [12, 101], when applying the total concept of each term. In reality, there are gradation levels of SD and SWB. But this is true for almost every construct, such as anxiety or depression. We can say a person is anxious when perceiving a future threat but only has anxiety disorder when the anxious state is out of proportion to the event and significantly impacts everyday life and performance [87]. We can say a person is sad because something negative happened and is a normal reaction, but we say a person is depressed if the sadness is out of proportion to the event and impairs daily functioning [87]. Applying this reasoning, we can hypothesize that experiencing SD-DC (**Table 2**), such as anger (towards oneself/ others/God), lack of hope or serenity, can be expected as part of the Human spiritual journey of growth and transformation; however, there is a point, above which, it harms the person causing a state of suffering. At this stage, we might diagnose SD.

A cross-sectional study in primary health care with PC adult patients showed a link between depression and the SD-DC 'expresses lack of MIF' but not with the SD-DC 'expresses suffering' [6]. More research is desirable to address this issue.

The standard features of all depressive syndromes are sad, empty, or irritable mood with somatic or cognitive symptoms that disrupt everyday life [87]. Anhedonia and the absence of positive affect are specific to depression [76]. In the terminally ill, after impeccable pain control, worthlessness, guilt, and suicidal ideation strongly suggest depression [89, 90]. The core features of SD are SD-DC [49], including a perceived loss of MIF and the expression of suffering [2, 49]. SD and depression diagnoses are clinical and can only be ascertained through a client-therapeutic relationship and complete anamnesis. Questionnaires can be helpful for screening or corroboration purposes.

Spiritual suffering seems to be a key component in the differential diagnosis between SD and depression and might be relieved with anxiolytic medication (instead of antidepressants). In PC patients, anger, grief, regret, the need for forgiveness, receiving terminal care, and relevant traumatic life events might indicate SD [2, 6, 49]. On the other hand, depression is based on somatic or cognitive symptoms, where antidepressive medications play a crucial role [90]. SWBQ, FACIT-Sp, and HADS scales are effective screening tools [50–52, 60, 93].

6. SD treatment

Spiritual care embraces all religious, existential, cultural, and philosophical backgrounds. All health care team members at all levels of care are responsible for delivering spiritual care as they address the biopsychosocial-spiritual model of holistic care [58, 102], with complete respect towards the patient's and family's beliefs, traditions, values, and practices [25, 35].

Spiritual care comprises spiritual screening, history, and assessment. Spiritual needs, strengths, and resources must be registered in the patient's health records [35]. Whenever a patient presents spiritual issues but no SD, non-chaplain clinicians can provide generalist spiritual care [60].

Following Stein, being Empathy an extent of Leib (soul), Frank stated that a genuine client-therapist relationship based on Empathy is therapeutical [103]. The healing process is complex and simple at the same time. Healing from within requires the healer to be genuine and non-judgemental, putting their reactions and prejudices aside to be with the patient compassionately and respectfully. However, the healer also needs to nurture their spirituality. Training in spiritual care and mindfulness clinical congruence is desirable for all health care professionals [104]. Primarily, impeccable control of pain and other symptoms is necessary [34].

Also, addressing the patient's spiritual, cultural, and emotional needs, reinforcing positive spiritual/religious coping mechanisms and spiritual strengths (such as the use of spiritual/cultural symbols and practices and support from the religious leader and religious community), meaning-centred psychotherapy, dignity-centred psychotherapy, legacy creation, art and music therapies, yoga, and mindfulness meditation, are therapeutical [60].

SD diagnosis demands spiritual assessment from a board-certified chaplain (BCC) trained to deal with spiritual and emotional issues and a spiritual care plan with interventions and expected outcomes discussed within the PC team. BCC is part of the PC team and trained in PC. Referral to the nearest PC team might be necessary whenever no BCC is available [60, 105].

If the SD diagnosis is uncertain or the patient has spiritual concerns such as anger (towards God or others), sense of abandonment (by God or others), need for forgiveness and reconciliation, concerns about death and the afterlife, and conflict between religious beliefs and recommended treatment, amongst others, referral to a BCC is indicated [27, 102].

Referral to mental health care can also be required [60]. Although medication is not the core treatment of SD [21], it can be a supportive measure until the patient overcomes SD. In that case, anxiolytics seem more prone to relieve SD than antidepressive medication [6].

7. Depression treatment

The first step in treating depression is relieving uncontrolled symptoms, particularly pain [71, 74, 75, 86], providing social support, and addressing psychological and spiritual issues such as anger related to diagnostic delay and SD [90].

Terminally ill patients with depression benefit from holistic, patient-centred, and compassionate care. Psychotherapies include dignity therapy, meaning-centred psychotherapy, therapeutic life review, and cognitive behavior therapy. If the diagnosis is uncertain, there is suicidal ideation (passive or active), the patient who requests assisted suicide or euthanasia, is psychotic or unresponsive to therapy, there is an indication for a mental health specialist referral [67, 90].

Antidepressants effectively treat depression in PC patients. As PC patients have a short life expectancy, especially in the terminally ill, drugs with rapid onset of action are helpful, such as psychostimulants which have shown to be effective in PC patients [106]. Drug choice also depends on the duration and severity of symptoms, comorbidities, side effects, possible drug-drug interactions, and the availability of liquid or orodispersable formulations [67, 90].

Although there are no guidelines on first-choice antidepressants in PC, selective serotonin reuptake inhibitors (SSRIs) are well tolerated, have fewer side effects and drug-to-drug interactions, and are usually the first choice. Start with 50% of the standard dose and then titrate based on the efficacy and side effects balance. Psychostimulants benefit patients with fatigue and depressive patients weeks from dying or with severe depression. Psychostimulants are usually well tolerated, used alone or with tricyclics or SSRIs until these begin to work. It is advisable to know well and use one medication of each class of antidepressants. **Table 3** summarizes the advantages and disadvantages of each antidepressant [67, 71, 90].

Drug class	Advantages	Side effects & disadvantages
Antidepressant		
SSRIs	• Well tolerated • A wider margin of safety	• Common: headache, restlessness, anxiety, agitation, headache, sexual dysfunction, GI symptoms (diarrhea and nausea), insomnia, and activation (mainly with fluoxetine and sertraline) • Rare: SIADH, increased bleeding risk, extrapyramidal symptoms, serotonin syndrome (in combination with other serotonergic drugs)
Fluoxetine		• Inhibits P450 (CYP): possible DDIs
		• Long half-life
Paroxetine	• Fewer active metabolites	
Fluvoxamine		
Sertraline	• Fewer DDIs than the other SSRIs	
Citalopram		
Escitalopram		
TCAs	• Useful in neuropathic pain	• Sedating and anti-ACh effects, including dry mouth, blurred vision, constipation, urinary retention, tachycardia, orthostasis, impaired memory, confusion, hallucinations or delirium, cardiotoxicity
Desipramine	• Less anti-ACh than other TCAs	
Nortriptyline*		• Sinus tachycardia, severe angina, and an increase in ventricular ectopy
Imipramine*		• Exacerbate the sedating effects of other medications
Amitriptyline		
Doxepin		
SNRIs		• Similar to SSRIs plus increased BP
Venlafaxine	• Generally well tolerated	• The use in terminally ill has not been studied
Atypical antidepressants		
Mirtazapine*	• Effective for improving depression, QOL, insomnia, nausea, anxiety, appetite, and weight gain	• Sedating
		• Risk of serotonin syndrome (if co-administration with SSRIs)
Trazodone	• Good for insomnia	• Sedating
	• Analgesic effects	• Priapism
Nefazodone		• Should not be used (liver failure)

Drug class	Advantages	Side effects & disadvantages
Bupropion	• Energizing effects	• Seizures, insonmia, anxiety, decreased appetite
		• Avoid in Child-Pugh C cirrhosis
Mianserin	• Adjuvant analgesic properties	• Effective in cancer patients
MAOIs		• Large number of DDI
Triazolobenzodiazepine		
Alprazolam	• Mildly effective antidepressant and anxiolytic	
Psychostimulants	• Rapid onset of action	• Agitation, insomnia, tremor, anxiety, dry mouth, anorexia, headache, nausea, diarrhea, seizures psychosis, arrhythmia, nightmares • Cardiac decompensation (in older patients with heart disease) • Rarely: hallucinations, delirium
	• Energizing	
	• Improve cognitive impairment	
	• Useful in dysphoric mood associated with opioid-related sedation, appetite, weakness, and fatigue	
	• Promote a sense of well-being	
Dextroamphetamine, Methylphenidate		
Modafinil	• Less sympathomimetic effects	

No efficacy data on chronic kidney disease; BP, blood pressure, CYP, cytochrome; DDI, drug-drug interactions; GI, gastrointestinal; MAOIs, monoamine oxidase inhibitors; SIADH, syndrome of inappropriate antidiuretic hormone secretion; SNRIs, serotonin and norepinephrine reuptake inhibitors; SSRIs, selective serotonin reuptake inhibitors; TCAs, tricyclic antidepressants.
Sources: *Refs. [67, 71, 107–109].*

Table 3.
Antidepressants advantages and disadvantages in palliative medicine.

8. Conclusions

SD and depression are common diagnoses in PC patients and share common symptoms. Both have a substantial impact on the patients and their families QOL. However, although interrelated, SD and depression belong to different dimensions, 'spirituality' and mental, respectively. Depression, in PC, should be diagnosed based mainly on cognitive symptoms, and SD diagnosis relies on a state of suffering related to a perceived loss of MIL. Impeccable pain and symptom control are mandatory for SD and depression. Spiritual care is fundamental in treating SD, whereas pharmacologic and psychotherapy are united in treating depression.

Conflict of interest

The author declares no conflict of interest.

Appendices and nomenclature

BCC	board-certified chaplain
DC	defining characteristic
DSM	diagnostic and statistical manual of mental disorders
FACIT-Sp	functional assessment of chronic illness therapy—spiritual well-being scale
HADS	hospital anxiety and depression scale
MIL	meaning in life
NANDA-I	North American Nursing Diagnosis Association-International
PC	palliative care
QOL	quality of life
SC	spiritual coping
SD	spiritual distress
SSRIs	selective serotonin reuptake inhibitors
SWB	spiritual well-being
SWBQ	spiritual well-being questionnaire

Author details

Teresa Velosa
Northern Regional Health Administration, Dr. Vale Lima Health Unit, Braga, Portugal

*Address all correspondence to: teresavelosa@gmail.com

References

[1] Caldeira S, Timmins F, de Carvalho EC, Vieira M. Nursing diagnosis of "spiritual distress" in women with breast Cancer: Prevalence and major defining characteristics. Cancer Nursing. 2016;**39**(4):321-327. DOI: 10.1097/NCC.000000000000 03103

[2] Caldeira S, Timmins F, de Carvalho EC, Vieira M. Clinical validation of the nursing diagnosis spiritual distress in cancer patients undergoing chemotherapy. International Journal of Nursing Knowledge. 2017; **28**(1):44-52. DOI: 10.1111/ 2047-3095.121053

[3] Schultz M, Meged-Book T, Mashiach T, Bar-Sela G. Distinguishing between spiritual distress, general distress, spiritual well-being, and spiritual pain among Cancer patients during oncology treatment. Journal of Pain and Symptom Management. 2017; **54**(1):66-73. DOI: 10.1016/j. jpainsymman.2017.03.0183

[4] Hui D, de la Cruz M, Thorney S, Parsons HA, Delgado-Guay M, Bruera E. The frequency and correlates of spiritual distress among patients with advanced cancer admitted to an acute palliative care unit. The American Journal of Hospice & Palliative Care. 2011;**28**(4): 264-270. DOI: 10.1177/10499091 103859173

[5] Delgado-Guay MO, Chisholm G, Williams J, Frisbee-Hume S, Ferguson AO, Bruera E. Frequency, intensity, and correlates of spiritual pain in advanced cancer patients assessed in a supportive/palliative care clinic. Palliative & Supportive Care. 2016; **14**(4):341-348. DOI: 10.1017/ S147895151500108X3

[6] Velosa T, Caldeira S, Capelas M. Depression and spiritual distress in adult palliative patients: A cross-sectional study. Religions. 2017;**8**(8):1-18. DOI: 10.3390/rel80801563

[7] Roze des Ordons AL, Sinuff T, Stelfox HT, Kondejewski J, Sinclair S. Spiritual distress within inpatient settings-a scoping review of Patients' and Families' experiences. Journal of Pain and Symptom Management. 2018; **56**(1):122-145. DOI: 10.1016/j. jpainsymman.2018.03.0093

[8] Huey NS, Guan NC, Gill JS, Hui KO, Sulaiman AH, Kunagasundram S. Core symptoms of major depressive disorder among palliative care patients. International Journal of Environmental Research and Public Health. 2018;**15**(8): 1-9. DOI: 10.3390/ijerph150817583

[9] Antunes B, Murtagh F, Bausewein C, Harding R, Higginson IJ, Euro I. Screening for depression in advanced disease: Psychometric properties, sensitivity, and specificity of two items of the palliative care outcome scale (POS). Journal of Pain and Symptom Management. 2015;**49**(2):277-288. DOI: 10.1016/j.jpainsymman.2014.06. 0143

[10] Hotopf M, Chidgey J, Addington-Hall J, Ly KL. Depression in advanced disease: A systematic review Part 1. Prevalence and case finding. Palliative Medicine. 2002;**16**(2):81-97. DOI: 10.1191/02169216302pm507oa3

[11] Walker J, Holm Hansen C, Martin P, Sawhney A, Thekkumpurath P, Beale C, et al. Prevalence of depression in adults with cancer: A systematic review. Annals of Oncology. 2013;**24**(4):895-900. DOI: 10.1093/annonc/mds5753

[12] Caldeira S, Carvalho EC, Vieira M. Spiritual distress-proposing a new definition and defining characteristics. International Journal of Nursing Knowledge. 2013;**24**(2):77-84. DOI: 10.1111/j.2047-3095.2013.01234.x3

[13] Noorani NH, Montagnini M. Recognizing depression in palliative care patients. Journal of Palliative Medicine. 2007;**10**(2):458-464. DOI: 10.1089/jpm.2006.00993

[14] Wilson KG, Chochinov HM, de Faye BJ, Breitbart W. Diagnosis and management of depression in palliative care. In: Chochinov H, Breitbart W, editors. Handbook of Psychiatry in Palliative Medicine. New York: Oxford University Press; 2000. pp. 25-49

[15] Stein E. Finite and Eternal Being: An Attempt at an Ascent to the Meaning of Being. Washington DC: ICS Publications Institute of Carmelite Studies; 2002. 625 p

[16] Chan C, Ho PS, Chow E. A body-mind-spirit model in health: An Eastern approach. Social Work in Health Care. 2001;**34**(3–4):261-282. DOI: 10.1300/j010v34n03_023

[17] Dhar N, Chaturvedi SK, Nandan D. Spiritual health, the fourth dimension: A public health perspective. WHO South East Asia Journal of Public Health. 2013; **2**(1):3-5. DOI: 10.4103/2224-3151.1158263

[18] Online Etymology Dictionary. Spirit (v) [Internet]. 2023. Available from: https://www.etymonline.com/word/spirit [Accessed: May 26, 2023]

[19] Wallenfang DL. The heart of the matter. Edith Stein on the substance of the soul. Logos: A Journal of Catholic Thought and Culture. 2014;**17**(3): 118-142

[20] Teichman J. The Mind and the Soul. London: Routledge; 2014. 116 p. DOI: 10.4324/97813157402563

[21] O'Neill MT, Mako C. Addressing spiritual pain. Health Progress. 2011; **92**(1):42-45

[22] Rawlins RP, Williams SR, Beck CK. Mental Health-Psychiatric Nursing: A Holistic Life-Cycle Approach. 3rd ed. London: Mosby Year Book; 1993. 980 p.

[23] Swinton J. Spirituality and Mental Health Care. London: Jessica Kingsley; 2001. 224 p

[24] Frankl VE. Man's Search for Meaning. New York: A Washington Square Press Publication of Pocket Books; 1985. 221 p

[25] Puchalski CM, Vitillo R, Hull SK, Reller N. Improving the spiritual dimension of whole person care: Reaching national and international consensus. Journal of Palliative Medicine. 2014;**17**(6):642-656. DOI: 10.1089/jpm.2014.94273

[26] Benito E, Oliver A, Galiana L, Barreto P, Pascual A, Gomis C, et al. Development and validation of a new tool for the assessment and spiritual care of palliative care patients. Journal of Pain and Symptom Management. 2014;**47**(6): 1008-18 e1. DOI: 10.1016/j.jpainsymman.2013.06.0183

[27] Puchalski C, Ferrell B, Virani R, Otis-Green S, Baird P, Bull J, et al. Improving the quality of spiritual care as a dimension of palliative care: The report of the Consensus Conference. Journal of Palliative Medicine. 2009;**12**(10): 885-904. DOI: 10.1089/jpm.2009.01423

[28] Bethesda (MD): National Cancer Institute. Spirituality in Cancer Care (PDQ®): Health Professional Version

[Internet]. PDQ Supportive and Palliative Care Editorial Board, editor2002 2022-10-26. 2002. Available from: https://www.cancer.gov/about-cancer/coping/day-to-day/faith-and-spirituality/spirituality-hp-pdq [Accessed: May 28, 2023]

[29] Pargament K, Feuille M, Burdzy D. The brief RCOPE: Current psychometric status of a short measure of religious coping. Religions. 2011;**2**(1):51-76. DOI: 10.3390/rel201005123

[30] Steinhauser KE, Fitchett G, Handzo GF, Johnson KS, Koenig HG, Pargament KI, et al. State of the science of spirituality and palliative care research Part I: Definitions, measurement, and outcomes. Journal of Pain and Symptom Management. 2017; **54**(3):428-440. DOI: 10.1016/j.jpainsymman.2017.07.0283

[31] Balboni TA, Fitchett G, Handzo GF, Johnson KS, Koenig HG, Pargament KI, et al. State of the science of spirituality and palliative care research part II: Screening, assessment, and interventions. Journal of Pain and Symptom Management. 2017;**54**(3): 441-453. DOI: 10.1016/j.jpainsymman.2017.07.0293

[32] Panzini RG, Mosqueiro BP, Zimpel RR, Bandeira DR, Rocha NS, Fleck MP. Quality-of-life and spirituality. International Review of Psychiatry. 2017;**29**(3):263-282. DOI: 10.1080/09540261.2017.12855533

[33] Saunders C. The evolution of palliative care. Journal of the Royal Society of Medicine. 2001;**94**(9): 430-432. DOI: 10.1177/014107680109400904 3

[34] World Health Organization. WHO Definition of Palliative Care [Internet]. 2020. Available from: https://www.who.int/news-room/fact-sheets/detail/palliative-care [Accessed: June 25, 2023]

[35] National Coalition for Hospice and Palliative Care. National Consensus Project for Quality Palliative Care Clinical Practice Guidelines for Quality Palliative Care. 4th ed [Internet]. Richmond, VA: National Coalition for Hospice and Palliative Care; 2018. Available from: https://www.nationalcoalitionhpc.org/wp-content/uploads/2020/07/NCHPC-NCPGuidelines_4thED_web_FINAL.pdf [Accessed: June 24, 2023]

[36] National Consensus Project for Quality Palliative Care. Clinical Practice Guidelines for Quality Palliative Care. 3rd ed [Internet]. Pittsburgh, PA: National Consensus Project for Quality Palliative Care; 2013. Available from: https://www.nationalcoalitionhpc.org/wp-content/uploads/2017/04/NCP_Clinical_Practice_Guidelines_3rd_Edition.pdf [Accessed: June, 26, 2023]

[37] Riley BB, Perna R, Tate DG, Forchheimer M, Anderson C, Luera G. Types of spiritual well-being among persons with chronic illness: Their relation to various forms of quality of life. Archives of Physical Medicine and Rehabilitation. 1998;**79**(3):258-264. DOI: 10.1016/s0003-9993(98)90004-13

[38] Perez JE, Chartier M, Koopman C, Vosvick M, Gore-Felton C, Spiegel D. Spiritual striving, acceptance coping, and depressive symptoms among adults living with HIV/AIDS. Journal of Health Psychology. 2009;**14**(1):88-97. DOI: 10.1177/13591053080979493

[39] Noor A, Bashir S, Earnshaw VA. Bullying, internalized hepatitis (hepatitis C virus) stigma, and self-esteem: Does spirituality curtail the relationship in the workplace. Journal of Health Psychology. 2016;**21**(9):1860-1869. DOI: 10.1177/13591053145672113

[40] Bekelman DB, Havranek EP, Becker DM, Kutner JS, Peterson PN, Wittstein IS, et al. Symptoms, depression, and quality of life in patients with heart failure. Journal of Cardiac Failure. 2007;**13**(8):643-648. DOI: 10.1016/j.cardfail.2007.05.0053

[41] Abdi A, Doulatyari PK, Mahmodi M, Torabi Y. Relationship of spiritual wellbeing with life expectancy and quality of life for patients living with heart failure. International Journal of Palliative Nursing. 2022;**28**(6):262-269. DOI: 10.12968/ijpn.2022.28.6.2623

[42] Bai M, Lazenby M. A systematic review of associations between spiritual well-being and quality of life at the scale and factor levels in studies among patients with cancer. Journal of Palliative Medicine. 2015;**18**(3):286-298. DOI: 10.1089/jpm.2014.01893

[43] McCoubrie RC, Davies AN. Is there a correlation between spirituality and anxiety and depression in patients with advanced cancer? Supportive Care in Cancer. 2006;**14**(4):379-385. DOI: 10.1007/s00520-005-0892-63

[44] Nelson CJ, Rosenfeld B, Breitbart W, Galietta M. Spirituality, religion, and depression in the terminally ill. Psychosomatics. 2002;**43**(3):213-220. DOI: 10.1176/appi.psy.43.3.2133

[45] McClain-Jacobson C, Rosenfeld B, Kosinski A, Pessin H, Cimino JE, Breitbart W. Belief in an afterlife, spiritual well-being and end-of-life despair in patients with advanced cancer. General Hospital Psychiatry. 2004;**26**(6):484-486. DOI: 10.1016/j.genhosppsych.2004.08.0023

[46] McClain CS, Rosenfeld B, Breitbart W. Effect of spiritual well-being on end-of-life despair in terminally-ill cancer patients. Lancet. 2003;**361**(9369):1603-1607. DOI: 10.1016/S0140-6736(03)13310-73

[47] Schneiderman N, Ironson G, Siegel SD. Stress and health: Psychological, behavioral, and biological determinants. Annual Review of Clinical Psychology. 2005;**1**:607-628. DOI: 10.1146/annurev.clinpsy.1.102803.1441413

[48] Lazarus RS, DeLongis A. Psychological stress and coping in aging. The American Psychologist. 1983;**38**(3): 245-254. DOI: 10.1037//0003-066x.38.3.2453

[49] NANDA International. In: Herdman TH, Kamitsuru S, Lopes CT, editors. NANDA International Nursing Diagnoses: Definitions and Classification 2021–2023. 12th ed. New York: Thieme Medical Publishers, Inc.; 2021. 590 p. DOI: 10.1055/b0000005153

[50] Peterman AH, Fitchett G, Brady MJ, Hernandez L, Cella D. Measuring spiritual well-being in people with cancer: The functional assessment of chronic illness therapy–Spiritual well-being scale (FACIT-Sp). Annals of Behavioral Medicine. 2002;**24**(1):49-58. DOI: 10.1207/S15324796ABM2401_063

[51] Gomez R, Fisher JW. Domains of spiritual well-being and development and validation of the spiritual well-being questionnaire. Personality and Individual Differences. 2003;**35**(8):1975-1991. DOI: 10.1016/s0191-8869(03)00045-x3

[52] Caldeira S, Timmins F, de Carvalho EC, Vieira M. Spiritual well-being and spiritual distress in Cancer patients undergoing chemotherapy: Utilizing the SWBQ as component of holistic nursing diagnosis. Journal of Religion and Health. 2017;**56**(4): 1489-1502. DOI: 10.1007/s10943-017-0390-43

[53] Grant E, Murray SA, Kendall M, Boyd K, Tilley S, Ryan D. Spiritual issues and needs: Perspectives from patients with advanced cancer and nonmalignant disease. A qualitative study. Palliative Support Care. 2004;**2**(4):371-378. DOI: 10.1017/s14789515040404903

[54] Flannelly K, Galek K, Bucchino J, Vane A. Relative prevalence of various spiritual needs. Scottish Journal of Healthcare Chaplaincy. 2006;**9**(2):25-30

[55] Piderman KM. On these holy mountains. Journal of Health Care Chaplaincy. 2022;**28**(1):63-68. DOI: 10.1080/08854726.2020.17454883

[56] Villagomeza LR. Spiritual distress in adult cancer patients: Toward conceptual clarity. Holistic Nursing Practice. 2005; **19**(6):285-294. DOI: 10.1097/00004650-200511000-000103

[57] Brown AE, Whitney SN, Duffy JD. The physician's role in the assessment and treatment of spiritual distress at the end of life. Palliative & Supportive Care. 2006;**4**(1):81-86. DOI: 10.1017/s14789515060600933

[58] Sulmasy DP. A biopsychosocial-spiritual model for the care of patients at the end of life. The Gerontologist. 2002; **42**:24-33

[59] Fitchett G. Screening for spiritual risk. Chaplaincy Today. 2014;**15**(1):2-12. DOI: 10.1080/10999183.1999.107671023

[60] Puchalski CM, Otis-Green S, Handzo G. Overview of spirituality in palliative care [Internet]. UpToDate. 2022. Available from: https://www.uptodate.com/contents/overview-of-spirituality-in-palliative-care [Accessed: May 28, 2023]

[61] Carpenter JS, Brockopp DY, Andrykowski MA. Self-transformation as a factor in the self-esteem and well-being of breast cancer survivors. Journal of Advanced Nursing. 1999;**29**(6): 1402-1411. DOI: 10.1046/j.1365-2648.1999.01027.x3

[62] Delgado-Guay MO. Spirituality and religiosity in supportive and palliative care. Current Opinion in Supportive and Palliative Care. 2014;**8**(3):308-313. DOI: 10.1097/SPC.00000000000000793

[63] Silvestri GA, Knittig S, Zoller JS, Nietert PJ. Importance of faith on medical decisions regarding cancer care. Journal of Clinical Oncology. 2003;**21**(7):1379-1382. DOI: 10.1200/JCO.2003.08.0363

[64] Peteet JR, Balboni MJ. Spirituality and religion in oncology. CA: A Cancer Journal for Clinicians. 2013;**63**(4): 280-289. DOI: 10.3322/caac.211873

[65] Carey LB, Newell CJ, Rumbold B. Pain control and chaplaincy in Australia. Journal of Pain and Symptom Management. 2006;**32**(6):589-601. DOI: 10.1016/j.jpainsymman.2006.06.0083

[66] Loosen PT, Beyer JL, Sells SR, Gwirtsman HE, Shelton RC, Baird P, et al. Mood Disorders. In: Ebert MH, Loosen PT, Nurcombe B, editors. Current Diagnostic and Treatment in Psychiatry. Lisbon: Lange Medical Books/McGraw-Hill; 2000. pp. 290-327

[67] Breitbart W, Dickerman AL. Assessment and Management of Depression in Palliative Care [Internet]. UpToDate. 2014. Available from: https://medilib.ir/uptodate/show/2205 [Accessed: July 04, 2023]

[68] Shakin EJ, Holland J. Depression and pancreatic cancer. Journal of Pain and Symptom Management. 1988;**3**(4): 194-198. DOI: 10.1016/0885-3924(88)90030-93

[69] Brown JH, Paraskevas F. Cancer and depression: Cancer presenting with depressive illness: An autoimmune disease? The British Journal of Psychiatry. 1982;**141**:227-232. DOI: 10.1192/bjp.141.3.2273

[70] Gottlieb SS, Khatta M, Friedmann E, Einbinder L, Katzen S, Baker B, et al. The influence of age, gender, and race on the prevalence of depression in heart failure patients. Journal of the American College of Cardiology. 2004;**43**(9):1542-1549. DOI: 10.1016/j.jacc.2003.10.0643

[71] Kissane DW, Doolittle M. Depression, demoralization, and suicidality. In: Cherny NI, Fallon MT, Kaasa S, Portenoy RK, Currow DC, editors. Oxford Textbook of Palliative Medicine. 5th ed. Oxford: Oxford University Press; 2015. pp. 1074-1084

[72] Belsher G, Costello CG. Relapse after recovery from unipolar depression: A critical review. Psychological Bulletin. 1988;**104**(1):84-96. DOI: 10.1037/0033-2909.104.1.843

[73] Cooper SG, Whyte S, Hansell C, Horvath K, Mahr CW, Mokadam NA, et al. Abstract 212: Incidence of depression and anxiety in patients with durable left ventricular assist device. Circulation: Cardiovascular Quality and Outcomes. 2017;**10**(Suppl. 3):A212-A212. DOI: 10.1161/circoutcomes.10.suppl_3.2123

[74] Lloyd-Williams M, Dennis M, Taylor F. A prospective study to determine the association between physical symptoms and depression in patients with advanced cancer. Palliative Medicine. 2004;**18**(6):558-563. DOI: 10.1191/0269216304pm923oa3

[75] Glover J, Dibble SL, Dodd MJ, Miaskowski C. Mood states of oncology outpatients: Does pain make a difference? Journal of Pain and Symptom Management. 1995;**10**(2):120-128. DOI: 10.1016/0885-3924(94)00073-t3

[76] Olie E, Guillaume S, Jaussent I, Courtet P, Jollant F. Higher psychological pain during a major depressive episode may be a factor of vulnerability to suicidal ideation and act. Journal of Affective Disorders. 2010;**120**(1–3):226-230. DOI: 10.1016/j.jad.2009.03.0133

[77] Goldberg RJ, Cullen LO. Depression in geriatric cancer patients: Guide to assessment and treatment. The Hospice Journal. 1986;**2**(2):79-98. DOI: 10.1080/0742-969x.1986.118825603

[78] Frasure-Smith N. Depression following myocardial infarction. JAMA. 1993;**270**(15):1819-1825. DOI: 10.1001/jama.1993.035101500530293

[79] Lloyd-Williams M, Shiels C, Taylor F, Dennis M. Depression–An independent predictor of early death in patients with advanced cancer. Journal of Affective Disorders. 2009;**113**(1–2):127-132. DOI: 10.1016/j.jad.2008.04.0023

[80] Kessler RC. The costs of depression. The Psychiatric Clinics of North America. 2012;**35**(1):1-14. DOI: 10.1016/j.psc.2011.11.0053

[81] Chochinov HM, Wilson KG, Enns M, Mowchun N, Lander S, Levitt M, et al. Desire for death in the terminally ill. The American Journal of Psychiatry. 1995;**152**(8):1185-1191. DOI: 10.1176/ajp.152.8.11853

[82] Breitbart W, Rosenfeld B, Pessin H, Kaim M, Funesti-Esch J, Galietta M, et al. Depression, hopelessness, and desire for hastened death in terminally ill patients with cancer. Journal of the American Medical Association. 2000;**284**(22):

2907-2911. DOI: 10.1001/jama.284.22.29073

[83] Haugan G, Innstrand ST. The effect of self-transcendence on depression in cognitively intact nursing home patients. ISRN Psychiatry. 2012;**2012**:1-10. DOI: 10.5402/2012/3013253

[84] Lloyd-Williams M, Dennis M, Taylor F, Baker I. Is asking patients in palliative care,"are you depressed?" appropriate? Prospective study. British Medical Journal. 2003;**327**(7411):372-373

[85] Chochinov HM, Wilson KG, Enns M, Lander S. "Are you depressed?" screening for depression in the terminally ill. The American Journal of Psychiatry. 1997;**154**(5):674-676. DOI: 10.1176/ajp.154.5.6743

[86] Mitchell AJ. Are one or two simple questions sufficient to detect depression in cancer and palliative care? A Bayesian meta-analysis. British Journal of Cancer. 2008;**98**(12):1934-1943. DOI: 10.1038/sj.bjc.66043963

[87] American Psychiatric Association. DSM-5 Task Force. Diagnostic and Statistical Manual of Mental Disorders: DSM-5™. 5th ed. Washington DC: American Psychiatric Publishing, Inc; 2013. 1000 p. DOI: 10.1176/appi.books.97808904255963

[88] Endicott J. Measurement of depression in patients with cancer. Cancer. 1884;**53**:2243-2249

[89] Block SD. Psychological issues in end-of-life care. Journal of Palliative Medicine. 2006;**9**(3):751-772. DOI: 10.1089/jpm.2006.9.7513

[90] Rayner L, Price A, Hotopf M, Higginson IJ. The development of evidence-based European guidelines on the management of depression in palliative cancer care. European Journal of Cancer. 2011;**47**(5):702-712. DOI: 10.1016/j.ejca.2010.11.0273

[91] De Cassia Lopes Chaves E, De Carvalho EC, De Souza Terra F, De Souza L. Clinical validation of impaired spirituality in patients with chronic renal disease. Revista Latino-Americana de Enfermagem. 2010;**18**(3):309-316. DOI: 10.1590/s0104-1169201000030 00033

[92] Mitchell AJ, Chan M, Bhatti H, Halton M, Grassi L, Johansen C, et al. Prevalence of depression, anxiety, and adjustment disorder in oncological, haematological, and palliative-care settings: A meta-analysis of 94 interview-based studies. The Lancet Oncology. 2011;**12**(2):160-174. DOI: 10.1016/S1470-2045(11)70002-X3

[93] Zigmond AS, Snaith RP. The hospital anxiety and depression scale. Acta Psychiatrica Scandinavica. 1983;**67**(6): 361-370. DOI: 10.1111/j.1600-0447.1983.tb09716.x3

[94] Bornet M-A, Rochat E, Dürst A-V, Fustinoni S, Büla C, von Gunten A, et al. Instruments to assess depressive symptoms and spiritual distress investigate different dimensions. Clinical Gerontologist. 2015;**39**(2):104-116. DOI: 10.1080/07317115.2015.11202553

[95] O'Connor TSJ, Meakes E, McCarroll-Butler P, Gadowsky S, O'Neill K. Making the most and making sense: Ethnographic research on spirituality in palliative care. Journal of Pastoral Care & Counseling. 1997;**51**(1):25-36. DOI: 10.1177/002234099705103

[96] Martsolf DS, Mickley JR. The concept of spirituality in nursing theories: Differing world-views and extent of focus. Journal of Advanced

Nursing. 1998;**27**(2):294-303. DOI: 10.1046/j.1365-2648.1998.00519.x3

[97] Chow EO. The role of meaning in life: Mediating the effects of perceived knowledge of stroke on depression and life satisfaction among stroke survivors. Clinical Rehabilitation. 2017;**31**(12): 1664-1673. DOI: 10.1177/02692155177086043

[98] Bernard M, Strasser F, Gamondi C, Braunschweig G, Forster M, Kaspers-Elekes K, et al. Relationship between spirituality, meaning in life, psychological distress, wish for hastened death, and their influence on quality of life in palliative care patients. Journal of Pain and Symptom Management. 2017; **54**(4):514-522. DOI: 10.1016/j.jpainsymman.2017.07.0193

[99] Yanez B, Edmondson D, Stanton AL, Park CL, Kwan L, Ganz PA, et al. Facets of spirituality as predictors of adjustment to cancer: Relative contributions of having faith and finding meaning. Journal of Consulting and Clinical Psychology. 2009;**77**(4):730-741. DOI: 10.1037/a00158203

[100] Bamonti P, Lombardi S, Duberstein PR, King DA, Van Orden KA. Spirituality attenuates the association between depression symptom severity and meaning in life. Aging & Mental Health. 2016;**20**(5):494-499. DOI: 10.1080/13607863.2015.10217523

[101] Georgesen J, Dungan JM. Managing spiritual distress in patients with advanced cancer pain. Cancer Nursing. 1996;**19**(5):376-383. DOI: 10.1097/00002820-199610000-000073

[102] Handzo G, Puchalski C. The role of the chaplain in palliative care. In: Cherny NI, Fallon MT, Kaasa S, Portenoy RK, Currow DC, editors. Oxford Textbook of Palliative Medicine. 5th ed. Oxford: Oxford University Press; 2015. pp. 170-176

[103] Frank JD. Psychotherapy: The restoration of morale. The American Journal of Psychiatry. 1974;**131**(3): 271-274. DOI: 10.1176/ajp.131.3.2713

[104] Hutchinson TA, Hutchinson N. Healing and whole-person care. In: Chochinov HM, Breitbart W, editors. Handbook of Psychiatry in Palliative Medicine: Psychosocial Care of the Terminally ill. 3rd ed. New York: Oxford University Press; 2022. DOI: 10.1093/med/9780197583838.001.00013

[105] Spiritual Health Association. Guidelines for Quality Spiritual Care in Health. Abbotsford, Australia: Spiritual Health Association; 2020 [Accessed: June 20, 2023]

[106] Johnson JR, Burnell-Nugent M, Lossignol D, Ganae-Motan ED, Potts R, Fallon MT. Multicenter, double-blind, randomized, placebo-controlled, parallel-group study of the efficacy, safety, and tolerability of THC: CBD extract and THC extract in patients with intractable cancer-related pain. Journal of Pain and Symptom Management. 2010;**39**(2):167-179. DOI: 10.1016/j.jpainsymman.2009.06.0083

[107] Mullish BH, Kabir MS, Thursz MR, Dhar A. Review article: Depression and the use of antidepressants in patients with chronic liver disease or liver transplantation. Alimentary Pharmacology & Therapeutics. 2014; **40**(8):880-892. DOI: 10.1111/apt.129253

[108] Shirazian S, Grant CD, Aina O, Mattana J, Khorassani F, Ricardo AC. Depression in chronic kidney disease and end-stage renal disease: Similarities and differences in diagnosis, epidemiology, and management. Kidney International

Report. 2017;**2**(1):94-107. DOI: 10.1016/j.ekir.2016.09.0053

[109] Zambrano J, Celano CM, Januzzi JL, Massey CN, Chung WJ, Millstein RA, et al. Psychiatric and psychological interventions for depression in patients with heart disease: A scoping review. Journal of the American Heart Association. 2020;**9**(22):e018686. DOI: 10.1161/JAHA.120.0186863

Chapter 19

Pets in Palliative Care

María Sabina Ah. Chu Sánchez de Spengler

Abstract

Although human interaction with domesticated animals has existed since time immemorial, it has recently been in the spotlight to make it a candidate for improving health. This is a chapter dedicated to reflecting on what characteristics of the human-pet nexus can constitute new and better ways to care for patients in palliative care. We review basic concepts in animal-assisted interventions and therapies and reflect on the characteristics of pets that serve to incorporate palliative care integrally into health. Observations and recommendations are mentioned to be considered in future studies.

Keywords: animal-assisted interventions, palliative, pets, dog, cat, horse

1. Introduction

The reason for writing this chapter is to analyze what role the human-animal relationship plays in palliative care. In these pages, we will review the different roles that animals occupy and the different ways in which pets can be seen from the point of view of palliative care.

First, one could ask, "What do pets have to do with Palliative Care?"

Palliative care as a philosophy has existed since humanity became aware of the importance of caring for a vulnerable partner, attending to the sick or helpless with dignity, and accompanying the terminally ill in solidarity with them through the process of dying.

Later, palliative care as a discipline in the field of health was objectified to ensure the interdisciplinary quality of life of human beings affected by diseases for which there is no cure, considering physical, psychic, social, and spiritual contexts, while at the same time addressing pain and other symptoms that cause severe suffering in the health system.

I will review what things in this human-animal nexus can be instruments in palliative care. The writer is a pediatrician who is in daily contact with patients in palliative care and who approached the world of therapies assisted by dogs rescued from the street that now keep company with patients and staff in palliative care.

2. Background

2.1 The relationship of humans with animals

The hominid species, by virtue of its superior brain power owing to the shape of the skull, evolved towards ever more sophisticated neural functions. Among many other abilities, humans can organize thoughts and share them with others.

 IntechOpen

Pets, which are the subject of this chapter, also have a level of neural sophistication. Phylogenetic characteristics and instinct, among other factors, brought dogs, cats, and other species into domestication [1]. The ability of pets to survive, coupled with their innate ability to learn, led humanity to regard dogs, cats, and the like as life partners.

The search for food, shelter, and companionship, which are merely basic biological functions, are particularly similar in mammals. Evolution, seen as a dynamic process, would sooner or later make humans and their pets co-workers.

In recent years, attempts have been made to include pets in the solution of health issues [2].

The integration of animals to solve health problems is a concept that today offers both opportunities and challenges. The One Health concept recognizes the link between animals and human beings in the same survival environment [3].

2.2 The dog and the human

Interactions between companion dogs and humans date back to the Ancient Neolithic period. Dogs were the first domesticated animals [4].

The dog in particular for its physical capabilities (its smell allows it to snoop and search with purpose; its muscular strength allows it to fight to defend its territory) and neuronal (ability to learn and distinguish) can be trained for the benefit of human work from the beginning of man-animal coexistence. In today's times, man should also think about updating the defense of the quality of life of our animal co-workers.

For the ancient Egyptians, it was the god Anubis, a companion of souls and bodies during their passage to the afterlife. In this civilization, they gave the divine characteristic to the qualities of companionship, protection, and fidelity that the dog has [5]. The deity who watches over health, the healing of diseases, funeral honors, and life beyond death has the head of a jackal.

2.3 Horses as healers

Since the Pleistocene, horses and humans have worked together, in transportation and cargo, in hunting and in war, in sport, in the commonplace of life, and in occasions of greatness.

Now let's fast forward in time to ancient Greece, the time of Plato, where long horseback rides were used to heal people suffering from incurable diseases to lift their spirits and restore their self-esteem [6].

The latter confirms what modern equine therapists know that the horse is a creature that is evolutionarily sensitive to the sensations of other living beings, captures the entire range of emotions, perceives different moods, and is capable of communicating with the other being [7].

2.4 Cat ownership and its effect on the health of the most vulnerable patients

Owning pets, specifically cats, is related to a decrease in stress levels and secondarily to a decrease in the risk of strokes. Cat purring can be a factor that lowers blood pressure, and catecholamine levels, and facilitates relaxation in humans. This may have an evolutionary explanation because purring is part of the natural sounds that cats produce to communicate that they are happy [8].

Cats require relatively less care than dogs or horses, they do not need to be taken for a walk, their size makes them fit on the lap, and they are agile, which makes them a good candidate to accompany an elderly person, someone who is ill, or a child.

With the company of the cat, the human being in a state of vulnerability and who feels alone learns to accept the other as they are. The cat is an animal that does not make value judgments when it seeks company, and this makes its presence special.

In palliative care, we find a universe of patients who feel alone, are marginalized, and for whom communication with their fellow human beings is difficult or impossible. Some examples are advanced dementia, degenerative neurological diseases, frail elderly people, and children with seizures or problems that affect their behavior and socialization. In these cases, the cat, as a companion animal, offers its tameness, its ease of care, and its portability.

2.5 The birth of animal-assisted goal- oriented Interventions with animal

Biophilia: Product of evolution and development that proposes that human beings deserve to affiliate with other forms of life [9].

Vernooij did an analysis of Human-Animal Interactions (HAI) following psychoanalytic theory and conceptualized that the function of the animal is to identify, protect, motivate, and serve as a catalyst in cases where humans encounter emotions that are difficult to handle [10].

When the initiative arose among the different associations interested in promoting the concept of visualizing animals as part of the range of therapies that should be at the service of health, it became clear that they should work on the definitions [11, 12].

Animal-Assisted Interventions (AAI) are interventions structured to achieve a goal, in which a service animal is intentionally incorporated. Achievements can be in the fields of health, education, social, or any area that promotes the improvement of life. The AAI is subdivided into three categories [13]:

Animal-Assisted Therapy (AAT) are structured intervention whose purpose is to achieve recovery, rehabilitation, or improvement of a health problem by increasing the patient's quality of life through the intervention of a professional human and animal team and includes documentation and acting in the management of this health achievement.

Animal-Assisted Education (AAE): these are activities whose objective is to achieve the acquisition of knowledge or skills that can be used in the service. The achievement that uses the presence or interaction of animals.

Animal-Assisted Activities (AAA): unlike the previous ones, they are informal activities. They have in their favor spontaneity in achieving achievements under the condition of pleasure in the company of an animal.

Pet therapy: It is synonymous with AAI. Which pets are used when defining pet therapy? It usually refers to the following species [14] (although they are not the only ones) the dog (Canis familiaris), the cat (Felis catus), the rabbit (Oryctolagus cuniculus), the horse (Equus caballus), and the donkey (Equus asinus). There are experiences with dolphins and birds used for AAI, but for the purpose of this article, we will discuss dogs, cats, and horses.

2.6 The one health concept

Before analyzing what role, animals play with people in palliative care; we will take a pause to discuss the One Health concept.

The One Health concept identifies the human-animal bond as a way to improve mental and physical well-being. The AAI is a set of interventions that incorporate a human-animal team whose objective is to contribute to the health of the patient (IAHAIO.IAHAION White paper). One Health proposes that the work of the human therapist with the animal therapist for global quality of life is a low-cost wellness alternative in this world where procedures to augment health are expensive. Thus, the relationship can result in sustainable benefits in time [15].

However, due to the recent arrival of animal-assisted interventions (AAI) in the health field, it is a subject of study. A determination must be made as to the true reasons why animals can cooperate with the healing process. Specifically, what type of patients will they best serve and what is the best way to integrate them into conventional therapies to provide advantages for both parties? The novel issue is to study how and why the presence of the animal can be in some ways beneficial for the recovery of people's health. This is how AAI emerged as a subject of study, protocolization, indications, and contraindications. In short, to discover if it fits into all the categories that other treatments do [16].

The advantages provided by the presence of an animal in an AAI are mental, physiological, social, and neurological, and probably modulated by a common neurological pathway that involves emotion, memory, reward, and affiliation. That is connected to the production of oxytocin in both the animal and the person [17]. Researchers are looking for the common factors that should be investigated to try to reach conclusions in a standardized and repeatable way.

2.7 Pets in palliative care: the topic of this chapter

Palliative care, given its holistic approach, with the help of pharmacology to treat symptoms, makes use of therapies that have a lot to do with psychological and personal well-being, drawing from disciplines such as mental health and social sciences [18].

The early contributions from parts of the medical community such as nursing, psychology, and social work, from the moment of diagnosis of an incurable disease result in improvement of the quality of life and initiate the healing process.

In addition to sciences such as physiotherapy, respiratory therapy, occupational therapy, and sensory conductive psychological therapy, there are alternative therapies such as music therapy, meditation, mindfulness, art therapy, and what is featured in this chapter, a therapy in which animals participate.

Let's look at some properties of our relationship with pets that help us incorporate the philosophy of palliative care into health care.

2.8 Pets as significant beings

Living with pets allows us to better understand the nature of all beings, and our pets provide us with significant life lessons. Many of us have memories of our years of raising a pet, which endured the passage of time.

As part of the education of children in the principles of behavior, fables are used in which the protagonists are animals. This makes animals wise and special beings within the teaching and understanding of existence.

Many times, in my experience as a pediatric and palliative oncologist, hospitalized patients have wished to return home for the company of their family, and that includes pets. For a patient who is going through a process of resilience, a pet accompanying them can be a factor that increases resilience. A beloved dog or cat, unconditionally giving affection, is a source of joy for a patient.

It is worth mentioning that, in the survey on which palliative care professionals base our management plans, we consider family members and significant pets; a fact that makes a difference in the management of the emotional, mental, and social aspects of the families we serve.

Animals have had symbolic meaning in different times and cultures, as we have seen.

Those of us who work with patients in palliative care might inject into our conversations with them narratives featuring animals that are enshrined in personal beliefs, in the current social reality, or in traditions.

For example, to explain to a child the different stages of life, we often refer to dogs that started as puppies and then grew up. In fact, the rapid reproductive cycle of rodents used as pets, such as hamsters, illustrates to children the dynamics of life in just a few weeks. Spiritual themes closely linked to palliative care are illustrated with natural metaphors, such as the metamorphosis of butterflies.

An event that recently occurred in Colombia [19] in the aftermath of a plane crash, in which children survived in the jungle. An army dog that put the search teams on alert played a fundamental role in the rescue. Fortunately, the children were found alive, but the Belgian shepherd was never found. With a moving story, the aborigines who are natives of that Guaviare jungle explained the loss of the dog according to their aboriginal worldview: "the dog's being is really a warrior guardian and he has gone with his mission accomplished". This ancient narrative relates to what often helps us as palliative care professionals and that is to reach the most symbolic part of our patients.

2.9 Pets as a reason to reflect physically psychically and spiritually

A wound or infection heals because the living organism has the ability to regenerate. And health science practitioners give the best of themselves to initiate or facilitate this process. Healing in palliative care is more than a physical process. Complete healing includes awareness of vulnerability, resilience in the face of adversity, and the realization that we all value our inner selves above our material body.

Experiences that have left their mark on the psyche also help this process of healing in palliative care. Also, of such great importance are relationships with other beings that have contributed to our lives; our human and animal companions.

The presence of a pet has healing value in that it can lower blood pressure and alleviate glycemia. Also, a pet that remains sitting next to the bed of a sick person is company, love, and presence. In a word, it is healing.

The concept of the "*Wounded Healer*", is one in which every person who works caring for the sick, through their lived experience as a human being and their compassionate companionship, can help a patient who cares, to find their own healing. This is both a spiritual and a scientific concept.

Animals can also be "wounded healers". I remember a teenage amputee whose company was her amputee dog.

An article by a medical colleague entitled "The Death of My Dog: Lessons Learned from the Palliative Care of an Animal" reminded me that I had learned a lot from my own experience of the death of my cat, Ursula. She suffered seizures at the end of her life. Because of my beloved pet, I have a better understanding of the subject of the approach to death of patients with terminal neurological disease, such as the author says in his reflections about his canine friend [20].

2.10 Could pets sense when death is near?

There are numerous cases in which a cat or dog literally detects death through its sense of smell. In the well-studied and described case of the cat Oscar, it is hypothesized that the feline, due to its natural sensitivity to changes in body temperature, "predicted" with better than clinical accuracy, which patient had a few hours left to live, and this was useful to the hospital/hospice staff in complying with getting notices to family members [21]. The case of Oscar is well known, a cat who lived in a hospice and who took long naps next to the beds of patients who were in their final hours of life. This phenomenon was observed and described by the hospice geriatrician and was the subject of a medical article in the New England Journal of Medicine [22].

After repeated and methodical observations, the hypothesis was raised that the feline could perceive the lack of heat in the patient's body and thus know that death was near. The cat's approach to the human being, as if it were its feline way of giving palliative care and individualized attention to those for whom the end was near, was the subject of an episode of the series "Dr. House" (18th episode of the 5th season) [23].

In any case, Oscar the hospice cat gave rise to serious medical discussions about the role of an animal in the search for high-quality palliative care.

Ethology, which is a part of zoology that studies animal behavior and its relationship with biological evolution, may have an explanation for that pet's uncanny ability. During the evolution of the species, canids and felines developed their sense of smell not only for hunting, reproduction, and survival but also as a way to detect which member of the pack was weak or sick.

The mammalian sense of smell can perceive ketones, which are biochemically derived from cells undergoing cell death.

2.11 Do dogs have a place in palliative care?

A dog that serves as a stimulus to perform therapy is not only a therapeutic incentive but a healing presence. There are physiological benefits for humans in interaction with dogs: it decreases the level of stress and blood pressure, and in diabetic children, the blood sugar level. In the field of mental health, it has been found that pet ownership is related to decreased stress levels in owners especially if they take them for walks and engage in physical activity.

At a time when the world was under the effects of the pandemic, interesting experiences were published such as an article based on observations in rural populations of Sri Lanka, where it was observed that dog ownership is related to family behaviors that promote their health and that of their communities [24]. Rathish et al. conclude that it is essential to have background information on the effects of a pet dog on personal and family health to implement One Health via human-animal interaction.

Despite the benefits, biosecurity and infection prevention precautions must be ensured in all interventions involving animals. In addition, there is much to study in terms of the characteristics of patients that can actually benefit (Dalton, 2022) [25]. At the forefront of these challenges is the concern for potential exposure to and spread of infectious disease agents, which was particularly relevant during the COVID-19 pandemic.

Human–dog interaction improves the mental well-being of participants as suggested by [26]. Prefrontal brain activation in healthy subjects increased with the rise in interaction and closeness with a dog. In their controlled trial, the observations suggest that interactions with a dog can activate stronger attentional processes in palliative care with animals.

More and more experiences are published in terms of animal-assisted therapy. Diabetes, post-traumatic stress, physical and emotional rehabilitation, and Alzheimer's are some pathologies with published articles in which the benefits of the presence of pets during therapy are evaluated. However, it is still a challenge to see a pet as a member of the palliative care team.

Palliative care units for symptom control have modified their policies so that significant beings for patients, including pets, can spend time with them, yielding improved quality of care, improvement in the patient's functionality scale in palliative care, and significantly better results on the Edmonton Symptom Assessment [27].

Schmitz et al., nursing professionals, published a publication on patients with advanced and incurable diseases in Dusseldorf at the Center for Palliative Medicine of the University of Dusseldorf [28].

In June 2014 at the Interdisciplinary Centre for Palliative Medicine of the University Hospital Dusseldorf, they performed animal-assisted therapy sessions and to date only very limited scientific data is available. In the field of Palliative Care, future research should focus on its possible benefits. In this study they described AAT in the company of dogs, recalling the writings of Florence Nightingale who wrote in her Nursing Notes that a small pet was excellent company for a chronically and long-ill patient (Nightingale) [29].

The indications for AAT were: severe tension, adjustment disorder, depression, demoralization syndrome, terminal delirium, and anxiety of fear. The AAT was determined by the doctor, or by the psycho-oncologist. Contraindications were patients allergic to animals, fear of the animal, or severe psychological distress (**Table 1**).

In the observations, it was notable that during the observation of the therapy dog, when they verbalized, they showed mirrored behavior and some individuals reflected their own emotions.

The most observed achievement in well-being was achieving relaxation, inducing an environment of good humor, and increasing the patient's rapport by allowing him/her to pet the dog. The authors make a recommendation for future studies to better formulate therapeutic indications and also to video record the sessions for monitoring purposes.

Since March 2020, the world of health services has experienced changes in the way it provides its services. There was an experience in Panama to be published as a poster in the SIOP Congress, that focused on the role a dog's company could have during the pediatric palliative care home visit [30].

The team visited pediatric patients in their homes during the COVID-19 pandemic. Two female dogs rescued from the street and rehabilitated, who were the pediatrician's pets, were incorporated into the team that made the visits. The author

1. Greeting of the Patient
2. Introducing the dog and motivational conversation. Opportunity to observe dog
3. Patient-dog activities: games, giving treats, physical activities
4. Farewell ritual, arranging for another therapy

Table 1.
The content of the AAT was.

observed that the pets entertained patients and family members, facilitated the spontaneity of conversation, and let two dogs, one per visit, accompany them to the patients' home. The observations were documented in order to make a list of activities that would make these visits an organized health service.

There was 99% compliance with routine activities programmed by the basic team, which were:

- Examine the child-patient
- Talk to the caregiver about the child's activities, health issues, or caregiving education
- Do procedures that do not require anesthesia at the patient's bedside
- Collect emotions and mental state of the patient and family members at home

This experience concludes that when visiting a child who is severely ill with a terminal illness, the presence of properly trained pets within the health team adds novelty to the family environment, can contribute to rapport between the team and the family, and can even promote an environment for conversation. On palliative care issues such as disease progression, limitation of efforts, and grief for the loss, since the animal fulfills its role as a catalyst, and while the pet is accompanying the child; the other members of the team may be interacting with the animals. Caregivers.

A detailed work from the Barretos Hospital in São Paulo, Brazil gives us details about the characteristics of the animal and specific care, it also mentions some cases in which this therapy is not indicated [31].

2.12 Characteristics of therapy animal

1. Docile in character and trained in obedience and socialization
2. That it has approval given by a veterinary professional and/or trainer
3. Have your vaccination and deforming card up to date
4. Have a bi-annual laboratory examination (hematological and biochemical) reviewed by a veterinarian
5. That it is a pet in good nutritional status and that it eats only animal food

The handler must have AAI training (**Table 2**).

2.13 Basic requirements for AAI

1. If present, contact a veterinarian and suspend contact with patients until the veterinary authority orders it.
2. The animal should not enter the kitchen or areas where food is prepared.

3. 24 hours before the presence of the animal in the AAI, it must: bathe, brush, groom, and cut nails, approval of the absence of ticks, fleas, lice, and other ectoparasites. Their paws will be disinfected with 70% alcohol before and after the session (**Tables 3** and **4**).

2.14 The presence of animals that assist in therapy not only benefits patients, but health personnel, as well

A study held at the Central Military Hospital in the Czech Republic observed nursing staff that had the opportunity to play, feed, or give water to a dog that was already working as a therapeutic pet in the long-stay ward and in the internal medicine room.

Salivary cortical levels and perception of stress were measured and it was observed that both showed a decrease with a single intervention. The recommendation is to

Stress, fatigue, agression
Estrus
Immunodepression
Infections
Open wounds
Episodes of diarrhea and/or vomiting
Fecal or urinary incontinence

Table 2.
Rule out the following circumstances in the animal.

Regarding which patients should not be visited by an animal, and therefore would not benefit from AAI
1. Patients with isolation precautions
2. Patients with complications of surgical wounds
3. Patients with ostomies
4. Patients with neutropenia of 1000/mm^3 with the possibility of dropping even further
5. Patients who are scheduled for surgery in the next week
6. Patients with sepsis or severe infection
7. Patients with the presence of resistant bacteria

Table 3.
The human-animal team must comply with biosafety standards.

1. Patients who verbally do not want the presence of animals or are scared and have expressed this in the presence of an animal
2. Patients with severe mental disorders can cause stress or harm to the animal and this could trigger unfortunate situations
3. Allergies to animals

Table 4.
Other exclusion categories include.

consider including the interaction of health personnel with animals as a means of mitigating the consequences of work stress [32].

2.15 Equine therapy: how it helps patients live better

There are some basic concepts of equine therapy that are important in the field of chronic patient health.

Equine therapy or equestrian therapy is the set of treatments aimed at improving the quality of life of people suffering from some type of disability that affects their motor, cognitive, and emotional function. In this type of therapy, horses intervene as directed by health professionals or equinotherapists to apply the natural qualities of horses to help the patient regain their health [33].

Horse riding is an activity that requires neuromuscular coordination. The horse's back in contact with the pelvis, and its components, the lower extremities, which are the parts by which the riders support themselves, produces a neurological, sensory, motor, and psychological interaction [34].

In the time of Hippocrates, he recommended in his medical and academic texts the practice of horse riding to cure physical disabilities and mental pathologies (460 BC).

Chaisaignacc (1805–1895) described how muscle strength, voluntary control of movements, and coordination improved in neurological patients with the help of horseback riding [35].

The study of the Horse-Patient relationship began as a modern science after World War II, in Scandinavia and Germany. In 1953, Max Reichenbach carried out the first studies with numerous patients in Germany, developing the method of equine therapy [36].

In modern times, patients who congenitally suffer from neurological pathologies or their sequelae live for many years, with a good quality of life, as long as complications are avoided, rehabilitation begins early and the patient and their caregivers are mentally empowered in self-care.

This is why horse therapy has a lot to do with palliative care and health in general.

2.16 Helping to dispel doubts about the methodology of AAI and future recommendations

In the past, AAI has been criticized for its "inaccurate methodology, dubious analyses, conclusions that leave questions" [37].

In this regard, Holder and collaborators made a recent systematic review of the different therapies in which animals participated. These included activities facilitated by animals, pet therapy, and equine therapy in pediatric patients. They sought to summarize the information and compare conclusions [17].

This review proposes three mechanisms through which AAI obtained results in terms of the perception that it did improve the patient's quality of life. The mechanisms are:

1. Compatible Animal Personality Mechanism

2. Distraction and Entertainment Mechanism

3. Physical Touch Mechanism

4. Increased Human Interaction Mechanism

They concluded that AAI has an important place in improving the quality of life, but that theoretical frameworks are still at the forefront of the discussion since mechanisms often overlap. However, they do agree that everyone acting in coordination offers substantial well-being benefits.

2.17 Working mechanism of AAI and the planning of study questions

A systematic review published in Frontiers in Psychology, by authors Wagner et al. (2022) points out that in previous research on AAIs, the question to be answered was, “Do AAIs work?” However, the matter of, “How do they work?” has been practically ignored and to this day there is no answer [38].

This systematic review used well-known databases (PsychINFO, PSYNDEX; ERIC; MEDLINE; Embase, PubMed, Cochrane; Scorpus, Science, CINAHL, PTSDpubs) to identify 2001 reports and scanned 1893 abstracts on AAI.

The factor most mentioned in the citations found in the database is Human-Animal Interaction. This is what researchers most frequently point to as an AAI mechanism of action. What is it about this interaction that can reduce human stress or anxiety and increase oxytocin levels?

The next most indicated element is Movement by Animals. What is it about the dynamics of the movement of a horse during equine therapy that is beneficial for humans riding the horses?

The factors can be divided into specifics such as the presence of the animal, or the interaction with an animal, or non-specific such as the social interaction of a human with other humans when the animal is present. For each component, it is necessary to determine how it functions socially, psychologically, biochemically, and maybe even in some ways we have not considered to improve the condition of the patient in different ways.

The authors suggest that future research will establish which of these hypothetical factors can be clearly observed and measured.

2.18 Zoonosis and AAI

You must always consider the risk of diseases whose contagion cycle occurs between animals and humans.

Of course, the first thing that must be taken into consideration is the characteristics of the patient that make them vulnerable to infections. As in any therapy, a balance must be made between the risks of infection and the benefits. Strict control of conditions is necessary to avoid infections [39].

One Health analyzes this and warns that in all cases in which you plan to involve an animal in therapy, biosafety measures must be taken. Not all animals can participate in AAI and we already mentioned clinical situations where it is risky to interact with animals (neutropenic patients, with complicated wounds and drainage) those suitable must be subjected to an evaluation to consider whether the veterinary standards of biosafety, vaccination, grooming and compliance with import requirements [40].

3. Conclusion

Animal-assisted interventions have been used since their formal beginnings as an alternative therapy, to improve chronic conditions, restore mental health, and reduce cortisol levels. In other words, they aid in reducing stress, strengthening the musculoskeletal and neuronal systems, and treating mental illnesses.

Consider that the range of palliative care spans children with neurodegenerative pathologies, patients with cerebral palsy, patients with sequelae of surgeries to remove tumors or those who live with tumors, children, and adolescents who go to school under the stress of knowing that they have or have had cancer. As caregivers, whose lives are subject to caring for people with diseases that cannot be cured, the topic of animal-assisted interventions, activities, or education is of great interest to us.

They have their place in complementary therapy for incurable patients or those who live with chronic illness, by providing benefits such as stabilization of the disease, regulation of stress, and social improvement. All of this has its roots in people-to-animal contact that has never ceased to amaze us since the first human domesticated the first animal.

Our relationship as providers of palliative care working side-by-side with companion animals as we strive for the best quality of care has been harmonious, inspiring, and respectful and has been destined to endure since prehistoric times because animals have occupied the imagination of all peoples in all periods of history. As we look towards the future of this human-animal nexus that began when both species met, we propose taking it as an opportunity to view life with true and sincere Biophilia: working together for life and with respect for everything created, while not abandoning or fearing death, but rather accompanying it.

Thus, we will say in future years that by respecting our animal co-therapists, man is that much more human and the animals turn out to be true healers (**Figure 1**).

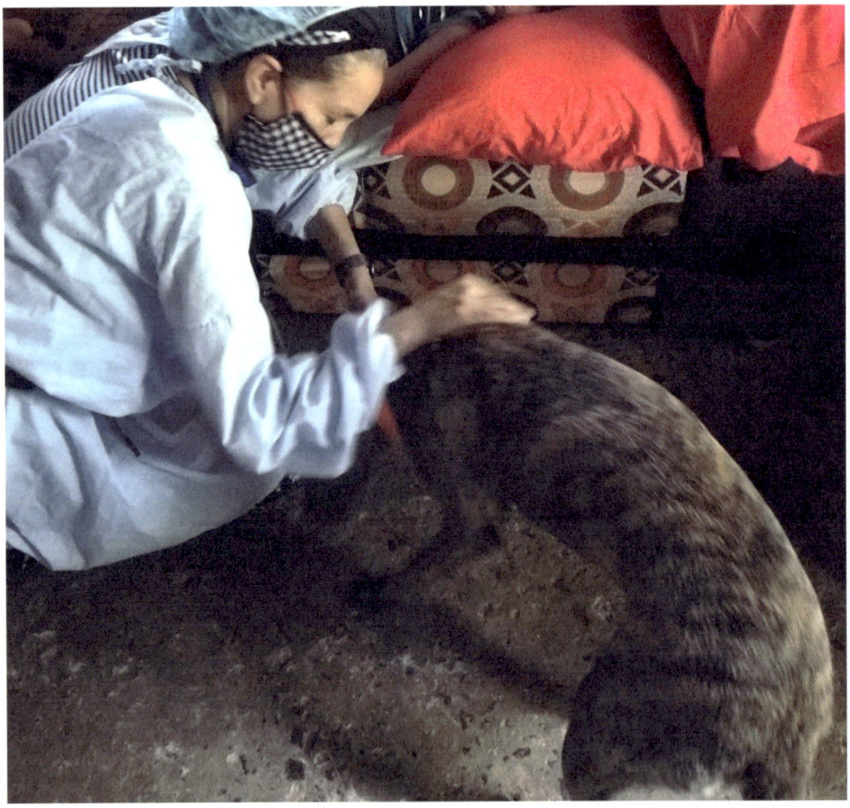

Figure 1.
The author with her dog Tosca visits a patient.

DOI: http://dx.doi.org/10.5772/intechopen.1003762

Author details

María Sabina Ah. Chu Sánchez de Spengler
Panama National Program of Palliative Care/Hospital Del Niño de Panamá Doctor José Renán Esquivel, Panama

*Address all correspondence to: mahchu@minsa.gob.pa

References

[1] Beck A. The biology of human-animal bond. Animal Frontiers. 2014;**4**:32-36. DOI: 10.2527/af.2014-0019

[2] Menna LF, Santaniello A, Todisco M, Amato A, Borrelli L, Scandurra Moretti A. Concept Paper The Human–Animal Relationship as the Focus of Animal-Assisted Interventions: A One Health Approach. International Journal of Environmental Research and Public Health. 2019;**16**:3660. DOI: 10.3390/ijerph16193660

[3] Hediger K, Meisser A, Zinsstag J. A One Health Research Framework for Animal-Assisted Interventions. International Journal of Environmental Research and Public Health. 2019;**16**:640. DOI: 10.3390/ijerph16040640

[4] Sundman A. Dog Behavior, Intricate Picture of Genetics, Epigenetics and Human-Dog Relationship. LiU-Trunk: Linköping; 2019

[5] Britannica, The Editors of Encyclopedia. Anubis. Great Britain: Encyclopedia Britannica; 2023. Available from: https://www.britannica.com/topic/Anubis [Accessed: September 23, 2023]

[6] Vecino AP. Psychology With Horse. (Psicología a través del Caballo). Norte de Salud Mental. 2016;**14**:84-87

[7] Benito SM. Equine Therapy as Complementary Therapy to Favor the Development of Mental Disability Patients. Valladolid: Universidad de Valladolid; 2019

[8] Muñoz GB. Animal-Assisted Therapy Applied in a Rural Geriatric Residency. Murcia: Universidad de Murcia; 2013

[9] Wilson E. Biophilia. United States: Harvard University Press; 1984

[10] Vernooij M, Schneider S. Handbuch der Tierstützen Interventionen Grundlagen Konzepte Praxisfelder. Germany: Quelle & Meyer Verlag; 2018. ISBN: 978-3-494-01751-8

[11] International Association of Human-Animal Interaction Organizations. 2023. Available from: https://iahaio.org/wp/wp-content/uploads/2018/04/iahaio_wp_updated-2018-final.pdf

[12] Association AVAVMA. Animal Assisted Intervention Definitions 2023. Available from: https://www.avma.org/resources-tools/avma-policies/animal-assisted-interventions-definitions

[13] Lundqvist et al. Patient benefit of dog-assisted interventions in health care a systematic review. BMC Complementary and Alternative Medicine. 2017;**17**:358. DOI: 10.1186/s12906-017-1844-7

[14] Liguori G. Human-animal interaction in animal-assisted interventions: Zoonosis, risks, benefits and future directions. Animals. 2023;**13**:1592

[15] Zinsstag J, Hediger K, Osman YM, Abukhattab S, Crump L, Kaiser-Grolimund A, et al. The promotion and development of one health at Swiss TPH and its greater potential. Diseases. 2022;**10**(3):65. DOI: 10.3390/diseases10030065. PMID: 36135221; PMCID: PMC9497760

[16] Chalmers D. Applying one health to the study of animal-assisted interventions. EcoHealth. 2015;**12**(4):560-562

[17] Holder TRN, Gruen ME, Roberts DL, Somers T, Bozkurt A. A systematic literature review of animal-assisted

interventions in Oncology (Part II): Theoretical mechanisms and frameworks. Integrative Cancer Therapies. 2020:19. DOI: 10.1177/1534735420943269

[18] Miccinesi G, Caraceni A, Garetto F, et al. The path of cicely Saunders: The "Peculiar Beauty" of palliative care. Journal of Palliative Care. 2020;**35**(1):3-7. DOI: 10.1177/0825859719833659

[19] Wilson the rescue dog who helped find the amazon children is missing. Wall Street Journal. 15 June 2023. Available from: https://waj.com/articles/colombian-military-calls-off-search-for-wilson-the-rescue-dog-801d05db

[20] Wallace M. The death of my dog: Lessons learned from the palliative care of an animal. British Journal of General Practice. 2013;**63**(611):317. DOI: 10.3399/bjgp13X668366

[21] Szawarski P. Classic cases revisited: Oscar the cat. Journal of the Intensive Care Society. 2016;**17**(4):341-345. DOI: 10.1177/1751143716646123

[22] Dosa D. A day in the life of oscar the cat. The New England Journal of Medicine. 2007;**357**:328-329. Available from: https://www.nejm.org [Accessed: July 30, 2007]

[23] Blake P. In: Lauri H, editor. Here Kitty. United States: YouTube; 2009

[24] Rathish D, Rajapakse J, Weerakoon K. In times of stress, it is good to be with them: experience of dog owners from a rural district of Sri Lanka. BMC Public Health. 2022;**22**(1):2380. DOI: 10.1186/s12889-022-14863-6. PMID: 36536373; PMCID: PMC9761628

[25] Dalton KR, Altekruse W, Campbell P, Ruble K, Carroll KC, Thorpe RJ Jr, et al. Perceptions and practices of key worker stakeholder groups in hospital animal-assisted intervention programs on occupational benefits and perceived risks. People Animal. 2022;**5**(1):4

[26] Marti R, Petignat M, Marcar VL, Hattendorf J, Wolf M, Hund-Georgiadis M, et al. Effects of contact with a dog on prefrontal brain activity: A controlled trial. PLoS One. 2022;**17**(10):e0274833. DOI: 10.1371/journal.pone.0274833

[27] Quintal V, Reis-Pina P. Animal-assisted therapy in palliative care. Acta Médica Portuguesa. 2021;**34**(10):690-692. DOI: 10.20344/amp.13164 Epub 2020 Sep 15

[28] Schmitz A. Animal-assisted therapy at a university centre for palliative medicine- A qualitative content analysis of patient records. BMC Palliative Care. 2017;**16**:50. DOI: 10.1186/s12904-017-0230-z

[29] Nightingale F. Notes of Nursing: What is and What isn't. London: Harrison and Sons; 1859

[30] Ah Chu MS. Who is the New Furry Member on the Home-Palliative-Care-Team? Ottawa: SIOP International Congress; 2023

[31] Silva NB, Osorio FL. Impact of an animal-assisted therapy programme on physiological and psychosocial variables of paediatric oncology patients. PLoS One. 2018;**13**(4):e0194731. DOI: 10.1371/journal.pone.0194731

[32] Machová K, Součková M, Procházková R, Vaníčková Z, Mezian K. Canine-assisted therapy improves well-being in nurses. International Journal of Environmental Research and Public Health. 2019;**16**(19):3670. DOI: 10.3390/ijerph16193670

[33] Zhao M, Chen S, You Y, Wang Y, Zhang Y. Effects of a therapeutic

horseback riding program on social interaction and communication in children with autism. International Journal of Environmental Research and Public Health. 2021;**18**:2656. DOI: 10.3390/ijerph18052656

[34] Cairns K. Inpatients' experiences with equine therapy: A qualitatively driven mixed-method exploratory study. International Journal of Advanced Nursing Education and Research. 2022;**7**(1):19-38. DOI: 10.21742/ijaner.2022.7.1.02

[35] Services SM. History of Equine Therapy. 2023. Available from: https://www.spiritmountainhealing.com/blog/a-history-of-equine-assisted-therapy#:~:text=The%20therapeutic%20benefits%20of%20spending.similar%20to%20human%20movement%20patterns

[36] López RL. Hippotherapy as a technique of habilitation and rehabilitation. Revista Ciencias de la Salud. 2015:271-279

[37] Kazdin A. Methodological standards and strategies for establishing the evidence base of animal-assisted therapies. In: Handbook on Animal-Assisted Therapy: Theoretical Foundations and Guidelines for Practice. United States: Elsevier Academic Press; 2010. pp. 519-546

[38] Wagner C, Grob C, Hediger. Specific and Non-specific Factors of Animal-Assisted Interventions Considered in Research: A Systematic Revie. Frontiers in Psychology. 2022;**13**:931347. DOI: 10.3389/fpsyg.2022.931347

[39] Shaheen MNF. The concept of one health applied to the problem of zoonotic diseases. Reviews in Medical Virology. 2022;**32**(4):e2326. DOI: 10.1002/rmv.2326 Epub 2022 Jan 20

[40] Lönker NS, Fechner K, Abd El Wahed A. Horses as a Crucial Part of One Health. Veterinary Sciences. 2020;**7**(1):28. DOI: 10.3390/vetsci7010028

Section 5

Future Perspectives

Chapter 20

Predicting High Need End-of-Life in Medicare Patients through Machine Learning

Ian Duncan and Tamim Ahmed

Abstract

Patients are often at risk of consuming significant medical resources during the last 6 to 12 months of life, without improving their life expectancy. We develop a model for predicting patients likely to die within the next 6 to 12 months based on administrative claims and demographic data. Standard statistical models as well as newer machine learning approaches are used to identify target patients. Patients identified through the model are candidates for palliative care of hospice care. Timely intervention with appropriate care has been shown to both improve the quality of life of such patients while also reducing resource consumption. We demonstrate the use of the model by incorporating in an economic model of an intervention program, showing that intervention in the highest predicted probability cohort can provide a positive return on investment, provided the program is targeted at the highest-risk patients.

Keywords: end-of-life, predictive analytics, hospice care, machine learning, program planning

1. Introduction

As the Medicare program struggles to control expenditures, there is increased focus on opportunities to manage patient populations more efficiently and at lower cost. A major source of expense for the Medicare program is beneficiaries at end of life. A recent paper by the same authors [1] concludes, using the Medicare Limited Dataset files that the full cost of Medicare decedents in 2015 amounted to 21% of Medicare's expense in that year. A Kaiser Family Foundation study by Cubanski et al. [2] found the average cost per decedent in 2014 to be $34,500, or about 3.5 times the cost of the average Medicare beneficiary. A well-known paper by Finkelstein et al. [3] has been interpreted to imply that patients in the last year of life account for only 5% of spending. This interpretation is incorrect, because the authors were looking at the cost of patients *predicted to die,* rather than those who actually died. Because risk-taking entities such as Medicare Advantage plans and Accountable Care Organizations[1] (ACOs) need to reduce costs while improving the quality of care of

[1] A risk-taking physician or medical group.

IntechOpen

terminally-ill patients, they should initiate programs to better manage the care of patients with serious or advanced illness [4, 5]. There is evidence in the literature that such programs both improve quality of care and provide savings to the payer [6–8]. With limited resources available to manage high-need patients, it is important to identify early those patients who are at risk of death within 6 to 12 months. Using available claims data and newer statistical methods it is possible to identify patients who are at risk of end of life and who are candidates for intervention.

2. Prior predictive models of end-of-life risk

It is important to understand the value of models for prediction either to supplement or replace the judgment of medical professionals. On the accuracy of clinician predictions, see Christakis and Lamont [9] or Selby et al. [10]. Models to identify patients at risk may be classified into three types:

- Rules-based models

An example of a rules-based model is that of Amy Kelley [11, 12]. Dr. Kelley stratifies patients merging different data sources. A challenge with such models is ranking patients according to urgency of intervention when multiple different scales are integrated.

- Parametric models

There are numerous examples of parametric models, both commercial and in the literature. A sample of publications may be found at [13–16].

- Machine learning and Artificial Intelligence models

The remainder of this chapter discusses the development of Machine Learning and AI models.

3. Machine learning and AI models

There are various machine learning algorithms that can be used to solve complex problems. Using a data set, called Training Data (TD) we can look at various important characteristics behind a desired outcome. Developing a TD dataset requires subject matter knowledge so that there are fewer chances of spurious outcomes. See Duncan Chapter 3 [17] for an extensive discussion of administrative data and their use. We discuss some of the most compelling machine learning algorithms that can enhance our approach model development.

1. Decision Tree A decision tree is a non-parametric estimation procedure where the process begins with splitting choices progressively to identify the best options available for attaining the outcomes, predictions, or reduced residual noises. When splits are made progressively the process emulates tree branches and leaves. This is strictly a hierarchical model as shown in **Figure 1** where the process starts from the top and then branches out along various conditional

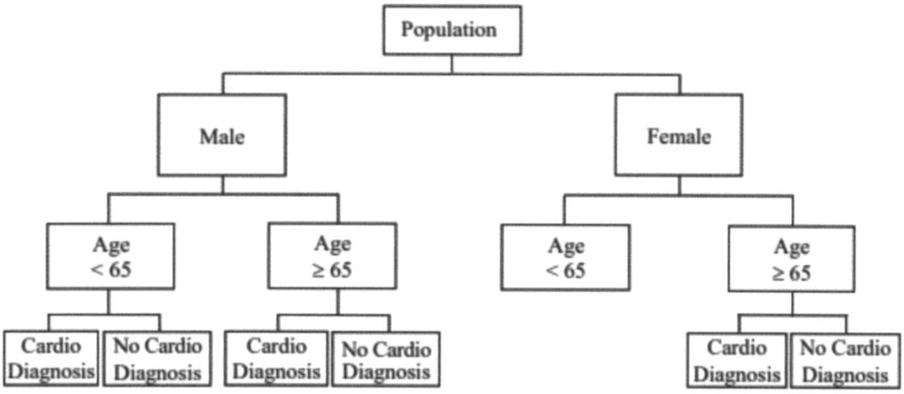

Figure 1.
Decision tree example (from Duncan [15]).

statements. Expected outcomes are measured at the end of the process by looking at the probability of each branch or node and then calculating expected outcomes. The decision tree approach is satisfactory for simplistic scenarios but fails in complex estimation problems.

In the image above nodes indicate branching logic at which the tree splits into branches/edges. The end of the branch occurs when no further split is possible (in this case whether or not there was a Cardio diagnosis). The model uses two features/attributes from the data set, namely sex and age. The outcome is either a cardiac diagnosis or not.

2. Random Forest A Random Forest is simply an extension of the decision tree approach where multiple decision trees are assembled. The final estimation is done by tracking the mean outcomes from various trees included in the model. Random Forests assume that the learning from a single tree is much weaker than when a result gathered from multiple trees of unequal size. Final outcomes are derived as an average of various trees, resulting in lower variance and better predictions of the target outcomes (**Figure 2**).

   Random Forest (strong learner) is built as an ensemble of Decision Trees (weak learners) to perform different tasks such as regression and classification. Unlike Decision Trees, only one tree Random Forest generates n-trees randomly from training data.

3. Gradient Boosting Trees (GBT) Gradient boosting is a machine learning technique which uses decision tree models, called weak learners, and creates a composite model. Each successive tree in this model improves its prediction from the previous one by minimizing the error residuals from previous tree. This technique is also an ensemble method which combines multiple weak models. Based on using previous constructs of trees and their weighted residuals, the models attempt to slowly build more and more trees and in that process reduce noise (residual error) from successive builds. When ultimately the marginal (gradient) reductions in error becomes small or zero, the model completes the total construct (**Figure 3**).

In the example *blue dots (left) plots are input (x) vs. output (y). The red line (left) shows values predicted by decision tree. Green dots (right) show residuals vs. input (x) for i-*

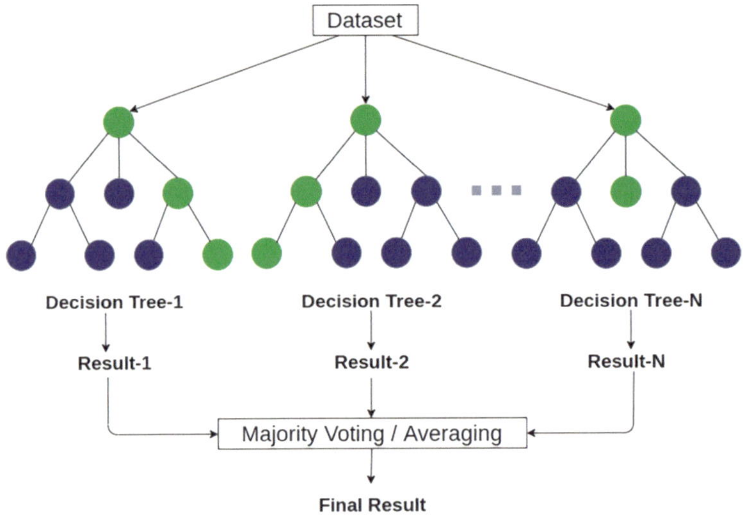

Figure 2.
Random Forest – Simplified [18].

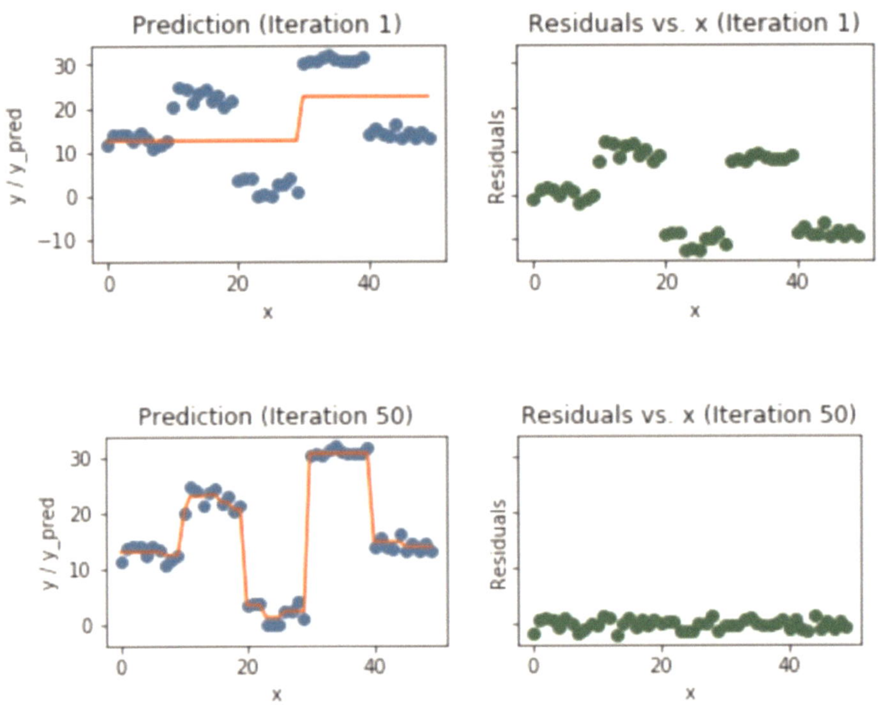

Figure 3.
Gradient boosting trees [19].

th iteration. Each iteration represents the fitting of a gradient boosting tree. With more iterations we see that the residuals become smaller and smaller. At some point we consider that the model has come up with a prediction much robust compared to the first set of iterations.

4. Logistic Regression Model (LRM) Logistic regression is the appropriate regression analysis to conduct when the dependent variable is either dichotomous (binary) or may have multinomial (multiple) outcomes but at discrete levels. Like all regression analyses the logistic regression can be used as a predictive analysis. In our approach

   - Linear Model: $y = b_0 + b_1x$.
   - Logistic Model: $p = \frac{1}{1+e^{-b_0+b_1x}}$.

When there are limited dependent variables, the appropriate technique is not to use procedures like regression estimation due to the following disadvantages.

a. Prediction of linear regression will allow the expected value to fall outside the range of 0 to 1.

b. Due to the dichotomous nature of the dependent variable, the residuals of the linear regression method will not be normally distributed.

c. Logistic regression produces predicted values which are bound between 0 and 1 range.

d. In the case where the outcome variable has more than two outcomes, multinomial logistic regression may still be applied. In that case, every outcome is assigned a probability whose sum must be between values of 0 to 1.

1. Naïve Bayes The Naïve Bayes machine language technique borrows from Bayes' Rule, which is applied to estimate probability of certain outcomes of interest based on our a priori knowledge of certain events preceding it. The 2nd aspect of this technique is Naïve which means independence of events. Applying Naïve Bayes' approach is to figure out probabilities of given attributes and then estimate posterior probability of various outcomes of interest.

2. Deep Learning A subset of machine learning algorithms called Deep Learning is based on artificial neural networks. Such algorithms are based on functionality similar to a human brain, learning from large amounts of data. Deep Learning algorithms perform a task repeatedly, each time tweaking it a little to improve the outcome. We refer to "deep learning" because the neural networks have various (deep) layers that enable learning.

3. Neural Net Neural Net is another AI technique which has been growing in importance. There has been many applications in various sectors but we are mostly interested as they apply to improvements in predicting target outcomes in healthcare. There are various layers in this technique—input, hidden and output. The complex model may have multiple hidden layers. When Neural Net receives data via the input layer, it passes on that input to the hidden layers. Each input node may pass that information to one or multiple hidden layer's nodes. The hidden nodes then create weights which is then applied to various combinations of inputs based on hidden connections and correlations which have been built in the hidden part of the model. When trained data is applied to the model, it goes via the input layer to various nodes of the hidden layer and then gets transformed

in its journey to the output layer. During the training process, various weights and thresholds are continuously adjusted and readjusted so that training data consistently yield similar outputs (**Figure 4**).

4. Random Tree The Random Tree technique is similar to the Random Forest but deviates from that process by selecting attributes from a subset of trees instead of using all the trees. There are various types of stochastic processes that could be applied to randomly choose trees for an ensemble set of weak learners (trees). The model uses bootstrap sampling with replacement to generate sample data. The sample data is then used to grow a tree model. The model then proceeds to select part of the predictors and uses the best ones to split a tree node. This process is repeated in splitting various other tree nodes.

5. Generalized Linear Model (GLM) Generalized Linear Models are a family of regression models using maximum likelihood estimation techniques to generate parametric estimators including error distribution. This model can accommodate various distribution functions of the dependent variable—normal, binomial, Poisson, exponential, gamma, logistic, probit, fixed-effects, random-effects, nonlinear regression, quantile regression—to develop unbiased estimators. There is an assumption that the Link function is linearly related to the independent variables in the model. Unlike ordinary least square (OLS) or multi-variate least square (MLS), GLM uses the maximum likelihood estimator (MLE).

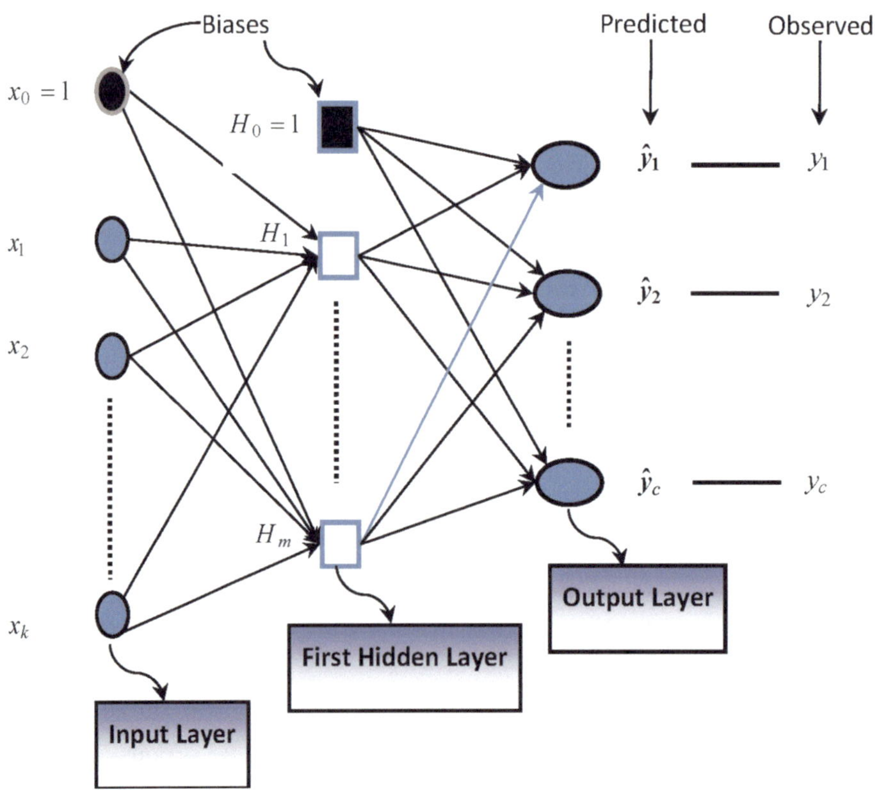

Figure 4.
Network diagram for a feed-forward NN model with one single hidden layer (from Duncan [17] chapter 12).

4. Objective

For the purpose of managing the utilization and cost of a population it is useful to identify those patients who, at end of life, are likely to be high utilizers of healthcare services. While in many cases such services are important and contribute to patient health, in other cases alternative treatments such as palliative care or hospice may be more appropriate and lead to higher quality outcomes.

Our objective in modeling is to identify members of an insured population that are at high risk, not just of mortality but of consuming considerable medical resources over a short time period (for example the last 6 months of life). An example of such a member might be a terminally ill cancer patient treated with certain modern biological drugs, or a patient admitted for an extended period to the ICU. We refer to these patients in the following discussion as "high need" patients. They represent a subset of patients for whom different treatment modalities exist (palliative care; hospice) that may contribute to high quality of life while reducing resource needs.

5. Data

We used CMS's Limited Data Set (LDS)[2] for the years 2015–2016 to develop a data file for this analysis. In order to analyze data coded according to the same coding structure, we also restricted the analysis to the period October 1, 2015 through December 31, 2016 during which the ICD-10 coding structure was used. The mortality rate in our sample data is 4.5%, consistent with other studies of Medicare mortality rates as reported in Duncan [1]. Medicare managed care (HMO, Medicare Advantage) members are excluded because the reported data in the Medicare LDS dataset is not always complete.

We selected members who were enrolled in fee-for-service Medicare between October 1, 2015 through December 31, 2016 and those who died between April 1 and December 31, 2016. This more limited timeframe allows us to have at least 6 months of claims experience for both survivors and decedents. Starting with a sample size of 1.67 million members with both Part A (hospital) and Part B (Major Medical) coverage we revised with certain selections of conditions in order to screen members at low-risk of mortality. We required all members in our sample to have one or more of a list of conditions[3] which reduces sample size slightly but improves the percentage of decedents. The selection at Step 2 in **Table 1** reflects an attempt to capture members at risk of death. In Step 3 we extracted a 10% stratified random sample. These steps generated a test group consisting of 4983 deceased and 84,604 survivors and a validation group consisting of 2135 deceased and 36,027 survivors.

---

[2] https://www.cms.gov/research-statistics-data-and-systems/files-for-order/limiteddatasets

[3] Members are required to experience one or more of the following conditions: Septicemia, Sepsis, Systemic Inflammatory Response Syndrome/Shock, Cardio-Respiratory Failure and Shock, Congestive Heart Failure, Specified Heart Arrhythmias (SRA), Chronic Obstructive Pulmonary Disease, Acute Renal Failure, various cancers, patients using anticoagulants, depression, GERD, kidney diseases, malaise, metal, nicotine, orthopedic conditions, pneumonia, CHF % renal and CHF & SRA.

Sample Description	Test Sample			Validation Sample		
	Deceased	Survived	% Deceased	Deceased	Survived	% Deceased
Step1: Medicare 5% FFS Sample with Parts A & B	52,194	1,116,665	4.5%	22,369	478,571	4.5%
Step2: Step1 minus Select Conditions	49,823	840,631	5.6%	21,353	360,271	5.6%
Step3: 10% Stratified Random Sample of Step2	4983	84,064	5.6%	2135	36,027	5.6%

Table 1.
Sample selection details.

5.1 Dependent variable

This model has a binomial dependent variable (survived or deceased). From the demographic data from the Medicare LDS dataset we are able to work with indicators of death and date of death.

5.2 Independent variables

1. The independent variables available for analysis are:
2. Age/Sex Bands—5 bands for male and 5 bands for female
3. Race—6 flags
4. Region—5 flags
5. HCC—79 flags based on CMS Medicare risk grouper[4]
6. Additional 5 HCC conditions[4]
7. 15 comorbid conditions
8. Additional 24 clinical conditions
9. Discharge indicator to Home/Self-care
10. Hospital readmission
11. ICU before death flag in 30 days
12. ICU before Hospice admission
13. Charlson Co-morbidity Index [20]
14. Hospice Admission count 3-month and 6-month prior to death

[4] For explanation of Grouper Models, see Duncan [15] Chapter 5.

15. Inpatient Admission count 3-month and 6-month prior to death

16. SNF Admission count 3-month and 6-month prior to death

17. Transition of Care count 3-month and 6-month prior to death

18. 30-day Readmission counts over 6-month prior to death

19. ER Visit count 3-month and 6-month prior to death

20. ER Trauma Admissions 3-month and 6-month prior to death

21. Hospital Admission via ER flag

22. Total PMPM of Patient, square root of PMPM and square of PMPM

23. Percent cost of patients in last 3-month prior to death

24. Homecare DME

6. Results

We used RapidMiner™ software[5] to develop various models. We used the test sample to explore various relationships between the dependent variable and the list of independent variables above. The validation sample was used to score the prediction of members' outcomes into 2 possible categories - survival and death (**Figure 5**).

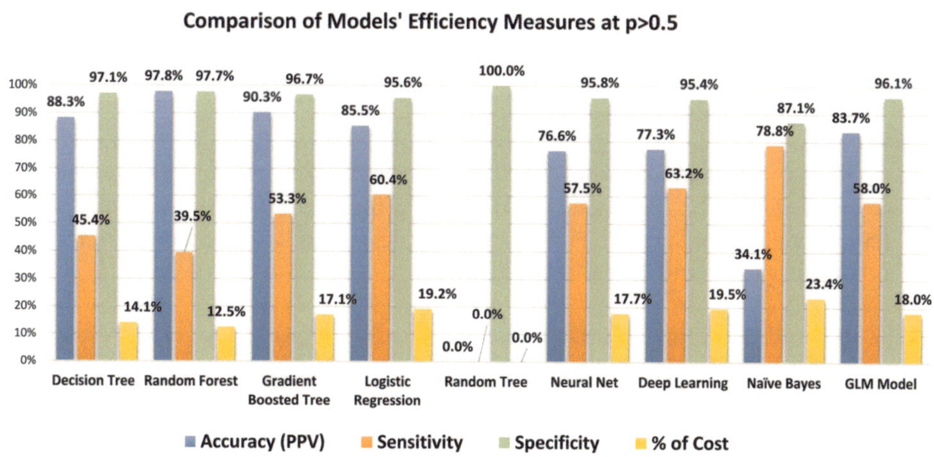

Figure 5.
Performance of models for predicting high need members.

5 Rapid Miner Software https://rapidminer.com/products/

There are three key measures we used to determine relative performance of the model, all for predicted probabilities >0.5. Specificity is the ability of the model accurately to predict the negative outcome (in this case survival). Sensitivity is the ability of the model accurately to identify the positive outcome (in this case death). Sensitivity measures how many of the High Need members did indeed consume considerable resources prior to death. Positive Predictive Value (PPV) measures accuracy for cases where prediction >0.5, how many members were correctly identified as experiencing high need death. The higher the probability, the more accurate the prediction. The findings can be summarized below:

1. Invariably almost all the models exhibited high specificity, meaning that members who were predicted to survive, actually survived. This is unsurprising given the high frequency of survival relative to death. This observation is true for most models (specificity >90%); the exception is Naïve Bayes (87.1%) which has the lowest specificity of all the models.

2. Sensitivity shows the proportion of those members with probabilities exceeding 50% (i.e., $p > 0.50$) who were predicted to experience high need. Naïve Bayes' has the best score (78.8%), followed by Deep Learning (63.2%), Logistic Regression (60.4%), GLM (58.0%), Neural Net (57.5%), and followed by Gradient Boosted Tree (53.3%) being the Top 6 models. High sensitivity score is very important because it generates a higher proportion of people for expected deaths.

3. Regarding the positive predictive accuracy (PPV), most models perform well, with a few exceeding 90% accuracy. This measure is a ratio of people predicted to die with a $p > 0.50$ as a proportion of all members (e.g., survivors and decedents) in that range. This measure shows the accuracy of the model in predicting high need (or deceased) people as a proportion of all members in that probability range. Some models have high PPV but low sensitivity. That reduces the model's overall efficiency, that is, it is only accurate on a small number of people. The Top 6 models are Random Forest (97.8%), Gradient Boosted Tree (90.3%), Decision Tree (88.3%), Logistic Regression (85.5%), GLM (83.7%) and Deep Learning (77.3%).

4. We also created percentage of cost (i.e., % of Cost) measure which shows cost of high need members who were predicted (at $p > 0.50$) to die as a percentage of all costs for those who deceased or survived. Performance is mixed with the Naïve Bayes model doing well at 23.4%. Deep Learning and Logistic models being the other two at 19.5 and 19.2% respectively.

The appropriate choice of attribute from Sensitivity, Specificity and PPV is an art. For example, we could pick a model with high sensitivity like Naïve Bayes (78.8%) as best performer, but we have a problem because its PPV is very low (34.1%)! Since specificity is relatively high for all models, we can choose best performers based on only PPV and Sensitivity attributes.

How do we weigh sensitivity and PPV? It depends on the proposed use. For example, one may weigh PPV higher than sensitivity or vice versa. If PPV is weighed higher than sensitivity, then Random Forest and GBT could be possible candidates. However, if sensitivity is more important than PPV, then possibly Naïve Bates and Deep Learning models could be good performers.

Models	Accuracy (PPV)	Sensitivity	Specificity	% of Cost	Equal Weight PPV, Sensitivity	Product of PPV and Sensitivity
Logistic Regression	85.5%	60.4%	95.6%	19.2%	73.0%	51.6%
Deep Learning	77.3%	63.2%	95.4%	19.5%	70.3%	48.9%
GLM Model	83.7%	58.0%	96.1%	18.0%	70.9%	48.5%
Gradient Boosted Tree	90.3%	53.3%	96.7%	17.1%	71.8%	48.1%
Neural Net	76.6%	57.5%	95.8%	17.7%	67.1%	44.0%
Decision Tree	88.3%	45.4%	97.1%	14.1%	66.9%	40.1%
Random Forest	97.8%	39.5%	97.7%	12.5%	68.7%	38.6%
Naïve Bayes	34.1%	78.8%	87.1%	23.4%	56.5%	26.9%
Random Tree	0%	0%	100.0%	0%	0%	0%

Table 2.
Summary of model PPV, sensitivity and specificity at $p > 0.5$.

Finally, if we assume equal weights for both sensitivity and PPV from the list of all models, then the following rankings could be made (with the top 4 performers all clustered just above 70%): Logistic Regression (73.0%), GBT (average 71.8%), GLM (70.9%), Deep Learning (70.3%), Random Forest (68.7%), Neural Net (67.1%), Decision Tree (66.9%) and Naïve Bayes (56.5%). Random Tree model has zero sensitivity and thus not included for any consideration.

Lastly, if we take product of PPV and Sensitivity, the ranking remains in favor of logistic regression (51.6%), followed by Deep Learning (48.9%), GLM (48.5%), Gradient Boosted Tree (48.1%) and Neural Net (44.0%). The new ranking based on the product of sensitivity and PPV measures the dual impact of accuracy and how much of an impact it can have on the underlying eligible population, especially those who were predicted to be of high need (deceased). **Table 2** shows various measures of model efficiency. Product of PPV and Sensitivity changes the ranking compared to equal weights placed on PPV and Sensitivity measures although Logistic Regression model comes out on the top of both considerations.

7. Application to population management

7.1 Program development

The development of a model such as that developed in this chapter, while interesting theoretically, has important practical applications. The ability to identify early in an insured member's course of illness that the patient is likely to be a high need, end-of-life patient allows care managers to begin discussions about palliative care earlier. This section develops a simple economic model to demonstrate the application of the model in the context of care management programs.

We were able to estimate the impact of identifying members who are predicted to die within a period of 6–12 months and moving those members to palliative care. Based on the 2021 Medicare budget of $829 billion dollars [21] the potential of savings as a percent of total cost is provided in **Figure 6** below. Given that the Naïve Bayes model has a low PPV, we would prefer to apply either the Logistic model or the Deep

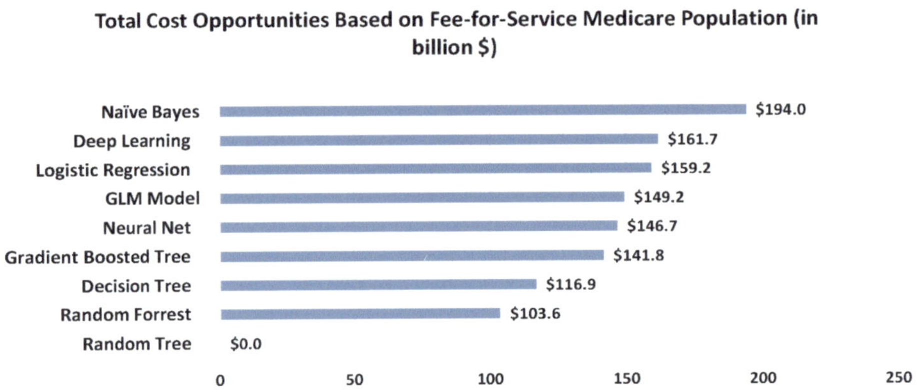

Figure 6.
Predicted impact of EOL model on cost of Care for Medicare Population in 2021.

Learning model, or other models like GLM, Neural Net or GBT to identify members at risk of high need death. **Figure 6** basically shows potential costs associated with the high need population that could be targeted for end-of-life planning. The cost estimate shows the proportion of total cost (excluding pharmacy) at risk. The extent of savings depends upon the early target and providing palliative care for the willing patients.

7.2 Using the model for program planning

Table 3 shows the application of the model in combination with program economics to plan an intervention program.

We first divide the population by decile according to predicted deaths (we further divide the top decile into sub-cohorts in order to illustrate the method). Applying the probability of death to the population by decile allows us compare predicted and actual deaths. The model performs well overall in terms of total predicted deaths; by decile the model also performs reasonably accurately with members identified with a high predicted score dying at a high rate. Importantly, the model allows the program planner to identify that cohort of members in which there is likely to be a high probability of death, and other cohorts with a low probability that are not as likely to justify an intervention program. Said differently, focusing on the highest predicted risk members captures the largest proportion of members.

The question that we address: if the model is to be used for planning an intervention program, how should this be done? We incorporate some data into the decile table about the number of nurses required to intervene with patients in a palliative care and hospice program, the cost of the program and the likelihood of patient engagement. Combined with a "success" rate (actual number of deaths from the model together with likelihood of cost avoidance) we are able to estimate a Return on Investment (ROI) in such a program. For more information about program design, operation and outcomes see Yosick et al. [6].

Noticeably the program returns a positive ROI only in the top sub-population. The ROI in this sub-population is, however, substantial. It is sufficiently high that if a program sponsor were interested in *total savings* rather than *ROI,* it would be economically efficient to manage a larger cohort of patients. If, for example the program sponsor were to manage the top 2 cohorts (top decile in total) the total savings would be $13.5 million at an ROI of 2.325, vs. total savings of $10.9 million at an ROI of 3.76 in the top cohort.

Decile	No. Members	Death Probability	Expected Deaths	Actual Deaths	Nurse Case-load (annual)	No. Nurses	Nurse cost (fully-loaded)	Program Cost	Est. Cost/ Patient 2023; 90 days)	Expected Total Cost of sub-set	Estimated engagement (40%)	Estd. Cost Avoided (40%)	ROI
1	3817	0.2%	7.6	6	360	10.60	$550,000	$ 5,831,528	$ 19,435	$ 74,182,506	1527	$46,643	0.01
2	3817	0.3%	11.5	10	360	10.60	$550,000	$ 5,831,528	$ 19,435	$ 74,182,506	1527	$77,739	0.01
3	3817	0.4%	15.3	10	360	10.60	$550,000	$ 5,831,528	$ 19,435	$ 74,182,506	1527	$77,739	0.01
4	3817	0.5%	19.1	7	360	10.60	$550,000	$ 5,831,528	$ 19,435	$ 74,182,506	1527	$54,417	0.01
5	3817	0.6%	22.9	13	360	10.60	$550,000	$ 5,831,528	$ 19,435	$ 74,182,506	1527	$101,061	0.02
6	3817	0.8%	30.5	32	360	10.60	$550,000	$ 5,831,528	$ 19,435	$ 74,182,506	1527	$248,765	0.04
7	3817	1.2%	45.8	36	360	10.60	$550,000	$ 5,831,528	$ 19,435	$ 74,182,506	1527	$279,861	0.05
8	3817	1.8%	68.7	68	360	10.60	$550,000	$ 5,831,528	$ 19,435	$ 74,182,506	1527	$528,626	0.09
9	3817	4.0%	152.7	213	360	10.60	$550,000	$ 5,831,528	$ 19,435	$ 74,182,506	1527	$1,655,842	0.28
9.5	1908	14.4%	274.8	336	360	5.30	$550,000	$ 2,915,000	$ 19,435	$ 37,081,536	763	$2,612,033	0.90
10	1900	77.8%	1478.2	1404	360	5.28	$550,000	$ 2,902,778	$ 19,435	$ 36,926,058	760	$10,914,565	3.76
			2127.0	2135						$ 741,650,151			

Table 3.
Economic model for planning EOL intervention program.

8. Conclusion

In this chapter we have discussed the development of different machine learning and AI models to predict a specific outcome, the likelihood of high need death in a senior population (U.S. Medicare Fee-for-Service members 2015–6). We find that different models perform better on certain measures and that the choice of model depends on a balance of statistical tests and practical application. We combine the predictive model with assumptions about nursing costs and program efficiency to build an economic model for use in planning an intervention program. The economic model shows that a palliative care and hospice program could save substantial cost if applied to the right population.

Acknowledgements

Ian Duncan PhD FSA FIA FCIA FCA CSPA MAAA is Adjunct Professor of Actuarial Statistics at the Dept. of Statistics & Applied Probability, University of California, Santa Barbara, and President, Santa Barbara Actuaries Inc., Santa Barbara CA USA.

Tamim Ahmed is Director of Analytics, Santa Barbara Actuaries Inc. Santa Barbara CA USA.

RapidMiner™ is used with permission of Altair Engineering Inc. Altair is a global leader in computational science and artificial intelligence (AI) that provides software and cloud solutions in simulation, high-performance computing (HPC), data analytics, and AI. Altair enables organizations across all industries to compete more effectively and drive smarter decisions in an increasingly connected world – all while creating a greener, more sustainable future. For more information, visit https://www.altair.com/.

Author details

Ian Duncan* and Tamim Ahmed
Department of Statistics and Applied Probability, University of California Santa Barbara, USA

*Address all correspondence to: duncan@pstat.ucsb.edu

References

[1] Duncan I, Ahmed T, Maxwell TL, Dove H. Medicare cost at end of life. American Journal of Hospice and Palliative Care. 2019;**1**(6):705-710

[2] Cubanski J, Neuman T, Griffin S. And Damico a, Medicare Spending at the End of Life: A Snapshot of Beneficiaries Who Died in 2014 and the Cost of Their Care. Washington D.C: Kaiser Family Foundation; 2016

[3] Einav L, Finkelstein A, Mullainathan S, Obermeyer Z. Predictive modeling of U.S. health care spending in late life. Science. 2018;**360**:1462-1465

[4] Duncan I, Maxwell T, Dove H, Ahmed T. Medicare cost at end of life. American Journal of Hospice and Palliative Medicine. 2019;**36**(8):705-710

[5] Duncan I, Maxwell TL, Todd M, Huynh N. Polypharmacy, medication possession, and deprescribing of potentially non-beneficial drugs in hospice patients. The American Journal of Hospice & Palliative Care. 2020; **37**(12):1076-1085

[6] Yosik L, Crook RE, Gatto M, Maxwell TL, Duncan I, Ahmed T, et al. Effects of a population health community-based palliative care program on cost and utilization. Journal of Palliative Medicine. 2018;**22**(9): 1075-1081

[7] Luta X, Ottino B, Hall P, Bowden J, Wee B, Droney J, et al. Evidence on the economic value of end-of life and palliative care interventions: A narrative review of reviews. BMC Palliative Care. 2021;**20**:89

[8] Kelley AS, Deb P, Du Q, Aldridge MD, Carlson R, Morrison S. Hospice enrollment saves money for medicare and improves care quality across a number of different lengths-of-stay. Health Affairs. 2013;**32**(3):552-561

[9] Christakis N, Lamont EB. Extent and determinants of error in doctors' prognoses in terminally-ill patients: A prospective cohort study. BMJ. 2000; **320**(7233):469-472

[10] Selby D, Chakraborty A, Lilien T, Stacey E, Zhang L, Myers J. Clinician accuracy when estimating survival duration: The role of the patient's performance status and time-based prognostic categories. Journal of Pain and Symptom Management. 2011;**42**(4): 578-588

[11] Kelley AS, Bollens-Lund E. Identifying the population with serious illness: The "denominator" challenge. Journal of Palliative Medicine. 2018;**21** (S2):S7-S16

[12] Kelley AS, Covinsky KE, Gorges RJ, McKendrick K, Bollens-Lund E, Sean Morrison RS, et al. Identifying older adults with serious illness: A critical step toward improving the value of health care. Health Services Research. 2017; **52**(1):113-131

[13] Swerdel JN, Reps JM, Fife D, Ryan PB. Developing predictive models to determine patients in end-of-life care in administrative datasets. Drug Safety. 2020;**43**:447-455

[14] Reps JM, Schuemie MJ, Marc A, Suchard MA, Ryan PB, Rijnbeek PR. Design and implementation of a standardized framework to generate and evaluate patient-level prediction models using observational healthcare data. Journal of the American Medical Informatics Association. 2017;**25**(8): 969-975

[15] Murphree DH et al. Improving the delivery of palliative care through predictive modeling and healthcare informatics. JAMIA. 2021;**28**(6): 1065-1073

[16] Maley JH, Kerollos N, Wanis KN, Young JG, Celi LA. Mortality prediction models, causal effects, and end- of- life decision making in the intensive care unit. BMJ Health & Care Informatics. 2020;**27**:e100220

[17] Duncan I. Healthcare Risk Adjustment and Predictive Modeling. 2nd ed. New Hartford CT: Actex Publications; 2018

[18] Sharma A. Random Forest vs. Decision Tree: Which is Right for You? 2023. Available from: https://www.analyticsvidhya.com/blog/2020/05/decision-tree-vs-random-forest-algorithm/

[19] Grover P. Gradient Boosting from Scratch. ML Review; 2017. Available from: https://blog.mlreview.com/gradient-boosting-from-scratch-1e317ae4587d [Accessed: June 2023]

[20] Charlson ME, Kathy PP, Ales L, Ronald Mackenzie C. A new method of classifying prognostic comorbidity in longitudinal studies: Development and validation. Journal of Chronic Diseases. 1987;**40**(5):373-383

[21] Cubanski J, Neuman T. What to Know about Medicare Spending and Financing. San Francisco, CA, USA: Kaiser Family Foundation; 2023. Available from: https://www.kff.org/medicare/issue-brief/what-to-know-about-medicare-spending-and-financing/ [Accessed: July 15, 2023]

Chapter 21

The Last Aid Course as Measure for Public Palliative Care Education: Lessons Learned from the Implementation Process in Four Different Countries

Georg Bollig, Siobhan Neylon, Eva Niedermann and Erika Zelko

Abstract

This chapter provides an overview over the Last Aid Course (LAC) as measure for Public Palliative Care Education (PPCE) and the experiences from different countries on the implementation of Last Aid Courses. The concept of Last Aid and the public knowledge approach to teach Palliative Care for the public were first described by Bollig in 2008. Last Aid Courses can be seen as educational basis of compassionate communities and have now been spread to 21 countries worldwide. Experiences show differences and similarities in the national implementation process of LAC in four different countries.

Keywords: palliative care, education, citizens, public health, compassionate communities, last aid course, public palliative care education, worldwide

1. Introduction

Today most people want to die at home, but the majority actually die in institutions as hospitals, long-term care facilities and hospices. As the numbers of people who need palliative care at home will rise in the future [1] the healthcare system will not be able to meet the needs of those requiring palliative care without the support and contribution from members of the public. This includes relatives, friends, neighbors, colleagues and others in the community. Everybody, all parts of communities and societies have a responsibility to provide end-of-life care for others [2, 3]. Thus, it makes sense to prepare the public to participate in palliative care provision in the community. One measure that can assist with this is delivery of Last Aid Courses to the public in order to raise awareness on topics like palliative care, death, dying, grief and bereavement. Last Aid Courses have been introduced in different countries since 2014 and have been shown to help inform people, and to encourage and empower them to participate, in palliative care and end-of-life care [4–6]. Learning both First Aid and Last Aid should be part of the normal school education and be a part of ongoing life-long learning for everyone [4]. A six-step approach to education in Palliative Care for ALL including both the public and health care professionals has been described by Bollig [4, 7]. An overview over the Last Aid Movement and the experiences from the implementation of LAC in different countries will be described in more detail in the following parts of this chapter.

2. Last Aid International and the Last Aid Movement

The first description of the Last Aid Course and its curriculum and contents was presented by Bollig in a Masterthesis in 2008 and published as a book in 2010 [4]. The International Last Aid working group with representatives from Norway, Germany and Denmark established the first consensus about the Last Aid Course curriculum and slide set in 2014. Last Aid International was founded as a private organization to promote and implement Last Aid with the aim to enhance the public discussion about death, dying, grief and to improve Palliative Care in different countries in 2014 by its founder Georg Bollig. Mills et al. have in 2020 proposed to introduce a World Last Aid Day to raise awareness about the topics death, dying and Palliative Care [8]. During the course of the years from 2015 until today a variety of organizations from

2008	First presentation of the Last Aid Course in the Master Thesis of Georg Bollig
2009	Poster presentation 11th Congress of the European Association for Palliative Care, Vienna
2010	Masterthesis published as a book
2009–2011	Development of a Last Aid Course with 16 teaching hours in cooperation with the Austrian Red Cross and the IFF Vienna, University Klagenfurt/Graz
2012	Honorable mention for the lecture" The public knowledge approach as educational concept for bringing Palliative Care to the public" International Palliative Care Network conference
2013–2014	Development of a Last Aid Course with 4 teaching hours in cooperation of the Norwegian and Danish Associations for Palliative Care with Letzte Hilfe Deutschland
2014–2015	First pilot courses in Norway, Germany and Denmark
2015	Participation in the project startsocial - Invitation to Chancellor Angela Merkel
2015	Honorable mention for the poster presentation" Teaching Palliative Care to the Public: The Last Aid Course – An International Multicentre project from Norway, Denmark and Germany" International Palliative Care Network conference
2015	Reception of an award for Palliative Care from the German Association for Palliative Medicine and the pharmaceutical company Grünenthal
2016	Symposium of the Paula-Kubitschek-Vogel Stiftung München on Last Aid
2016	Publication of a German handbook for Last Aid Course participants
2016	Lecture on Last Aid on the International Palliative Care congress in Montreal, Canada
2017	1st German Symposium on Last Aid in Hamburg
2017	Lecture on Last Aid on the Scottish Palliative Care congress in Edinburgh, Scotland
2017–2019	Last Aid International as EUPCA project
2018	Last Aid courses recognized and recommended by German Hospice Association (DHPV) and the German Association for Palliative Medicine (DGP)
2018	Meeting of the International *Last Aid* working group in May in Frankfurt

2018	Relaunch of the German and English homepage www.lastaid.info
2018	Lecture on Last Aid on the 1. Baltic Palliative Care Conference in Liepaja, Latvia
2018	2nd German Symposium on Last Aid in Kassel
2018	Publication of a Danish handbook for Last Aid Course participants
2019	EAPC taskforce Last Aid and Public Palliative Care Education
2019	1stInternational Last Aid Conference Sønderborg, Dänemark
2019	3rd Letzte Hilfe Symposium München
2020	2nd International Last Aid Conference online
2020	Heinrich Pera prize for Georg Bollig
2021	4th Letzte Hilfe Symposium Frankfurt
2021	Order of merit of Schleswig-Holstein für Georg Bollig
2022	3rd International Last Aid Conference Maribor, Slovenia
2022	Workshop on Last Aid and Public Palliative Care Education 23rd Int. Palliative Care Congress Montreal, Canada
2023	Participation in the project startsocial - Invitation to chancellor Olav Scholz
2023	4th Letzte Hilfe Symposium Magdeburg
2023	Nomination for Schleswig Holsteinischer Bürgerpreis

Table 1.
The timeline of the development of last aid international and the last aid movement.

different countries and different backgrounds joined Last Aid International and Last Aid developed to become an international Last Aid Movement with many participating organizations, supporters and volunteers. The Last Aid Course concept is protected by an international trademark. Between 2017 and 2019 the implementation of Last Aid in different countries was promoted as part of Bolligs project in a European Palliative Care Academy (EUPCA) leadership course [9]. Today partner organizations from 21 countries from Europe, Brazil, Canada and Australia are part of Last Aid International and work together on the implementation of Last Aid Courses in different countries. Interestingly the national organizations that implement LAC in the different countries are not always the national Palliative Care organizations but can also be universities, hospices or the church. This will be addressed in the descriptions of different implementation models from different countries in part 3 of this chapter. In 2019 a Last Aid Research Group was established during the 1. International Last Aid Conference in Sønderborg, Denmark. The Last Aid Research Group International (LARGI) is led by Erika Zelko and Georg Bollig and is today a group of researchers from around the world working together to investigate the effects of Last Aid Courses and Public Palliative Care Education. The Last Aid Course project and its founder Georg Bollig have been nominated for and received a number of prizes. A summary of the timeline of the development of Last Aid International and the Last Aid Movement is shown in **Table 1**.

3. Implementation of Last Aid Courses in different countries

To implement and promote Last Aid Courses in different countries Last Aid International usually cooperates with one partner organization in each participating country. During the EUPCA-project to promote the international distribution of LAC, the first idea was to cooperate with the national Palliative Care organization. Interestingly the project has shown that not all Palliative Care organizations were interested or motivated to implement LAC and that different national organizations can be the best option to promote LAC in different countries [9]. For implementation and sustainability of the LAC, it is paramount that the participating national organization makes a commitment to keep to the agreed course rules, presentation and delivery guidelines provided by the International Last Aid working group. This can ensure that the Last Aid Course has the same content and learning outcomes in every country round the world. The only differences required are the national organizations of Palliative Care services, and explanation of national legislation and laws that concern Palliative Care provision and end of-life care for example rules for advance care planning and surrogate decision-making/power of attorney. Although physician assisted suicide or medical assistance in dying is legal in some countries, this is not a part of the curriculum. This decision was made as it was felt adequate Palliative Care does not usually include these options.

The LAC is in all participating countries based on the same standardized curriculum and slide set that is based on a consensus of the experts of the International Last Aid working group. This group consists of 1–2 experts from the field of Palliative Care from each of the participating countries. The group regularly meets every other year in connection with the International Last Aid Conference. The last meeting was held in Maribor, Slovenia in 2022 and the next meeting is planned to be held in

Module No.	Main topic and duration (minutes)	Course Content
Module 1	Dying as a normal part of life 45 minutes	• Welcome and introductions • First Aid and Last Aid • What you can do to care • The process of dying
Module 2	Planning ahead 45 minutes	• Networks of Support • Making decisions • Medical and ethical aspects • Advance care planning • Advance Directive • Medical Power of Attorney
Module 3	Relieving suffering 45 minutes	• Typical problems and symptoms • Caring/relieving suffering • Nutrition at the end of life • How to comfort
Module 4	Final goodbyes 45 minutes	• Saying goodbye/final farewell rituals • Funeral and various forms of burials • Grieving is normal • Grief and ways of grieving • Questions, Comments

Table 2.
The last aid course contents.

Cologne, Germany in September 2024. Additional meetings or subgroups may be established when needed and meet online when needed. The contents of the current LAC curriculum are shown in **Table 2**.

The implementation and distribution in the different countries is done by a national partner organization. The cooperation and work within the International Last Aid Movement is based on the following ethos and principles.

Ethos and Principles of Last Aid:

- Not for profit public awareness course: Last Aid should be delivered to members of the public with charges only being made to cover the cost of delivery (maximum 20 EUR per each course participant).

- The Last Aid course is a method of encouraging open discussions about the principles of death, dying and grief in order to improve the public's ability to cope with these aspects of life.

- The Last Aid Course provides a holistic overview of the human experience of death, dying and grief.

- The Last Aid Course aims to normalize the process of death, dying, bereavement and the aspects of care required.

- The Last Aid Course can be seen as educational basis of Compassionate Communities and aims to motivate and empower everyone to participate in Palliative Care and end-of-life care for everybody in need.

The national Last Aid partner organizations, also called national Last Aid hubs are responsible for the implementation and promotion of Last Aid Courses in the respective countries. The national Last Aid hubs can be supported by regional or local Last Aid hubs in the country if needed. The national Last Aid organizations have some general roles in their organization assigned. These include Last Aid Course instructor/facilitator; Last Aid Course Director and Last Aid Course Trainer in some regions supported by a local coordinator who works with the organization of the LAC and LAC instructor courses.

Last Aid Course Instructors/Facilitators

All Last Aid Course instructors/facilitators will deliver the Last Aid Course at least once per year (as per Last Aid International rules). They will attend facilitator training, by an approved Last Aid Trainer. Last Aid Course Instructors/Facilitators are required to have the following qualities:

1. Understanding of palliative/end of life care

2. Ability to commit to delivering the course with another Facilitator

3. Personal or professional experience with death, dying and bereavement concepts

4. A full understanding of the Last Aid course rules.

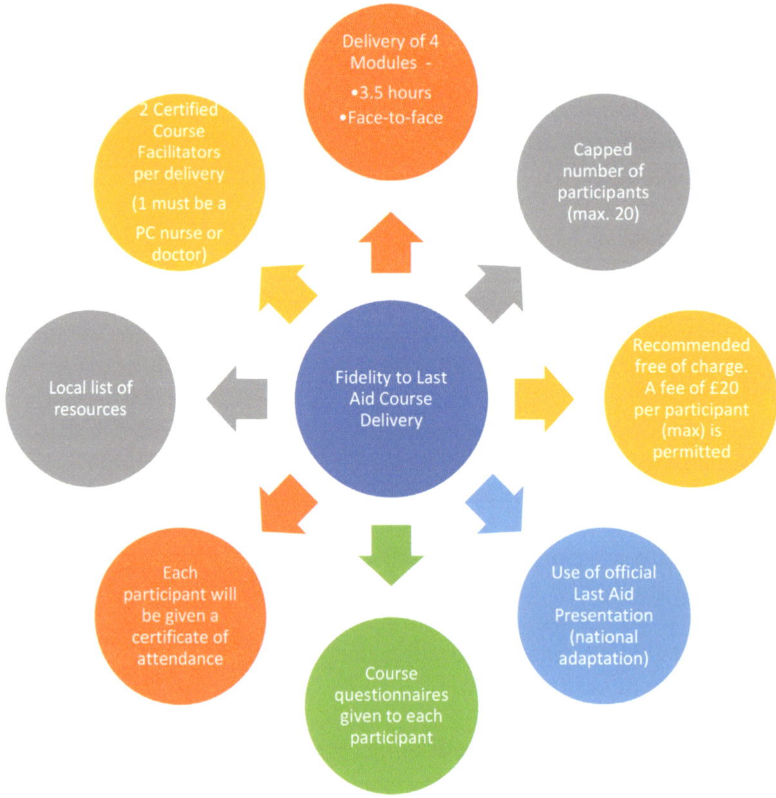

Figure 1.
Approach to Fidelity to the last aid concept.

In addition understanding of online video conferencing uses, and being prepared to learn how to facilitate Last Aid online is helpful. They must demonstrate fidelity to the Last Aid Course, and the course rules. The approach to fidelity within the Last aid Movement is shown in **Figure 1**.

The Local Last Aid Hub has the responsibility to recruit the appropriate facilitators to deliver Last Aid.

Last Aid Trainers

Last Aid Trainers have a dual role as Instructors/Facilitators of the Last Aid course and train the future Last Aid Course instructors/facilitators. They will deliver the one day Last Aid Instructor/Facilitator course together with a Last Aid Course Director.

The national Last Aid organization recruits Facilitator Trainers based on the points below:

1. Background in facilitation/teaching

2. Relevant clinical/educational experience in Palliative and End of Life Care services.

3. Awareness of local palliative care strategic development

4. Ability to attend train the trainers course

The national Last Aid organization will approve those recruited to be Facilitator Trainers, to ensure quality assurance and fidelity to the Last Aid Course.

Last Aid Course Directors

Last Aid Course directors are experienced trainers who lead the Last Aid Instructor/Facilitator course together with another trainer. They have the responsibility for the training. The Course Director must ensure the fidelity of the Last Aid Course, its ethos and principles.

The processes outlined below provide further guidance on preparing for the delivery of the Last Aid Courses. **Figure 2** illustrates the steps in the process of implementation of Last Aid Courses. Ongoing support and guidance will be provided by the National Last Aid Hub.

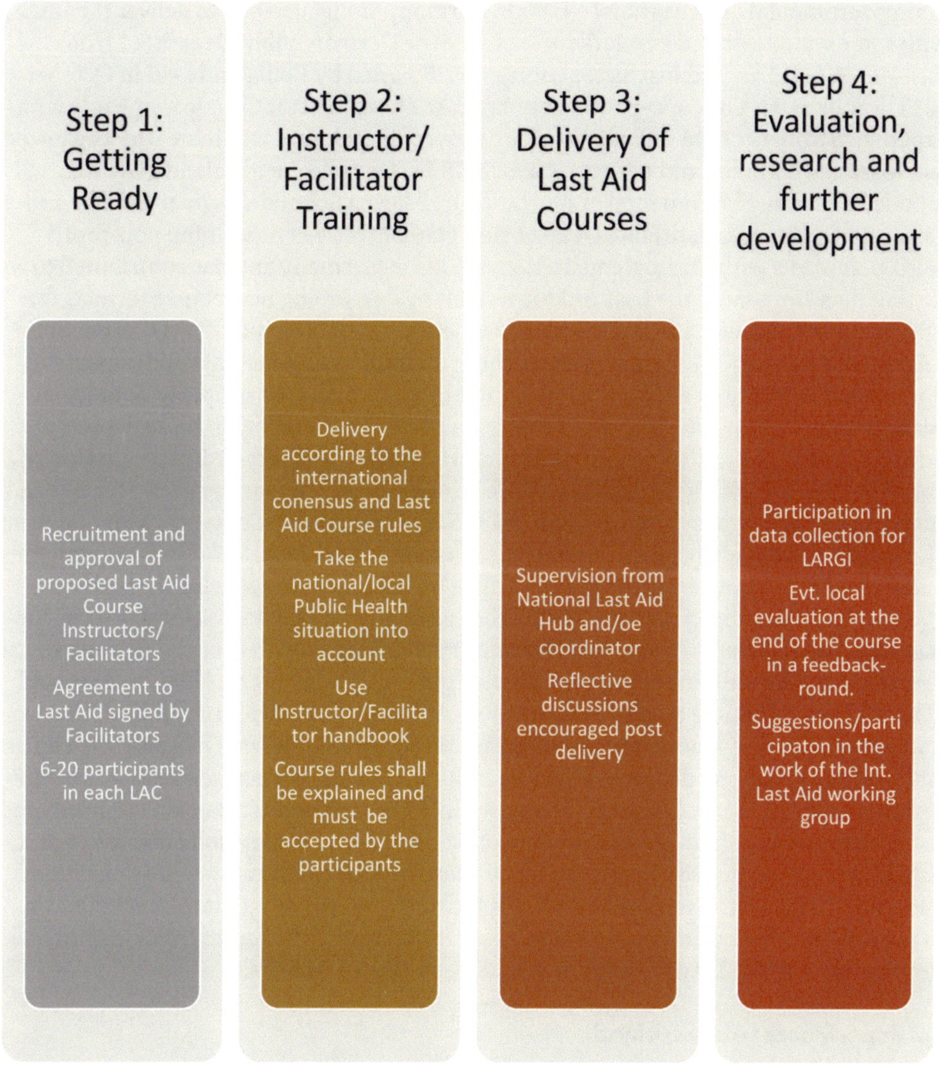

Figure 2.
Steps in the process of implementation of last aid courses.

In the following parts 3.1 to 3.4 the experiences from the implementation of LAC in four different countries will be described. In Germany LAC were started in 2015, in Scotland, Switzerland in 2017 and Slovenia in 2018.

3.1 Experiences from Germany

The first delivery of LAC in Germany was held in Schleswig in January 2015. It was the second LAC worldwide after the first course in Norway in November 2014. Led by Georg Bollig, the first LAC slide set was created by a group of Palliative Care experts, with a variety of professional backgrounds, from Germany, Norway and Denmark, as part of the International Last Aid working group in 2014. Courses in Germany were being delivered parallel with the work to establish a national organization that could take care of the further development of Last Aid in Germany. The process to start an organization proved to be complicated due to the complex rules for establishing a new non-governmental organization (NGO) in Germany. Bollig decided to deliver the LAC with some volunteers and co-workers to ensure the German public benefitted from the LAC. A first Last Aid instructor course was designed by Bollig and held in October 2015 in Schleswig. The concept of a one-day Last Aid instructor Course for people with experience from the field of Palliative Care proved feasible and was thereafter organized and managed by Bollig and co-workers. In 2018 Letzte Hilfe Deutschland gUG was founded as a non-governmental organization by Marina Schmidt, Ingmar Hornke and Georg Bollig. Today Letzte Hilfe Deutschland gGmbH is a self-sustaining non-profit NGO that works with the implementation of LAC in Germany and has contributed to the further development of the Last Aid Movement by developing new course formats for LAC for kids and teens; LAC online that was developed during the COVID-19 pandemic; LAC in easy language for people with learning disabilities and mental handicaps; LAC professional for health care professionals; and LAC Diversity for people with diverse backgrounds and the time to discuss cultural and other differences in more depth. Furthermore Letzte Hilfe Deutschland gGmbH engages in advocacy and promotion of Last Aid Courses and Public Palliative Care Education (PPCE) for the whole society and supports research projects on Last Aid and PPCE. The Last Aid Course for kids and teens (LAC-KT) has already been introduced in Switzerland and Austria. With these activities and a number of active working groups driven by volunteers Letzte Hilfe Deutschland gGmbH is a major contributor for the further development and testing of new LAC formats for special groups. Along with the countrywide implementation and delivery of the course, a need for fulltime employees became obvious. Today Letzte Hilfe Deutschland gGmbH has 1,5 fulltime employees (one of them being the CEO Marina Schmidt), a number of paid free-lancers for special tasks and many volunteers. There are several Last Aid working groups on different topics like course formats, advocacy, etc. that are working on a voluntary basis. The work of Letzte Hilfe Deutschland is financed via grants and income from fees of Last Aid Instructor Courses and LAC for the public that are in part paid by health-insurance companies. So far there have been educated more than 5000 Last Aid Course instructors and over 70,000 citizens. Germany is a major contributor in the nationwide implementation of LAC in Germany and the future development and improvement of the Last Aid Movement and new course formats.

3.2 Experiences from Scotland

The Highland Hospice, based in Inverness in the North of Scotland, is the main partner for the implementation of LAC in Scotland after a short period of cooperation with the Scottish partnership for Palliative Care Highland Hospice and Highland Hospice since 2017. The Highlands of Scotland has a geographical area similar to the country of Belgium, and a population of approx. 240,000 people. It has the lowest population density in Scotland, with around 8 people per sq. km. The Highland Hospice provides Pallaitive Care and outreach to this population. After an informational presentation from Georg Bollig, Highland Hospice CEO, Kenny Steele, felt that the public of the Highlands would benefit greatly from the Last Aid Course. In March 2019, the Facilitator course training was delivered by Georg Bollig to a group of 12 facilitators, many paid employees and volunteers with Highland Hospice, with a member of a charitable local agency also taking part in the training.

Led by Siobhan Neylon and Dr. Jeremy Keen, Consultant in Palliative Care from Highland Hospice, plans were made to connect with community groups to offer the LAC as part of a pilot delivery of the course. These groups were: Police Scotland, Church Groups and Community Centres. Each course had 3 members of the Facilitator group to ensure exposure to delivery as early as possible. The 4 pilot sessions received positive feedback, and the Hospice agreed to embed Last Aid Course delivery as part of their commitment to empowering and supporting the population of the Highlands. The engagement and delivery strategy for Last Aid required adjustment due to COVID-19, with online courses being well attended, not just with a Highland audience, but with a wider reach to all of Scotland, England, Wales, Northern and Republic of Ireland and even as far reaching as Poland and Canada. The courses were advertised online via Social Media platforms, and on the Highland Hospice website. However, the most influential advertising method was word of mouth and verbal dialog. A research study conducted with University of Highlands and Islands (UHI) and Highland Hospice using the Death Literacy Index as a guide, compared attendees' experiences before and after attending the Last Aid Course. Researchers also interviewed facilitators and examinded their experiences on delivering the course in person and online. The findings showed increased confidence in communicating about topics regarding death and dying, and planning ahead [10]. Facilitators expressed feelings of reduced confidence on delivering the course online and missing the in-person interaction with attendees. This study began a strong academic and research relationship with UHI and Highland Hospice for Last Aid and Public education initiatives. The Hospice adapted the Last Aid Course Handbook from German, and translated it to the English language, to ensure our new facilitators had more foundational knowledge behind the course and guidance on delivering the course online. An education website was also established, using the Moodle Platform. This allowed faciltiators to have links to further learning around each Module and topics within the Module, such as podcasts, YouTube videos, articles and website links. An adapted Facilitator Course was developed to enhance the confidence of the facilitator to deliver the course. This became a 2 day course, with an emphasis on the topics from expert speakers, such as Child bereavement officers, Occupational Therapists, MacMillan Citizen's Advice Bureau, Consultant Physicians and previous LAC Facilitators. This facilitator course was then delivered to members of the Fire Service, Scottish Ambulance Service (who would deliver to Tri-Services including Police Scotland) and Macmillan Cancer nursing team, along with Hospice Volunteers, who would become part of the Scottish Last Aid Course delivery to improve public knowledge and awareness of death, dying and bereavement. The course was being delivered in a hybrid method, with some attendees attending on Zoom platform, and others in person. This allowed for careers who were looking after their dying relatives to attend from their homes, people who lived further away in the Highlands to attend, and those who were hard of hearing to attend using the Closed Caption section of Zoom platform. This was oftentimes challenging for facilitators, and IT support was provided by the Hospice to ensure online attendees had positive experiences. Today, Highland Hospice has a dedicated Last Aid Development Officer who works with engagement of new hub development and outreach to rural communities in the Highlands. This role has become vital in the ongoing progress being made to ensure Last Aid is a widely recognized public education course. The Highland Hospice also provides leadership and support to the facilitators currently delivering the course and is committed to increasing public awareness and knowledge across the population.

3.3 Experiences from Switzerland

Since 2017, the Evangelical- Reformed Church of the Canton of Zurich has been a licensee for Last Aid Courses in Switzerland. Although this Church is the licencee, there are many other organizations that are involved in this project. These include: other Churches, sections of the Swiss professional association of Palliative Care, hospitals, nursing homes and foundations from 17 cantons of Switzerland. Through these organizations, Last Aid in Switzerland is being delivered in German, French and Italian languages. When developing the organizational structure, attention was paid to low-threshold, resource-saving processes. At the same time, emphasis was placed on the fact that there is a clear feedback relationship with the course leaders and the quality of the delivery of their courses. Up to time of writing, 360 course instructors are involved and more than 7000 people have attended the course. The national Last Aid structure has strong foundations that allows capacity for expansion or development as needed.

From the beginning, the Church Council of the Evangelical- Reformed Church of the Canton of Zurich was open to Last Aid Course and provided the necessary resources for nationwide development, management, and coordination. Funding was provided for 20% of the rolefor the project management/coordination of Last Aid Switzerland has been approved until further notice.

Accompanying people in dying, death and mourning is one of the church's core pastoral and diaconal tasks. In its actions, it actively participates in a discourse on good communal living and dying. In doing so, it also encourages dialog. After all, palliative and hospice care for chronically ill and dying people cannot succeed through professional services alone, but only with the commitment and participation of volunteers. The Evangelical- Reformed Church of the Canton of Zurich sees itself as jointly responsible for ensuring knowledge about dying, death and mourning is accessible to all people and encouraging them to seek support. It contributes to networking with other organizations around dying, death and bereavement. It thus shows itself to be a contributor to a caring community.

Switzerland will be known to some people for its liberal regulations in dealing with medically assisted suicide. One of the better-known euthanasia organizations is, for example, the association Exit. Although the number has increased, this is a rather small group, accounting for 1.8% of all deaths.

The title of the Last Aid Course is appealing and was correctly understood in Switzerland from the outset in accordance with the content of the course. There are no misunderstandings about assisted suicide.

In 2018, representatives from the French-speaking part of Switzerland, from Palliative Vaud, a section of the Swiss professional association of Palliative Care, contact project management in Zurich. They have translated all course materials, texts for the website and much more into French. They thus launched the version of "Derniers

Secours". Palliative Vaud cooperates in the French-speaking part of Switzerland, among others with the Reformed and Catholic Churches and mediates other organizations to Last Aid Course Switzerland. They are not only involved in networking for the Last Aid Course in the French-speaking regions of Switzerland, but also played a key role in enabling France to join the project in 2022.

In 2022, the Italian version "Ultimo Soccorso" was created. On behalf of the Evangelical- Reformed Church of the Canton of Graubünden, two Italian speaking course instructors translated all course materials into Italian. The first courses in Italian took place.

In 2023, 25 people were trained for the Kids & Teens Last Aid Course. The first courses are mainly run by parishes. It is expected that this offer will also become more widespread. Palliative Vaud has again agreed to translate and adapt the material into French.

3.4 Experiences from Slovenia

The Last Aid course, first organized in 2019 by the Institute for Palliative Medicine and Hospice Care at the University of Maribor's Faculty of Medicine Maribor, has undergone significant growth and adaptation over the past five years. In collaboration with the Slovenian Lions clubs and the Slovenian Hospice Association, this course has been delivered forty-five times, with eight of those deliveries transitioning to an online format during (six) and two after the COVID-19 pandemic. The organizers also developed a specialized online course (webinar) to cater to the deaf and hard of hearing community by utilizing sign language. To ensure effective interaction and active participation, each delivery of the Last Aid course accommodated a maximum of 15 participants. The participants' professional backgrounds span a wide spectrum, encompassing medical and healthcare students, nurses, physicians, teachers, social workers, business professionals, lawyers, engineers, priests, nuns, homemakers, and individuals without current employment. The course's content and materials were made possible through the Slovenian government-financed Assistance for a Better Quality of Life in the Last Phase of Life (PO-LAST) project, a collaborative effort involving Slovenian medical and healthcare professionals, hospice representatives, university teachers and students. The Slovenian Hospice Association and the University of Maribor's Medical Faculty and the Faculty of Arts were key contributors to the project, along with Alma Mater Europaea, an independent higher learning institution. The primary aim of the project was to provide comprehensive information and access to resources for individuals facing life-threatening illnesses and their caregivers. The project members, totalling thirteen, undertook various tasks to support this objective. They produced the Slovenian Atlas of Palliative Care, offering insights into support options and information sources for the terminally ill and their caregivers. Additionally, they translated the Last Aid instructor manual from German to Slovene and adapted its content to suit the Slovenian context. The team also created a brochure containing essential information about palliative care in Slovenia and organized and conducted dissemination workshops. All the materials generated during this project have been invaluable in facilitating the implementation of Last Aid courses in Slovenia. The courses have garnered high praise from participants. In 2022 the Medical Faculty Maribor organized also the third LAST AID Conference in presence, after the online Conference in 2020, which was also organized from the Slovenian LAST AID hub. The next challenge of the Slovenian hub is establishing a coordination and administration support for the LAST AID course providers and intensification of the research in this field. Some publications regarding the acceptance of the model were already done [11].

4. Lessons learned from the implementation process in different countries

In the starting phase of the international implementation a cooperation with national Palliative Care associations was sought but proved not to be a successful approach to promote LAC. Many national Palliative Care associations showed little or no interest to implement LAC in their countries. Many could not envisage the potential that the LAC has to raise awareness and to enhance the public dialog about death, dying, grief and Palliative Care. In contrast an approach that proved to be very successful was a cooperation with different national organizations that showed a great interest and commitment in bringing LAC to their countries. As the above four examples show this can be the formation of an own NGO as in Germany, the church as in Switzerland, a Hospice as in Scotland or a University as in Slovenia. That shows that an important factor for successful cooperation and implementation is to find people and organizations that support the ideas and aims of the Last Aid Movement and are willing to agree on common rules for implementation, further development and research to improve and adapt the LAC to the needs of the participants. In the countries that have successfully started LAC, there are always people who are willing to be the pioneers and the driving force for the implementation of LAC. Sometimes it seems most important to have a dedicated pioneer or small group of pioneers who show commitment to the idea of teaching the public by the use of LAC.

Experiences from all presented countries show that the promotion of the courses by word of mouth is a usual way of promoting and distributing the LAC. Media interest has been great in the participating countries. In Germany many reports have been published in newspapers, magazines, radio, podcasts and television. The media attention has in Germany led to the fact that many LAC are fully booked in advance after they are advertised on the homepage www.letztehilfe.info.

As described above the most important steps for the implementation of Last Aid in a country are:

1. An organization and dedicated people to start LAC

2. To establish a first Last Aid instructor/facilitator course

3. To run LAC and to gain experience

4. Establish a core group of trainers

5. Establish an organizational structure for the national Last Aid program and LAC and instructor/facilitator courses

6. Engage in media work and advocacy if possible

The international cooperation and collaboration has led to important improvements and the further development of the course contents as well as the development of new course formats. For example, delivering LAC for police officers, first carried out in Scotland, has gone on to inspire German colleagues to start such courses in Hessen, Germany where the courses were appreciated and will now be implemented more widely in other parts of Germany. In Germany a number of different course formats have been established. A LAC for deaf people has been tried out in Slovenia and the further work on that course format is still ongoing. The LARGI research group and the International

Last Aid Conferences are important meeting places for the exchange of experiences with LAC and the discussion of new ideas and new projects with international cooperation and participation. Many researchers and members of LARGI have contributed with a number of scientific articles about the experiences with and the effects of LAC at a national level and across different countries, ethnic and cultural backgrounds. A review of the research was published by Bollig and Bauer [12].

In summary, the collected experiences so far show that one of the most important learning points was that international cooperation and consensus on the LAC curriculum, as well as research, are important parts of the further development and sustainability of the Last Aid Movement.

5. Last Aid as learning system

As already pointed out above international cooperation and collaboration in the International Last Aid working group and the Last Aid Research Group International are the major factors for the worldwide success and implementation of LAC. Last Aid is viewed and perceived as a learning system where everyone can contribute to enhance knowledge and improve to better Palliative Care provision for everybody in need. Evaluation of the courses and research are an integral part of the implementation process of Last Aid. Evaluation and research results can be used in the communication with policymakers, media and the public to ensure public interest and support. **Figure 3** illustrates the different groups that interact and cooperate in order to make Last Aid a successful learning system and thereby ensure that the educational needs of the public are reflected and adapted in regular intervals with input from citizens, Last Aid Course instructors, experts from the field of Palliative Care and researchers.

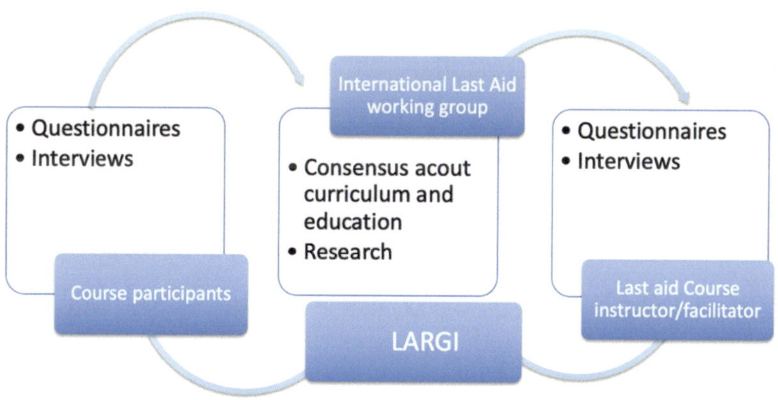

Figure 3.
Last Aid is a learning system.

6. Implications for the future development of Last Aid and the international distribution of PPCE and LAC

In the future the need for palliative care in the community will increase. According to the World Health organization lack of awareness of Palliative Care is a major barrier for Palliative Care provision [12]. Education about palliative care by *Last Aid courses* or other initiatives of Public Palliative Care Education in combination with a compassionate community approach may serve to improve both the awareness and the public discussion about death and dying as well as palliative care provision in the community [6, 13]. There is a need for more research about *Last Aid courses* and other measures to empower the public to engage in palliative care provision in the community.

Possible conflict of interest

GB receives financial compensation for teaching Last Aid Instructor courses. GB owns the trademarks "Last Aid" and "Letzte Hilfe". EN is working for the church in Switzerland and is responsible for the implementation of Last aid Courses in Switzerland. SN has no conflicts of interest.

Author details

Georg Bollig[1,2,3*], Siobhan Neylon[4], Eva Niedermann[5] and Erika Zelko[3,6,7]

1 Department of Anesthesiology, Intensive Care, Palliative Medicine and Pain Therapy, Helios Klinikum Schleswig, Germany

2 Department of Palliative Medicine, University of Cologne, Faculty of Medicine and University Hospital, Cologne, Germany

3 Last Aid Research Group International (LARGI), Schleswig, Germany

4 NHS Highland, Inverness, Scotland

5 Evangelical- Reformed Church of the Canton of Zurich, Switzerland

6 Medical Faculty, Institute for General Medicine, Johannes Kepler University Linz, Linz, Austria

7 Medical Faculty, Institute for Palliative and Hospiz Medicine, University Maribor, Maribor, Slowenia

*Address all correspondence to: georg.bollig@helios-gesundheit.de

References

[1] Etkind SN, Bone AE, Gomes B, Lovell N, Evans CJ, Higginson IJ, et al. How many people will need palliative care in 2040? Past trends, future projections and implications for services. BMC Medicine. 2017;**15**:102

[2] Kellehear A. Compassionate communities: End-of-life care as everyone's responsibility. The Quarterly Journal of Medicine. 2013;**106**:1071-1075

[3] Kellehear A. Compassionate Cities. Public Health and End-of-Life Care. Oxfordshire: Routledge; 2005

[4] Bollig G. Palliative Care für alte und demente Menschen lernen und lehren. Berlin: LIT-Verlag; 2010. Available from: http://www.lit-verlag.de/isbn/3-643-90058-6

[5] Bollig G, Kuklau N. Der *Letzte Hilfe* Kurs - ein Angebot zur Verbesserung der allgemeinen ambulanten Palliativversorgung durch Information und Befähigung von Bürgerinnen und Bürgern. Z Palliativmed. 2015;**16**:210-216

[6] Bollig G, Bauer EH. Last aid courses as measure for public palliative care education for adults and children: A narrative review. Annals of Palliative Medicine. 2021;**10**(7):8242-8253. DOI: 10.21037/apm-21-762

[7] Bollig G. Palliative care education for everybody. In: I Mollaoglu M, editor. Palliative Care. London, UK: InTechOpen; 2019. DOI: 10.5772/intechopen.85496

[8] Mills J, Rosenberg JP, Bollig G, Haberecht J. Last aid and public health palliative care: Towards the development of personal skills and strengthened community action. Progress in Palliative Care. 2020;**28**(6):343-345. DOI: 10.1080/09699260.2020.1829798

[9] Bollig G. Project Report: Last Aid International – The Last Aid Movement - Implementation of an International Working Group on Last Aid. Schleswig; 2019

[10] MacAden L, Broadfoot K, Carolan C, Muirhead K, Netlon S, Keen J. Last aid training online: Participants' and facilitators' perceptions from a mixed-methods study in rural Scotland. Healthcare. 2022;**10**(5):918. DOI: 10.3390/healthcare10050918

[11] Zelko E, Vrbek L, Koletnik M. Last aid course - the Slovenian experience. Healthcare. 2022;**10**(7):1-11. ISSN 2227-9032. Available from: https://www.mdpi.com/2227-9032/10/7/1154

[12] World Health Organization. Palliative Care. Available from: https://www.who.int/news-room/fact-sheets/detail/palliative-care

[13] Bollig G, Hjelm Brandt Kristensen F, Ciurlionis M, Knopf B. Last aid course. An education for all citizens and an ingredient of compassionate communities. Healthcare. 2019;**7**(1):19. DOI: 10.3390/healthcare7010019